HANDBOOK OF MOTOR SKILLS: DEVELOPMENT, IMPAIRMENT AND THERAPY

HANDBOOK OF MOTOR SKILLS: DEVELOPMENT, IMPAIRMENT AND THERAPY

LUCIAN T. PELLIGRINO
EDITOR

Nova Science Publishers, Inc.
New York

NOTICE TO THE READER

LIBRARY OF CONGRESS CATALOGING-IN-PUBLICATION DATA

Handbook of motor skills : development, impairment, and therapy / editor, Lucian T. Pelligrino.
   p. ; cm.
 Includes bibliographical references and index.
 ISBN 978-1-60741-811-5 (hardcover)
 1. Movement disorders. 2. Physical therapy. 3. Motor ability. 4. Motor learning. I. Pelligrino, Lucian T.
 [DNLM: 1. Motor Skills--physiology. 2. Human Development. 3. Movement--physiology. 4. Physical Therapy Modalities. WE 103 H236 2009]
 RC376.5.H348 2009
 616.8'3--dc22
               2009028881

Published by Nova Science Publishers, Inc. ✦ *New York*

CONTENTS

PREFACE

A motor skill is a learned series of movements that combine to produce a smooth, efficient action. Gross motor skills include lifting one's head, rolling over, sitting up, balancing, crawling, and walking. Gross motor development usually follows a pattern. Generally large muscles develop before smaller ones, thus, gross motor development is the foundation for developing skills in other areas. Development also generally moves from top to bottom. For example, the first thing a baby usually learns to control is its eyes. Fine motor skills include the ability to manipulate small objects, transfer objects from hand to hand, and various hand-eye coordination tasks. Fine motor skills may involve the use of very precise motor movement in order to achieve an especially delicate task. This new and important book gathers the latest research from around the globe in this field.

Chapter 1 - The purpose of this chapter is to discuss key concepts related to human motor development, especially as they pertain to childhood, and examine the application of this information in populations of children with and without disabilities. By definition, human motor development is "the changes in human movement behavior over the lifespan, the processes that underlie these changes and the factors that affect them" (Payne & Isaacs, 2008, p. 3). It is a process that we all undergo as a part of the gradually evolving maturation from inception through death, the qualitative change in our function that accompanies getting older. Because it is such a subtle and gradually emerging process, motor development often goes unnoticed and unappreciated. However, as you will see throughout this chapter, it is a critical process that impacts, and is impacted, by all other aspects of human development – physical, social-emotional, and intellectual development. It is a process that is integral to achieving our full maturity and potential as human beings.

Chapter 2 - Developmental Coordination Disorder (DCD) is a term used to describe a condition of motor incoordination found in children. Prevalence estimates for DCD obtained internationally indicate that about 6 to 10% of the school-aged population may be affected. Despite the high prevalence rates, a systematic review of the literature reveals that data have been mainly reported for north America and northern Europe. Recent evidence shows that DCD has a significant physiological impact on children's health and well-being. Specifically, it has been found that children with DCD are at increased risk for developing coronary artery disease at a later age. This has been attributed to the fact that children with DCD systematically avoid being active. Thus participation in physical activity has been suggested as a significant mediator in the relationship between clumsiness and coronary artery disease. These findings underline the necessity to identify individuals with DCD early in life, in order to prevent many of the secondary problems that may arise in later years. The factor contributing the most to the scarcity of DCD data is the challenge of screening/identification of children with this disorder. To date, no gold-standard has been universally recognized. Furthermore, widely accepted screening methods such as the Bruininks Oseretsky Test of Motor Proficiency, or the Movement Assessment Battery for Children, are neither practical nor cost-effective. A solution to this problem may be found in the Children's Self-Perceptions of Adequacy in and Predilection for Physical Activity (CSAPPA) scale. However, further investigation of the validity and precision of the CSAPPA scale in different populations is required.

Chapter 3 - Motor skills in an aquatic environment are typically defined with stroking parameters, in conjunction with the kinematic, kinetic and coordination profile of the swimmer. The collection and analysis of this data has followed the traditional processes of video and/or motion analysis of the entire body, followed by quantification of motor skill of specific body segments, such as the upper limbs. A similar process of analysis can be applied for able-bodied swimmers as well as swimmers with an impairment - with some variations. For example, if the swimmer does not have the use of their arms through disease or amputation the motor skill variable of arm stroke rate is not relevant. This chapter reviews motor skill development for both able-bodied and for swimmers with an impairment. By understanding the skill characteristics of both groups the unique process of aquatic motor skill development can be better understood. This profile is presented based on the established theories on aquatic motor skills, and is followed by practical examples based on data collected at elite competitions (Olympic and Paralympic Games) and motor skill profiles of unskilled swimmers.

Chapter 4 - Skill is a task-specific ability that is influenced by task demands to achieve a task proficiently. Motor skills consist of both movement and interactions as an observable, goal-directed action and have a sequence that constitutes a routine. While skills are performed in a routine sequence, they are linked together by individualized habits.

The assessment of skills has significant importance because, as with skills, task demands and physical and social environment can affect habits.

Motor skills may be evaluated with non-standardized and standardized methods. Nonstandardized methods are informal evaluation based on observation of the performing of any task. After the observation is completed, the relevant motor skill is investigated carefully and systematically. Standardized methods are objective and well documented.

This chapter aims to explain this wide variety of evaluation methods.

Chapter 5 - Stroke is a leading cause of adult disability and the number affected is increasing as the population ages and survival rates post-event improve. It is estimated that as many as 60% of stroke survivors live with significant physical deficits including muscle weakness, instability, poor motor coordination and cardiovascular compromise resulting in a loss of independence in performing activities required for daily living. This percentage has remained relatively constant over the past decades, which suggests that interventions to minimize or reverse the effects of stroke are not yet widely available. The authors propose that while most rehabilitation programs focus on reducing impairment they yield limited effect on mobility function because of inadequacies on two fronts. First, they often deal with impairments as isolated deficiencies and as such fail to consider stroke as a multisystem disorder that demands an integrated treatment approach for optimal restoration of function. Second, the minimum performance requirements of specific aspects of physical function including strength, balance, and aerobic capacity associated with every day activities are unknown. Consequently, clinicians are challenged to identify targets that if attained will translate into enhanced mobility. This chapter reviews the relevant literature and presents research findings to provide insight on these important issues.

The approach is to first discuss stroke related physical impairments and their association with mobility deficits. From our own research work and the growing body of literature examining the combined influence of muscle weakness, balance instability, and physiological cost on mobility the authors explore those factors that are important determinants of mobility function. Going a step further, the impact of reducing impairments on effecting positive change in mobility is discussed.

Stroke is a multisystem disorder and mobility is a complex construct dependent upon the integrity of individual physical systems as well as their capacity to work in concert. The research discussed in this chapter provides insight into the unique characteristics of these systems in stroke and their interactions which are fundamental to mobility.

Chapter 6 - Can one learn implicitly, that is, without conscious awareness of what it is that one learns? Daily life is replete with situations where our behavior is seemingly influenced by knowledge to which we have little access. Riding a bicycle, playing tennis or driving a car, all involve mastering complex sets of motor skills, yet we are at a loss when it comes to explaining exactly how we perform such physical feats. Thus, while it is commonly accepted and hence unsurprising that we have little access to the cognitive processes involved in mental operations, it also appears that knowledge itself can remain inaccessible to report yet influence behavior. Reber, who coined the expression "implicit learning" in 1967, defined it as "the process whereby people learn without intent and without being able to clearly articulate what they learn" (Cleeremans, Destrebecqz, & Boyer, 1998).

The research described in this chapter is positioned at the confluence of two different domains: Implicit Learning on the one hand, and Skill Acquisition on the other. The two domains have remained largely independent from each other, but their intersection nevertheless constitutes a field of primary import: the implicit motor learning field. The hallmark of implicit motor learning is the capacity to acquire skill through physical practice without conscious recollection of what elements of performance have improved. Unfortunately, studies dealing with implicit motor learning are not very abundant (Pew, 1974; Magill & Hall, 1989; Wulf & Schmidt, 1997; Shea, Wulf, Whitacre, & Park, 2001). These studies provide an apparently straightforward demonstration of the possibility of unconsciously learning the structure of a complex continuous task in a more efficient way than explicit learning allows. Nevertheless, other evidence seems to challenge this view. Indeed, recent studies (Chambaron, Ginhac, Ferrel-Chapus & Perruchet, 2006; Ooteghem, Allard, Buchanan, Oates & Horak, 2008) suggest that taking advantage from the repetition of continuous events may not be as easy as previous research leads us to believe. Indeed, these studies have suggested that sequence learning in continuous tracking tasks might be artefatctually driven by peculiarities of the experimental material rather than by implicit sequence learning per se.

Consequently, a central goal of this chapter will be to reconcile these discrepant results so as to better characterize the conditions in which implicit motor learning occurs. Moreover, understanding what facilitates or prevents learning of regularities in motor tasks will be useful both in sport and in motor rehabilitation fields.

Chapter 7 - This chapter reviews a growing number of studies that indicate it is difficult to predict fluctuations in the performance of professional golfers from their immediate preceding performance. Results indicate that the scores of professional golfers do not cluster together where successful performance follows successful performance ("hot streaks") and/or poor performance follows poor performance ("cold Streaks"). Professional golfers show little consistency in either their round-to-round performance or their hole-to-hole performance. Contrary to popular belief, choking under pressure is not a common occurrence among professional golfers. Evidence is presented that that the unreliability of golf scores for professional golfers is due to restriction of range. Professional golfers who play on professional tours are so nearly equal in ability that it is mainly a matter of chance who will have either better scores or the best score on any given day.

Chapter 8 - Background: Movement Related Brain Macropotentials (MRBMs) are electrical brain potentials occurring before, during and after skilled movements. Specific components of these potentials have been described and it has been reported that they can be recorded also during mental motor imagery and can be influenced by practice. To understand the exact relationship between MRBMs and skilled actions and to verify the hypothesis that motor training could modify MRBMs profile and influence specific components an experiment has been performed in which MRBMs were recorded during the execution of different skilled performance tasks and before and after a period of training.

Methods: The experiment has been carried out with 31 healthy male subjects, divided into three groups. Eleven performed the Alert test (A), a simple reaction time test, in which the subject had to press in a precise sequence three keys of a keyboard when a figure appeared on the computer monitor. Ten subjects performed the Choice test (CH), a complex reaction time test, in which they had to press the three keys in a different order when one of two different figures appeared randomly on the screen. Ten subjects performed the Choice test with the addition of a Go/No-Go paradigm (CHNG) in which participants had also to repress an unsuitable response. All subjects were tested before and after 10 days of training. During the trials EEG, EMG and other physiological parameters were recorded. The time of the recorded test was divided into three periods: prestimulus, motor (premotor, motor action, motor completion) and postmotor. Data were collected, averaged and compared by appropriate statistical methods.

Results: The time of EMG activation and Reaction Time (RT) were lower in A then in CH and CHNG. Training did not influenced A, but was followed by a significant reduction of RT in CH and CHNG. The profile of MRBMs was different in the motor period in the three tests. The duration of Premotor Potential (PMP), a positive wave recorded in the premotor component of the motor period, increased passing from A to CHNG, but after training, it was reduced only in the CHNG test. During motor action the duration of the negative wave Motor Cortex Potential (MCP) increased from A to CHNG and was reduced after training in all tests. In CHNG training reduced the latency of N1 and N2, the negative peaks recognizable in the MCP profile, and the latency of the Skilled Performance Positivity (SPP), a wave occurring in the postmotor period. Moreover, after training the period preceding the stimulus showed an increase of negativity in the last 200 msec.

Conclusions: MRBMs can change their profile in relation to the characteristics of the test and the skilled motor action. The increase of duration and latency of the motor period waves, passing from A to CHNG, can be considered as picture of increased information processing and response selection brain activity. Moreover, training can affect the profile of the waves, reducing their duration and latency, particularly when the performance requires high mental effort.

Chapter 9 - Cerebral palsy (CP) describes a group of movement and posture development disorders attributed to non-progressive disturbances in the developing fetal or infant brain, causing activity limitations and being the most common cause of severe physical disability in childhood. The motor disorders of CP are often accompanied by disturbances of sensation, cognition, communication, perception, behavior, and seizure disorders.

Oromotor dysfunction and oral-ingestive problems, as uncoordinated control mechanisms of orofacial and palatolingual musculatures, are often observed in CP individuals, and varies from mild to severe. These disabilities are expressed by drooling, coughing, choking, rejection of solid food, food loss, and spillage during eating. Difficulties in spoon-feeding, biting, chewing, cup drinking, straw drinking, swallowing and clearing are also observed.

Another nutritional issue to be considered is the common inability of severely oromotor impaired CP individuals to ingest solid food, which often leads to an exclusively liquid or semi-solid diet. In spite of contributing to some degree to growth and nutritional disturbances, especially at an early age, food consistency may also cause a significant impact on oral health. Therefore, a timely nutritional rehabilitation and preventive measures in oral health may significantly improve the quality of life of these individuals, as well as prevent deleterious and noxious habits such as bottle feeding. Performing an adequate oral hygiene on CP individuals however, can be a very difficult task for the caregivers, due to the patient's persistent pathological biting reflex.

Food consistency, sugared beverages, and long term oral medicines, associated with oromotor dysfunction and oral hygiene difficulties, may explain the high incidence of caries and periodontal diseases exhibited by the CP population.

The influence of oromotor impairment in CP individuals as a risk factor in caries experience was not studied yet. Therefore, this study aimed at evaluating the influence of oral motricity and diet consistency on caries experience and growth rate in CP individuals.

Chapter 10 - The authors describe Arthrogryposis Multiplex Congenita (AMC), the presence of multiple joint contractures at birth, and they analyze the capacities and limitations of the second author, Jennifer Border, who has this condition. In AMC, the joints (arthro) of hands, wrists, elbows, shoulders, hips, feet, and knees are often fixed in a curved (gryp) position. Characteristically, the thumbs are pinned in the palms, and the hands are bent toward the arms, which are turned toward the body. Range of motion is limited by these joint contractures and often by muscle weakness. The purpose of analyzing capacities and limitations is to lay a foundation for human-centered assistive technologies especially computer interfaces. Determining an optimal interface for Jennifer is timely because her physicians have asked her to stop using a stylus held in her mouth, which has been her main interface with computer keyboards. Jennifer developed a repetitive motion injury in her shoulders from frequent use of this interface throughout grade school, high school, college, and her current first year in a Human Factors Psychology graduate program. This injury is affecting not only her interface with computers, but also other important tasks such as preparing and eating meals for which she is heavily reliant on her shoulder muscles. To prepare meals, for example, she holds containers in her mouth and pours by tilting her head and shoulders. In order to maintain these essential abilities, she must find an alternative computer interface and work station. Alternative interfaces under consideration are voice, eye movements, and EMG signals from facial muscles. Preliminary evaluations of these alternatives and their combinations will be made, but the present focus will be on analyzing Jennifer's capacities and limitations as a step toward a human-centered final choice.

Chapter 11 - Manipulative activity is based on both manual motor skills and cognitive development. Humans and chimpanzees, the closest living relatives of human beings, share manual dexterity in manipulating objects in their daily lives. Chimpanzees are also known to use tools in their natural habitat to achieve a variety of goals. This chapter reports the findings gained by assigning tasks using identical objects conducted in a face-to-face situation for chimpanzees and human children. Manipulative skills in both species were analyzed as a non-verbal scale for direct comparison by focusing on their manipulative patterns. Tasks using blocks of different shapes were designed to test physical understanding involved in making a vertical stack. The subjects were required to selectively use appropriate orientation of differently-shaped blocks in order to stack them efficiently. The subjects acquired the solution of manually changing the orientation of the blocks to the appropriate one. The results illuminated a fundamental similarity between chimpanzees and humans. Tasks using nesting cups were originally designed to assess cognitive development in human children by analyzing the behavioral strategies of combining multiple cups into a nesting structure. The manipulation of nesting cups was described in a form of sequential codes in both chimpanzees and humans to illuminate the patterns of making a hierarchical combination among objects. Some of the subjects from both species succeeded in making a nesting structure with nine cups. The subjects tried to solve the task by reducing the number of cup units and by combining cups in an appropriate order. In sum, manipulative behavior revealed high levels of physical intelligence shared by chimpanzees and humans.

Chapter 12 - The aim of this chapter is to provide an overview of several aspects of TMT. Specifically, the chapter covers 3 topics, these being:

• Literature: what is known about TMT from published peer-reviewed reports of formal investigations of this strategy

• Recent research: an overview of 3 pilot projects conducted by the author and colleagues which each evaluate an aspect of TMT

• Clinical perspectives: a report of a pilot evaluation of how practising UK clinicians utilise TMT

Chapter 13 - This study investigated the effect of multi-modal imagery on anxiety and perceived stress levels in tennis players. The quasi-experimental design included pre- and post-treatment test subjects and a control group. Male tennis players (n=49) ranging in age from 16 to 18 years old (M=16.96, SD= 0.82) were divided into two groups: (1) a treatment imagery group and (2) a placebo imagery group used as the control group. The 27-item Competitive State Anxiety Inventory (CSAI-2) was used to assess anxiety and the Perceived Stress Scale (PSS10) to assess stress. The results showed a significant multivariate difference ($p < .05$) between the treatment imagery and control groups in terms of cognitive anxiety, self-confidence and perceived stress. The findings suggest that imagery is a powerful mental tool for overcoming some specific types of anxiety and stress.

Chapter 14 - Motor development research has experienced greater frequency in top-tier science journals over the past 25 years. While some dialogue has been of environmental factors, to a much greater extent, discussions of motor development have focused on the biological, psychological, cognitive, or movement aspects of change. Few would disagree that to truly understand the mechanisms and processes associated with change in human form and level of motor behavior, a more comprehensive and integrated approach is needed – one that links biological and environmental theory. One such approach and the focus of this chapter is the *Developmental Systems Perspective.*

Chapter 15 - The time between a stimulus and a response is commonly assumed to reflect the sum of the duration of a series of mental and motor processes. The source of the timing delay related to these processes has been determined by partitioning the total reaction time (RT) into premotor RT and motor RT components. The procedure of fractionating RT to the presentation of a stimulus has been applied to simple and choice RT tasks. However, people also commonly make a response to the omission of some regular stimulus. This chapter focuses on the omitted stimulus reaction time (OSRT) task, which presents a series of sensory stimuli that require an immediate response to the omission of the train of stimuli. Unlike the reaction to the presentation of a stimulus, the reaction to an omitted stimulus is triggered by an internal process and is considered to require additional cognitive loads. Research evidence suggests that during the premotor fraction, the mental processes underlying motor skills occur. The chapter describes independent changes in the two OSRT components when several factors are manipulated (e.g., sensory modality, inter-stimulus interval or training). The relation of premotor and motor components to the brain wave, known as the omitted stimulus potential (OSP), are also examined. The chapter address the evidence suggesting that the impairment of motor skills by a moderate dose of alcohol might be due to impaired activity located in particular brain areas related to cognition rather than actual motor processes.

Chapter 16 - Most validity and reproducibility studies on instruments to test muscle strength have been done in adults. There is need for data from children, because such instruments are frequently used on children in clinical practice. Our study on the performance of muscle strength instruments in children aged 4 to 11 years showed that a new Motor Performance Test had the highest validity and highest reproducibility compared to hand-held dynamometry and the Jamar dynamometer. The child-friendly Motor Performance Test can improve the diagnostic procedure in children suspected of having myopathy and spare more children from painful muscle biopsy. Moreover, it is a suitable instrument for monitoring purposes in children.

Chapter 17 - In 2007, the Centers for Disease Control and Prevention (CDC) estimated that approximately 1 in 150 children have an autism spectrum disorder (ASD) or a pervasive developmental disorder (PDD). In addition, autism ranked as the sixth most common category for children to receive services. These findings by the CDC suggest that ASD is no longer the rare condition it was once thought to be, but rather, many practitioners, both in medical and educational fields, will encounter children with suspected ASD in their practices. While the Diagnostic and Statistical Manual for Mental Disorders IV (DSM IV, American Psychiatric Association, 2000) criteria focus on the social and communication impairments of children with ASD, clinical practice and emerging literature indicate children with ASD also demonstrate a variety of motor impairments and deficits. However, a sparse number of studies have been conducted in the area of motor development and control in the past 30 years for children with ASD. The purpose of this chapter is to review literature exploring motor development and motor control abilities of people with ASD towards advancing our understanding of motor aspects in children with ASD. First, the authors review the existing motor related experimental and descriptive studies on motor disorder symptoms in children with ASD. Second, the authors will discuss both motor development and control in autism. Finally, the authors suggest directions for future research that integrate each of these areas.

From this chapter, clinicians and researchers alike may be able to gain insights and frameworks upon which they may base clinical intervention and future research methodology.

Chapter 18 - In this paper, the authors review research that examines associations between language-based learning disabilities (LD) and motor coordination. Driving this review is our belief that the theoretical concept of embodied cognition (Chiel & Beer, 1997; Thelen, 2000), which suggests a dynamic interdependence of perceptual, cognitive, and motor processes, may hold promise in providing both questions and solutions for those interested in understanding learning disabilities. Based on the literature, relationships appear to exist between language and motor development in children at risk for language-based learning disabilities, which are suggestive of motor skill acquisition delays and differences in fine and gross motor coordination. The relationship between learning disabilities and movement disorder suggest that decrements in motor coordination may indicate a child may be at risk for LD; potentially, standardized motor tests may be used as part of a battery of tests to identify young children at risk for language-based learning disabilities . The authors believe this line of inquiry holds promise, and calls for more empirical research into the quantitative nature of the learning disabilities-motor coordination association, and for more theoretical consideration into the heuristic value of embodied cognition as applied to language-based learning disabilities.

Chapter 19 - The present study was undertaken to follow the development of the capability to produce fast and precise movements reaching to visual targets, during childhood. One child (male) was tested repeatedly since age 6, until age 9. Accuracy increased progressively, while reaction and movemet times decreased, eventually approaching those typical of the adult. The most prominent finding is that our subject changed the strategy adopted for reaching to targets at different distances, from "width control" to "height control": when youngest, he scaled movement times of trajectories mainly (width control); when older, he scaled peak velocity of a stereotyped bell-shaped trajectory (height control), thus adopting a fully adult-like strategy. The results were confirmed in two groups of 5 children each, aged 6 and 9 respectively. It is concluded that, between age 6 and 9, children become capable of producing both quick and accurate trajectories to target, by implementing the optimized "height control" strategy typical of adults.

Chapter 20 - The often held view that motor control occurs largely as the final stage of cognitive processing is something that still needs to be dispelled. Granted that while there is a final level of motor control, all-be-it a lower level of motor control, this is only one level in the motor control hierarchy. Some inroads have been made in clarifying the different stages of motor control and its lateralization, however there is still a way to go with regards to delineating the various levels of motor control from the very highest or early inception/goal level to the final level of movement execution, as well as how each of these levels contributes to bimanual control, hand preference, hand proficiency and overall motor skill. Also, how exactly posture figures within the motor control hierarchy and its influence on final motor skill needs to be taken into account. Motor control is not separate from cognitive functioning, the two are intimately linked, and so the challenge within this area and one of the main directions for future research is the need to find the cognitive and language functioning associated with each respective level of motor control, thus clarifying the cognitive – motor skills link.

In: Handbook of Motor Skills
Editor: Lucian T. Pelligrino
ISBN: 978-1-60741-811-5
© 2009 Nova Science Publishers, Inc.

Chapter 1

HUMAN MOTOR DEVELOPMENT IN INDIVIDUALS WITH AND WITHOUT DISABILITIES: AN OVERVIEW

V. Gregory Payne[1], Jin H. Yan[2] and Martin Block[3]
[1] San Jose State University, San Jose, CA, USA
[2] The Chinese University of Hong Kong, Hong Kong, P. R. China
[3] The University of Virginia, Charlottesville, VA, USA

INTRODUCTION

We have all held a newborn with her head gently cupped in our hand to help maintain the head's upright position. Even a month or so after birth, many babies may need that supporting hand to compensate for the lack of muscle strength and control of their necks. However, by the second month of post birth life, babies have typically gained enough neck strength to raise and hold their heads upright. Many experts consider this to be the first major motor milestone of motor development in infancy. And, by two or three months of life, infants can normally hold their heads up and even turn them from side to side when lying on the floor in a prone position (Frankenburg, Dodds, Fandal, Kazuk, & Cohrs, 1992). By five months of life, the babies can raise their heads when in a supine position on the floor. This common and expected progression in controlling the head is just one example of early human motor development.

Human motor performance is one of the fundamental aspects of the sensory-motor system. Many questions appeal to researchers in the field of movement science and other areas such as neuroscience, psychology, physiology, education, pediatrics, and geriatrics. For example, how do humans learn and control movements? Considering that humans improve motor performance in childhood as a function of enriched experiences or maturation, developmental studies on motor performance inform our understanding of perceptual-motor skills (Thomas, Yan, & Stelmach, 2000; Yan, Thomas, Stelmach, & Thomas, 2000; Zelazo, Craik, & Booth, 2004). A developmental approach can answer questions like why children exhibit certain consistent motor behavior. When and how do these motor behaviors begin?

Are these behaviors learned behaviors or naturally developed? A better understanding of these questions has critical implications.

The purpose of this chapter is to discuss key concepts related to human motor development, especially as they pertain to childhood, and examine the application of this information in populations of children with and without disabilities. By definition, human motor development is "the changes in human movement behavior over the lifespan, the processes that underlie these changes and the factors that affect them" (Payne & Isaacs, 2008, p. 3). It is a process that we all undergo as a part of the gradually evolving maturation from inception through death, the qualitative change in our function that accompanies getting older. Because it is such a subtle and gradually emerging process, motor development often goes unnoticed and unappreciated. However, as you will see throughout this chapter, it is a critical process that impacts, and is impacted, by all other aspects of human development – physical, social-emotional, and intellectual development. It is a process that is integral to achieving our full maturity and potential as human beings.

THE SIGNIFICANCE OF THE STUDY OF HUMAN MOTOR DEVELOPMENT

Knowing and understanding the sequences of change in our motor development and the factors that affect these changes can be extremely important in education. Physical education teachers, for example, need to have an understanding of what children have done, what they are capable of doing, and what the likely next step in their development might be to be able to devise student learning outcomes for their classes as well as develop appropriate lesson plans. Without a thorough understanding of their students' motor development, creating developmentally appropriate lesson plans is difficult. Lessons are likely to be too simple and boring for their students or too difficult and frustrating. In short, teaching practices should be developmentally appropriate. According to the National Association for the Education of Young Children (NAEYC), this means that "Programs should be tailored to meet the needs of children rather than expecting the children to adapt to the demands of specific programs" (Bredekamp & Copple, 1997, p.1). The NAEYC suggests that developmentally appropriate includes two related dimensions, age appropriate and individual appropriate. Age appropriate relates to the importance of being knowledgeable of the relatively predictable growth and development sequences through which most children pass. These sequences are integral to the creation of viable learning opportunities for children. Though most children pass through these predictable sequences, they are still unique as they proceed through varying rates and patterns of development with their individual modes of learning, personalities, and out-of-school environments. These factors are critical to the term individual appropriateness and are also important considerations when creating educational experiences for young children.

Motor development is assumed to follow a specific or universal order, therefore, can be used in movement education or as a diagnostic tool. For instance, in terms of evaluating motor skill development, a teacher can report an individual's performance relative to that of other students of the same age, gender, or skill level or class (norm-referenced evaluation). On the other hand, a coach or teacher can evaluate someone's performance relative to a criterion or cutoff score that the coach or teacher wants the students to achieve (criterion-based evaluation). In choosing a particular approach to evaluate motor development in children, an important concern is whether it is developmentally appropriate. Motor development is age-related, not age-dependent. It is, therefore, necessary to evaluate motor performance of an individual or a group of individuals by comparing with others in the same age group (normative). However, it is equally important to consider individual differences in motor development and performance, because biological and environmental factors play a role in the development. Understanding motor development will allow a teacher or coach to know why a student is more or less movement proficient than his or her age-peers in motor performance. Understanding these developmental differences facilitates decision making related to enhancing motor ability in children.

UNDERSTANDING HUMAN MOTOR DEVELOPMENT: THE MOUNTAIN METAPHOR

To describe the complexities of human motor development in one chapter is a considerable challenge. Some might argue that a book would be insufficient. However, ways have been devised to help explain some of the most important aspects of human motor development in a more simplified, easily understandable, form. Clark and Metcalfe, 2002), for example, have proposed a "Mountain of Motor Development" as a metaphor for "the big picture" of the changes in human movement throughout life. This metaphor "emphasizes the cumulative, sequential, and interactive nature of motor skill development as an emergent product of lifelong changes within a multitude of constraints on our behavior" (p. 163). According to Clark and Metcalfe, previous metaphors devised in the examination of human motor development have focused on the product(s) of human movement where an emphasis was placed on describing the observed movement. Others have placed an emphasis on the process of the movement as they attempted to interpret the underlying explanations for the movement change. Clark and Metcalfe argue an opt for what they call an integrated metaphor where both the products and processes of movement are considered. It encompasses "periods" that one would pass through as they "climb the mountain" of life. Clark and Metcalfe believe their metaphor symbolizes the time it takes to learn the motor skills of life while showing the sequential nature and cumulative effect of the "climb." In addition, through their metaphor, these authors seek to symbolize the significant impact of factors like instruction, practice, and learning as well as inherent individual differences. Clark and Metcalfe also believe that human motor development is impacted by many constraints, factors that confine, or variously affect the way that we eventually move. These constraints are continually changing, thus having a variable impact on individual motor skill acquisition. They arise from the performer, the performer's environment, or may be related to the task in question. And, of course, we must also consider the interaction between all of these constraints and their relative effect on motor skill performance. Imagine, for example, someone climbing the metaphorical mountain. The climber is affected by his or her own personal strengths or limitations (e.g., endurance, strength, reach, motivation) the nature of the mountain (steep, high, number of handholds, number of passages), weather conditions (e.g., cold, icy, windy), and, of course, the interaction of all of these factors at any one time.

To illustrate the so-called products of motor development, Clark and Metcalfe also integrate six periods of motor development into their metaphor, the mountain. These periods begin during the prenatal state and are referred to as the reflexive, preadapted, fundamental patterns, context-specific, skillful, and compensation periods. The authors note that progression up the mountain is very individual with "climbers" accumulating skill in a sequential process as they go higher. Each period provides the "climber" with necessary prerequisites to assist the progression to the next period.

The journey up the hill begins during prenatal life when the body is forming. Immediately, constraints begin to impact development. For example, the fetus is affected by parental factors that may have far-reaching and long-term effects on the baby. For example, did the mother eat a healthy diet, exercise, smoke, drink excessive amounts of alcohol, experience excess stress, or contract a disease that could affect the fetus? The individual is also a product of their genetic makeup. All of these factors, and many more, will affect the climb up the mountain. Of course, the changing terrain encountered once the climb begins is symbolic of the varying paths we all take as we pass through life.

Reflexive Period

Clark and Metcalfe's first period, the Reflexive Period, generally exists for several weeks pre- birth and for a variable period of time after we are born. This period is particularly important as the reflexive movement exhibited in this period is important for sustaining survival while enabling beginning interactions with the surrounding world. The first year or year and a half of life is often referred to as infancy. The term infancy literally refers to the lack of speech that is one of the prime characteristics of this time of life (Piek, 2006). During the early weeks and months of infancy, one of the most fascinating human movement forms is prevalent. Infant reflexes are "involuntary movements that are generally elicited by an external stimulus specific to that particular reflex..." (Piek, 2006; p. 17). They are characterized by being stereotypical and subcortical. Stereotypical implies that they occur virtually the same each time they are elicited. For example, the well known palmar grasp reflex normally appears from slightly before birth to about four months of age. A stroke of the infant's palm will elicit a closing of the four fingers; usually the thumb is not involved. Each time the hand is stimulated, the reaction is virtually the same. Similarly, the sucking reflex is elicited upon a tactile stimulation of the baby's lips; the baby responds by a sucking action. Subcortical implies that the higher brain centers like the motor cortex are relatively uninvolved in the production of the movement. Thus, infant reflexes do not appear to be learned. Rather, they seem to be "prewired" in the normal infant. When a stimulus is applied, like the stroke of the hand, an impulse is sent to through the central nervous system to the lower brain or brain stem. Though the process is far from understood, we believe that the impulse is processed and sent back to the hand where a "close the hand" message is delivered (Payne & Isaacs, 2008).

Another very different example of an infant reflex is the labyrinthine reflex. This reflex can normally be elicited from approximately two to twelve months. It is elicited by holding the infant upright. As the baby is tipped to one side or the other, the head responds by tilting in the opposite direction. If the baby is tipped to the front or back, the head will respond by tilting backwards or forwards. Though little evidence is available to support the assertion, one might suspect that this reflex is primary in the establishment of eventual upright sitting and standing posture.

Because there are many infant reflexes, they have been categorized into the primitive and the postural types. The primitive reflexes are those which are believed to protect and nourish us when we are incapable of doing that for ourselves. Note, the sucking reflex mentioned above would be considered a primitive reflex, because of the role it plays in ingesting nourishment. The postural reflexes are those that are believed to play a role in the development of more advanced voluntary movement, learned movement that that is created as a result of an impulse from higher brain centers. An example of a postural reflex is the stepping or walking reflex. This reflex can be elicited by holding a baby upright with the floor or a tabletop applying a force to the bottoms of the feet. This stimulus will create an alternate stepping action of the legs that gives the appearance of a surprisingly mature walking action of the legs.

The exact relationship of the postural reflexes to ensuing voluntary movements like reaching, grasping, sitting, standing, or even walking, is unknown. However, researchers have examined the effects of manipulation of certain reflexes on the time of appearance of certain voluntary movements. One of the best examples of this type of research was conducted by Zelazo and associates (1993). In this classis research, the researchers repeatedly stimulated the stepping reflex with six-week-old infants. Compared to a control group, these infants were found to voluntarily step more on their own. The researchers speculated that the regular "practice" of the research may have enhanced the infant's equilibrium and strength of the stepping related muscles prompting the baby to more voluntary attempts at stepping.

In normal, healthy babies infant reflexes can be seen starting at birth and lasting past the first birthday. For example, the search or rooting reflex is typically present at birth. This reflex can be elicited by stroking the baby's cheek to the right or left of the mouth. The baby will turn the head toward the side of the stimulated cheek. This is a primitive reflex that is nourishment related. This reflex helps the baby locate the mother's nipple for sustenance. Once the nipple is located, the lips are stimulated to begin the sucking reflex for ingestion of breast milk. Like the search reflex, the sucking reflex is present at birth. However, both reflexes will subside at around three months of age.

The time of appearance of infant reflexes is somewhat variable individually, however, the reflexes are predictable enough to be used in pediatric diagnosis where they can be reasonably accurate predictors of a baby's neurological maturity (Malina, Bouchard, & Bar-Or, 2004). In such tests, pediatricians will look for significant deviations in the time of appearance, the strength, or the symmetry. Occasionally, a reflex may not appear at all. This, too, may be an indicator of a neurological impairment. Many of the infant reflexes are symmetrical in appearance. For example, children with cerebral palsy (a motor impairment rooted in early damage to the brain) often continue to demonstrate primitive reflexes such as the startle, grasping, and asymmetrically tonic neck reflex well into early childhood and even into their teens. The persistence of primitive reflexes into early childhood is an indication of neurological impairment, and additional testing should be requested (Zafeiriou, 2004).

While infant reflexes are a dominant form of movement over the first few weeks of life, the presence and significance of these movements gradually diminishes across the first year of life. Infant reflexes are gradually over-ridden or replaced by movements that are under voluntary control. This process gradually evolves until just after the first year of life when we are no longer able to elicit most of the infant reflexes. Despite the disappearance of these reactions, a number of reflexes remain and will be maintained throughout life in normal and healthy individuals. These reflexes, however, are not considered infant reflexes, because they are normal and expected beyond infancy. Examples of such lifelong reflexes are the knee jerk where the patellar tendon is abruptly tapped eliciting a sudden jerk of the leg into a partial extension at the knee.

Preadapted Period

Clark and Metcalfe's second period of their Mountain of Motor Development is characterized by the gradual "disappearance or inhibition" of the infant reflexes. During this period of time, voluntary movement becomes increasingly prevalent. By voluntary movement, we refer to movement that is intentionally, often consciously, initiated by the individual. This is in contrast to reflexive movement that is elicited by an external stimulus causing the individual to move. Clark and Metcalfe chose the term Pre-adapted Period to reflect the "progressive mastery of the body in a gravitational environment" (Clark and Metcalfe, 2002; p. 175). Clearly, the individual's genetic structure and environment create an extensive repertoire of possibilities for movement. Within that interaction, Clark and Metcalfe believe that the goal of this period of development is the achievement of an increased level of functional independence. This ranges from increased independence in feeding to exploring one's own environment via independent locomotion to increasing pursuit of social interactions as a result of the evolving independence of movement (e.g., crawling, walking).

Movements in this period of development are often divided into three categories, stability, manipulation, and locomotion (Gallahue & Ozmun, 2006). Stability involves those movements that enable us to control the body or place it in the desired position. Examples would include head control, rolling from front to back or back to front, sitting, and even standing. Manipulation involves the use of the hands and arms and locomotion involves the movement from one point in space to another (e.g., crawling, walking). Though all of these movements are critical to our existence and are clear examples of our developing movement, space limits our discussion of all of them. We will, however, focus on crawling as one example of the changes in movement behavior during this Pre-adaptive Period. Because the terms creeping and crawling are not consistently used and interpreted, some explanation is required. For our purposes, crawling is considered the less mature movement form that is often characterized by a pre-creeping movement that is highly variable, somewhat inefficient, usually low to the ground, and intending to propel the body forward. Creeping is the more mature locomotor pattern that generally follows by around 7 to 8 months of age. It is characterized by a higher, more efficient and upright, hand and knee form of locomotion with the torso elevated of the floor (Payne & Isaacs, 2008).

Adolph, Vereijken, and Denny (1998) studied 28 babies starting to crawl until they began to walk. The researchers were particularly interested in the effects of the baby's age, their body dimensions, and their previous experiences on crawling development. Generally, sequential and continuous improvement was seen in the way the babies crawled and how quickly they crawled. Despite many similarities in the way the babies crawled, there were also many differences demonstrating the individual variability in motor development at this time of life. Some of the babies skipped characteristics of crawling development that were quite common in others. One example was crawling on the belly or low-crawling where nearly half of the babies were found to "skip" this piece of the developmental progression. Characteristics that were encountered regularly included elevating the head and chest from the ground, pulling forward while the lower torso was still in contact with the supporting surface, and rocking rhythmically while in the crawling position. The progression of overall crawling development did not seem to be absolute, but rather, somewhat variable from baby to baby as many different crawling positions were exhibited. The earliest form of crawling was characterized by dragging the lower torso on the floor. Experience was clearly a factor as those babies with more exposure to crawling became more efficient and faster crawlers at an earlier age. Size was also a factor as smaller, leaner babies were found to crawl earlier than larger babies. Finally, hands and knees creeping (locomoting with the torso elevated off the floor on the hands and knees) was typically the final locomotor milestone before the onset of walking (Adolph, Vereijken, & Denny, 1998).

Fundamental Patterns Period

During the Fundamental Patterns Period of the Mountain, the young mover uses existing skill to advance to a level of movement that is often considered the base of many future movement skills. This period is formulated during infancy, but is often considered to last until approximately seven years of life (Clark & Metcalfe, 2002). At that time, these movements will gradually be applied to specific movement situations, like sports. Thus, these movements are often referred to as the "building blocks" of more context specific movements of later life (Clark & Metcalfe, p. 176; Payne & Isaacs, p.300). Without a solid base of ability in these fundamental movements, achieving a mature level of movement ability in the more complex and combined movements associated with later life will become more difficult or impossible to achieve. As in the previous periods of development, substantial differences may be noted in the skill levels of children based on their previous opportunity, experience, instruction, and practice of the skill in question.

The fundamental movements, or motor patterns, can be organized in several ways. Payne & Isaacs (2008) make reference to two types of fundamental movements: the fundamental locomotion skills and the fundamental object control skills. While locomotion, moving from one point in space to another (e.g., walking) really began in earlier periods of the mountain, it is during this time that real progress is typically noted, even to the extent of seeing nearly adult like skill evolving in many aspects of the child's ability in the fundamental locomotion skills like walking, running, jumping, hopping, leaping, skipping, and galloping. In addition, children commonly increase their interaction with objects (e.g., balls, rackets, bats) in their environment as they develop fundamental object control skills like throwing, catching, ball bouncing, kicking, and striking.

Research has indicated that fairly predictable development sequences exist in the fundamental movements (Roberton & Halverson, 1984). Though space will not allow for an examination of all of the fundamental movements, an examination of the relatively predictable sequences for one pattern will be useful as an example. Researchers (Roberton, 1983; Seefeldt, Reuschlein, and Vogel, 1972) have hypothesized that initial efforts to run are characterized by relatively flat-footed running as the feet generally contact the supporting surface with the entire foot. The legs are often abducted (i.e. swung out to the side) in immature runners as the leg recovers to the front position. Toes are often pointed out slightly and the angle (bend at the knee) of the recovering leg often exceeds ninety degrees during the recovery. In other words, the legs stay relatively straight compared to more mature runners. The stride is relatively short and inconsistent in both length and landing position. The arms are typically held in a high guard position and make little contribution to generating momentum for the run. They are held above the shoulders in a "high guard" position (Payne & Isaacs, 2008).

Gradually, with maturity, instruction, experience, and practice, the running pattern becomes more mature. This is illustrated by a more noticeable bend in the recovering leg, the amount of out-toeing is reduced, and the arms begin to lower into a position where they can assist in the generation of force for the run. The decreasing amount of abduction of the recovering leg is also a common characteristic of increasing maturity in the running pattern. With the onset of these more mature characteristics, we also note an increase flight time during the run. Flight time is the period in which no body part is touching the ground, one foot has just pushed off, but the opposite foot has not yet contacted the supporting surface. This is most likely a function of both the maturation of the movement technique as well as the child's increasing strength and power.

As the arms lower, the immature runner may exhibit a rotation of the upper body, or trunk, and a crossing of the body's midline with the slightly flexed arms as they swing through in the forward position. Also, noticeable when viewed from the rear, and perhaps a reaction to the upper body rotation, is the foot crossing the midline when behind the body. The stride gradually elongates and becomes more consistent in both length and foot placement.

A mature runner will assume a greater forward inclination and no longer exhibit the flat-footed characteristics described earlier. Typically, the heal of toe will make initial contact as the leg swings more directly straight forward and back with a significant flexion in each leg as it swings through in both the front and rear positions. However, once the rear leg reaches the full push-off position it will be nearing full extension in the mature runner. The amount of upper body rotation will diminish with the arms now swinging straight forward and straight back (sagittal plane) in a flexed position. The arms, swinging in opposition to each other, and in opposition to the same-side leg, drive through to provide additional force to achieve greater velocity in the run. Similarly, the legs will no longer cross the midline as they, too, swing straight forward and back with a minimum of excess motion (Payne & Isaacs, 2008).

Research has found that sixty percent of boys were able to perform at a mature level by four years of age. Sixty percent of girls were able to perform at a mature level by slightly more than five years of age (Seefeldt & Haubenstricker, 1982). Note, however, that these percentages were determined using a "total-body" assessment of movement. In other words, the observer makes an overall assessment of the general level of maturity of all aspects of the performer's movement. While this is a relatively simple and useful method of assessing the development of fundamental movement, it may not convey a completely accurate analysis of movement. This is because a child will often exhibit relatively mature characteristics in one aspect of the fundamental movement, like running, while others remain relatively immature. For example, a child may have a relatively mature arm action with the arms in the lowered position, flexed at nearly a ninety degree angle, and swinging through in opposition to the leg on the same side of the body. At the same time, however, the leg action may be characterized by a lack of leg flexion, a bent leg at push-off, and a slight abduction of the legs as they swing through – all relatively immature characteristics. For this reason, fundamental movement is often assessed by a "component" approach where individual assessment is made of the specific body parts involved in the movement. While this system is generally believed to provide more accurate information, it is less administratively efficient for many practitioners in a teaching setting.

Regardless of which assessment technique is employed, knowledge of the expected developmental trends in movements like running can be invaluable in making instructional decisions related to the student's level of maturity in a given movement pattern, assessing when a child might be able to achieve maturity in a given movement patterns, and designing educational programs to assist children in attaining higher levels of maturity in a given movement pattern. Thus, knowledge of motor development can yield informed decisions related to the education of children in physical education, sports, recreational, and fitness activities.

Context Specific Period

The Context Specific Period of the Mountain metaphor builds off of the skills developed in the previous period. The fundamental movement patterns (e.g., running, jumping, throwing, catching, kicking) are honed as the child's skill level improves. The mover gradually develops an ability to adapt these movements to new and different situations where the constraints may demand increased ability at adapting the movement to the demands of the movement setting. Achieving this level of ability in the fundamental movements varies widely from child to child. However, according to Clark and Metcalfe (2002), achieving this period of the Mountain could occur as early as four years of age in rare cases. More commonly, however, it would be expected closer to seven years of age. Nevertheless, more mature performers may also find themselves at this point on the Mountain, or below. For example, a young adult may decide to take-up tennis with little or no previous experience. Initially, as they begin to develop a more mature striking pattern (i.e., forehand, backhand, or serve), they may find themselves on the Fundamental Patterns Period of the Mountain working their way up to the Context Specific Period. This is a clear indicator that one's status on the Mountain is not just age related. It reflects much more than how much time has been spent "climbing." It is also affected by the array of one's unique life experiences like where and how they are raised. For example, we often find that children raised near a beach or an ocean may develop skills differently that those who are not. Aquatic activities like swimming, diving, surfing, or beach volleyball may be prevalent. In addition, certain geographic areas are more culturally predisposed to certain activities. For example, a child raised in the northeastern part of the United States would be more likely to play Lacrosse that a child raised in the Western or Southern United States where that sport is not as common.

As children "climb" up into this period of development, they will begin to use their fundamental movement abilities in more sophisticated ways. They will simultaneously combine one fundamental movement with another, or several others, while performing the movement in the face of increasing movement demands. They may begin to combine throwing with running as required in basketball or football, or catching while funning as required in baseball. They may seek to achieve greater accuracy or speed in the movement, or perform the movement with many more constraints than previously imagined. An example would be the progression from simply dribbling a basketball while standing to dribble the ball while running, even weaving, through a series of defenders on the basketball court. Obviously, this involves increasing perceptual-cognitive demands. The performer must more fully understand the constraints of the surrounding situation to achieve more success motorically. For example, when dribbling the ball down court, having a greater understanding of the possible defensive responses of the opposing team may signal a need to dribble right or left, or faster or slower.

Clark and Metcalfe believe that this period of time is particularly important, because one's level of success and feelings of competence in the performance of movements will impact future decisions governing their participation. Having a more fully developed skill level in the fundamental movements is integral to this success (Clark and Metcalfe, 2002).

Skillful Period

Not everyone will achieve this level of the Mountain, and this period is rarely achieved by a child. However, for many with sufficient instruction, practice, experience, and opportunity, an individual can climb from the Context-specific period of the Mountain to the Skillful Period. Skillful implies that a mover can perform with such a high level of ability that movement is performed confidently with the potential to integrate movements into situations requiring strategic analysis to enhance performance. Thus, like in the Context-specific Period, the cognitive component of movement is intertwined with the level of movement performance.

Interestingly, this period of the Mountain can be attained for one or more movement skills. In fact, some performers may even become quite skillful in many, though no one attains this level in most or all movement skills. This level of skill is rarely attained without considerable effort on the part of the performer and many people may never find the need or desire to achieve this level of skill. Seeking proper instruction or coaching and practicing that which has been taught are integral to skillful movement. Being motivated to achieve such a level is also critical. This suggests that the performer is in an environment where these opportunities are available. It may include having parents who are encouraging, friends who are supportive, and the surrounding culture that provides adequate incentive to improve. Of course, it also requires that inherent physical, cognitive, emotional, and motor capabilities are present. For example, performing a skilled back hand spring in gymnastics may not be possible if the performer lacks adequate strength, power, and agility to execute the movement. For some, even with instruction and practice, inherent characteristics may be too limiting to allow execution of the movement. That back handspring, for example, may be much more difficult, even impossible, for someone who is exceptionally tall, or dunking a basketball may be unachievable for someone who is exceptionally short regardless of their superior jumping ability.

According to Clark and Metcalfe (2002), this period of the Mountain often coincides with the onset of the adolescent growth spurt at puberty, though many exceptions exist. We have all seen evidence of elite level performers, like swimmers, tennis players, or gymnasts who have achieved superior levels of skill at very young ages. Similarly, many individuals may never be motivated to achieve such a level of skill until much later in life, even as late as middle adulthood or beyond. For some, this level of skill will simply never be achieved. However, when this level of expertise is achieved, it generally requires time, considerable practice, appropriate instruction, and the appropriate interaction of the performer's own biological characteristics with the surrounding environment. For that reason, exceptionally high levels of skill, expertise, often may not be achieved until early adulthood.

Compensation Period

Clark and Metcalfe's final period of the Mountain is referred to as the Compensation period (2002) where motor development continues to emerge. Our major emphasis in this paper is to provide an overview of movement during childhood. This period of the mountain is generally seen in the adult years. Nevertheless, because it is the last period of the metaphor, a brief examination of the major characteristics of the period is in order. As the name implies, compensation is integral to this period of development. According to the authors, this indicates that the human system may be interacting in a substandard way requiring adaptations for the movement in question to be performed. These adaptations may be necessary as a result of physical injury or as a function of the normal aging process. For example, a spinal cord injury may require considerable adjustments to re-learn sitting, standing, or walking. In severe cases, these behaviors may not be possible, so adaptations may focus on the use of the hands and arms in reaching and grasping movements. Similarly, children born with disabilities must learn to compensate for the disabilities. A child who is born with a visual impairment learns how to move relying on visual and tactile cues rather than visual cues, and a child born without legs learns to walk and run with prosthetics and crutches or perhaps learns to move and play sports using a wheelchair.

In the case of older performers, a gradual slowing with age, reduced strength or flexibility may similarly require adaptations to the way movements are performed, or decision as to which movements may no longer be possible. Regardless of whether the compensations are injury or age related, the system must reorganize or shift to accommodate a changing movement repertoire. Generally, this period involves the latter part of life when motor development is experienced or seen as a decline or regression occurring as the physical characteristics (e.g., strength, endurance, speed of movement). More positively, we can view this time of life as an adaptation or series of adjustments to the ever changing system that governs of motor development. In addition, considerable evidence points to the dramatic positive effect of physical activity and exercise on overcoming the rate of decline of the physiological systems that influence our motor development (Clark & Metcalfe, 2002). Nevertheless, regardless of the activity level one maintains, the regressive effects of the aging process are inevitable.

UNIQUE DEVELOPMENT CONSIDERATIONS FOR CHILDREN WITH VARIOUS DISABILITIES

The previous discussion of the Mountain of Motor Development outlined a typical course of development seen in most children without disabilities. However, there are certain types of disabilities that can affect how quickly children progress up the mountain and how high they progress up the mountain. For example, children with Down syndrome (a genetic cause of intellectual disabilities) are often delayed in walking by more than a year compared to children without intellectual disabilities, and some children with Down syndrome may never reach the context-specific period of motor development. The sections describe some of the more common types of developmental disabilities and how these disabilities can impact normal motor development. Note that due to space constraints and the diversity of characteristics children with physical disabilities were not included in this discussion.

Children with Intellectual Disabilities

The term intellectual disability (ID) is the new preferred term for what had been referred to as mental retardation (Schalock et al., 2007). The American Association for Intellectual and Developmental Disabilities (AAIDD) produced the definitive definition of ID for several decades now. The most recent definition is: "An intellectual disability is a disability characterized by significant limitations both in intellectual functioning and in adaptive behavior as expressed in conceptual, social, and practical adaptive skills. This disability originates before the age of 18" (Luckasson et al., 2002, p. 1). A significant limitation in intellectual functioning refers to an IQ two standard deviations or more (SD = 15) from the mean IQ of 100 (an IQ of 70 or below). In practical terms, this means a child will have significant problems in reading, writing, arithmetic, memory, attention, and problem solving (although individual children may have strengths in particular areas) (Luckasson et al., 2002). A significant limitation in adaptive behavior refers to how well people cope with common life demands and problems and how well they meet the standards of personal independence expected of someone about their age, community setting, sociocultural background. Adaptive behaviors include taking care of one self, handling money, living in the community, and displaying appropriate behaviors (APA, 2000; Luckasson et al., 2002).

Children with ID comprise a broad spectrum from relatively mild ID (IQ closer to 70) to those with more severe ID (those with IQ below 40). In addition, there a variety of causes of intellectual disabilities ranging from biological/genetic causes (e.g., Down syndrome, Fragile X syndrome), environmental causes (e.g., fetal alcohol syndrome), and educational/social causes (severely limited stimulation). As a result it is difficult to generalize functional abilities (including motor abilities and delays) across the generic classification of ID.

With regards to motor development, limited research shows children with mild ID tend to be one to three years delayed in motor development while children with more severe intellectual disabilities tend to have delays of four years or more (DiRocco, Clark, & Phillips, 1987; Rarick, 1980). These delays are both quantitative (Zhang, 2005; Yun & Ulrich, 1997) and qualitative (DiRocco et al., 1987). These motor delays tend to widen as children with ID grow older and motor performance relies on greater speed and movement control as well as the use of strategies (Sherrill, 2004; Wall, 2004). For example, Zhang (2005) found children ages 12-15 with mild intellectual disabilities scored between 6-10 years delayed compared to peers without ID on the Bruininks-Oseretsky Test of Motor Proficiency.

Children with ID, because of particular biological/genetic causes, often have physical anomalies that lead to specific and more pronounced motor delays and deficits. This is perhaps most notable in children with Down syndrome, a genetic disorder that causes pervasive developmental delays (Pueschel, 2000). Among many other issues, children with Down syndrome have hypotonia ((low muscle tone), increased flexibility in joints, decreased muscle strength, and medical problems such as heart and respiratory problems which all affect and limit motor development (Block, 1991; Pueschel, 2000; Winders, 1997).

Teaching and Coaching Children with Intellectual Disability

The combination of intellectual and adaptive behavior deficits coupled with motor delays in children with intellectual disabilities requires unique teaching methods. In most cases these unique teaching methods focus on presenting information so that individuals with ID will understand what to do and how to do it as well as staying focused on the task at hand. (Drane & Block, 2006; Krebs, 2005). *Communication* is the perhaps the most important teaching strategy. Children with ID may not understand verbal directions imitate demonstrations as well as their peers. This requires the teacher or coach to simplify verbal directions and highlight key components of a demonstration. For example, a coach may point to the inside of his foot, touch the child's inside foot, and then have the child touch a ball to the inside of his foot in order to make sure the child understand where to contact the ball when passing a soccer ball. When verbal and visual cues do not work, the coach or teacher may need to provide physical assistance.

"Attention" is another key teaching strategy when working with children with ID. Children with ID often do not have the attention span of their peers without ID, and as a result they have a difficult time staying focused when practicing a skill or staying focused on a key aspect of a skill (Drane & Block, 2006; Krebs, 2005). For example, a teacher may ask children to pick up a ball and practice their overhand throw against the wall. The teacher specifically tells children to focus on stepping with the opposite foot. The child with ID may throw a few balls remembering to step with the opposite foot, but quickly the student becomes distracted losing focus first on stepping with the opposite foot and eventually practicing the throw at all. To combat this problem, teachers and coaches need to organize the practice setting to help the child with ID stay focused. This includes making practice very concrete such as placing 20 balls in front of the child telling him to throw each ball one at a time until all the balls are gone. The teacher may place foot print or other visual cues on the floor to remind the child to focus on a particular component. The teacher may need to go to the child more often than to peers without ID to remind to keep him focused and provide extra instruction and reinforcement. Finally, a peer can assigned to the child during a particular activity to provide extra cues.

Finally, teachers and coaches should plan on dealing with *behavior problems* often displayed by children with ID. Behavior problems tend to be fairly mild (e.g., refusing to participate, walking away, playing with equipment inappropriately) revolving around frustration with lack of success, confusion with what to do, boredom, and wanting to exert some control. Strategies to combat behavior problems focus on understanding the root cause or the function of the problem (Block, 2007). For example, a child with an ID refuses to take his turn to hit a pitched baseball. This child may know from previous experiences that he cannot hit a pitched ball, and his refusal to participate is an indication of lack of confidence based on previous experience. In this situation the teacher or coach can offer a lighter, larger bat or allow the child to hit a ball off a tee. Similarly, a child with an ID tries to hit a peer after the teacher gives complex directions on how to rotate to various stations in the gym. The child is telling the teacher he does not know what to do, and this confusion lead to anxiety and acting out. Knowing ahead of time the child with ID may not understand directions; after directing the group the teacher immediately goes to this child and repeats the directions in a simpler form. The teacher may even walk the child over to the first station to help him get started.

Children with Learning Disabilities

Specific learning disability (SLD) defines a group of disabilities that affect a child's ability to learn which in turn affects a child's academic performance. Deficits are neurologically based, and damage to specific parts of the brain will determine specific types of learning disabilities (Lavay, 2005; Shapiro, 2001). For example, one child may have a learning disability in reading while another child may have a learning disability in math (see table 1 for a list of specific types of learning disabilities). Children with SLD do not have any intellectual disabilities and in some cases may even be quite gifted and do extraordinary things. Famous people with learning disabilities include Walt Disney, Albert Einstein, and General George Patton (LD Online, 2008). It is important to note that to have the label of learning disability a child cannot have other disabilities that might affect learning such as in intellectual disability, autism, deafness, blindness, and behavioral disorders. Also, a learning disability cannot occur suddenly by a lack of educational opportunities, attendance problems, or frequent changes of schools. Reported incidence of SLD ranges from as low as 5% of the school age population to as high as 15%. The discrepancy may be due to children who qualify for special education services (5%) compared to children who may have some type of a learning disability but who many not qualify for special education. Reading disabilities are the most common type of SLD comprising almost 80% of all learning disabilities (LD Online, 2008; Shapiro, 2001).

About 25 to 50% of children with SLD have other disabilities or problems. The most common related disability is attention deficit/hyperactive disorder (ADHD) (see discussion later in this chapter). Some children with SLD also have behavior or emotional problems. Behavior problems may be due to neurological impairments that may lead to depression or anxiety disorders. On the other hand, many children with SLD who display behavior problems may be reacting negatively to their academic difficulties (Shapiro, 2001). Imagine a 4th grade child with dyslexia who still struggles with reading. This child sees his peers moving to more advanced books while he still is barely able to read 1st grade material. It is not surprising that this child might have issues with self-esteem which in turn might lead to anxiety, depression, and withdrawal when faced with academic work. Or perhaps this child may get frustrated and angry with his struggles with reading which leads to acting out and conduct behaviors. In either case, behavior problems are directly related to the child's learning disability and how it affects academic performance. This is why it is so important to identify learning disabilities as soon as possible so a child does not struggle academically and can get some remedial help.

Table 1. Specific Types of Learning Disabilities*

Dyslexia – the most common type of learning disability, dyslexia refers to a language-based disability in which the child has trouble understanding written words including basic reading (decoding letters and words), reading comprehension (understanding what to read), spelling, and writing. Dyslexia is related to problems with visual perception, the ability to notice important visual details.
Dyscalculia – a mathematical disability in which a person has a difficult time with arithmetic problems and grasping math concepts. Specific mathematic problems can include math reasoning, memory of math facts, concepts of time and money, and musical concepts.
Dysgraphia – Also known as graphomotor disorder, dysgraphia is a writing disability where children finds it difficult to form letters and write within a defined space as well as the speed and precision in writing. Dyscalculia is often associated with dyslexia.
Dyspraxia **(apraxia)** – dyspraxia is a motor planning disability where the child had difficulty coordinating movements. These children appear awkward in their movements and may also have balance problems. Another term for dyspraxia is developmental coordination disorder (DCD).
Auditory Discrimination – auditory discrimination is an auditory disability in which a person has difficulty understanding language despite normal hearing. Auditory discrimination problems make it difficult for children to perceive differences between speech sounds then sequence sounds into meaningful words. Auditory processing also makes it difficult to understand the phonetics sounds of letters which is critical for learning to read.

From LD Online. *Common Learning Disabilities*. Retrieved November 10, 2008, from http://www.ldonline.org/ldbasics/whatisld.

Many children with learning disabilities do not have any gross motor problems and are actually quite athletic. Some famous athletes who had learning disabilities include Olympic gold medalist Bruce Jenner, basketball star Magic Johnson, football start Dexter Manley, and baseball star Pete Rose (Angle, 2007). However, some children with learning disabilities also have motor problems. Not surprisingly, motor problems are most notable in children with motor and sensory related learning problems such as dyspraxia and visual processing problems (Shapiro, 2001). For example, Miyahara (1994) found 25% of children with SLD scored poorly in a general motor ability test, and an additional 7% demonstrated significant balance problems. Similarly, Lazarus (1994) found children with SLD had greater levels of overflow (an inability to keep one arm or leg still while moving the other arm or leg) compared to same-age peers without SLD. Finally, Sherrill and Pyfer (1985) found 13 percent of children with LD scored 2-3 years below age level on perceptual motor tests. Again, these motor difficulties seem to be related to motor planning (dyspraxia) (e.g., Lazarus and Miyahara) and visual perception (Sherrill & Pyfer, 1985).

Teaching and Coaching Strategies for
Children with Specific Learning Disabilities

Special teaching and coaching strategies for children with learning disabilities are similar to those for children with ADHD. Strategies are designed to help these students stay focused on and understand the activity. Some additional strategies are needed to compensate for perceptual and movement problems. The following suggestions are adapted from Lavay (2005), Sherrill (2004), Drane and Block (2006):

1. Use a highly structured, consistent approach to teaching (i.e., establish a routine, have set places for children to sit, use a direct rather than exploratory approach when possible).
2. Include activities during warm-ups and cool downs that emphasize moving slowly to help control to decrease hyperactivity and impulsivity.
3. When necessary, teach in a quiet, less stimulating environment to decrease distractibility.
4. Assign a peer to provide extra instruction and assistance to a child who is having trouble moving correctly.
5. Encourage children to plan out loud and repeat directions to enhance motor planning. This is especially important for disorganized, distractible children.
6. Provide appropriate learning strategies to help disorganized learners focus on skill (tell class objective of lesson, ID critical elements of skill, use extra cues such as footprints on floor; teach students how to practice and use feedback).
7. Use a multisensory approach when giving instruction to students with perceptual problems. For example, give a direction verbally, demonstrate the skill, have the students mirror your demonstration, and even provide physical guidance as needed.
8. Eliminate embarrassing teaching practices that force comparison among students. For example, do not have a child with an SLD who is clumsy demonstrate in front of the class unless you know the child will be successful.
9. Use cooperative teaching styles to increase student's social interaction and self-concept.
10. Review previously acquired skills to make sure child has achieved mastery. Occasionally review previously mastered skills when introducing new skills to further enhance long-term retention.

Include perceptual and motor activities in the curriculum such as balance, body awareness, eye-hand coordination, and tactile/visual/auditory stimulation. P-M activities can easily be added as a station. For example, several soccer stations can be set up in the gym, and an additional station can be set up where children have to run through a rope ladder followed by leaping from one poly spot to another.

Children with Attention Deficit Hyperactivity Disorder (ADHD)

Attention Deficit/Hyperactivity Disorder (ADHD) is a disorder that makes it significantly difficult for children to pay attention, focus on a task, and sit still. There are two main types of ADHD. In the hyperactive-impulsive type children appear extremely energized and overactive (hyperactive) and unable to anticipate consequences of their behaviors (impulsivity). In the inattentive type children may be inattentive, have difficulty focusing, and may seem to be daydreaming or lack motivation. There is a third type (*combined*) in which both types of behaviors are present (APA, 2000; Glanzman & Blum, 2007). Table 1 presents the diagnostics criteria for ADHD from the American Psychiatric Association (APA, 2000).

ADHD affects approximately 1/20 children. It is 3 times more common in boys than girls, and usually appears when children start school and are asked to sit and pay attention for extending periods of time (NICHCY, 2001; Glanzman & Blum, 2007). ADHD characteristics can range from mild to severe with far more children being diagnosed with mild ADHD. An interesting note about children with mild ADHD is they seem to be able to focus and attend when they are participating in a highly motivating activity such as playing a video game or when they are given a novel activity (Glanzman & Blum, 2007).

As noted earlier, primary characteristics associated with ADHD revolve around problems with attention, impulsivity, and hyperactivity. However, children with ADHD often have problems that are directly related to these primary problems. In turn, these associated problems tend to be interrelated. For example, many children with ADHD have problems developing friendships and interacting appropriately with peers. Problems with peers are most likely related to the child's difficulty paying attention (e.g., not attending to peers) and hyperactivity (difficulty staying still or in one place). In addition, attention problems make it difficult for a child to pick up on peer's facial expressions, body language, and the flow of a conversation. As a result peers perceive the child with ADHD as uninterested in them and a nuisance, and as a result the child with ADHD may be isolated and even ostracized by peers. A child with ADHD who is isolated and not included may develop a lower self-esteem and becomes more susceptible to antisocial conduct disorders such as acting out, fighting, running away, and drug use. Some suggest as many as 30-50% of children with ADHD have these antisocial behaviors (Moffitt, 1990; Werry, Elkind & Reeves, 1987; Woolrich, 1994).

Somewhat surprisingly, motor delays are another characteristic often associated with ADHD. While many children with ADHD do quite well in physical education and sport, many others show signs of gross motor delays (Harvey & Reid, 2003). For example, Harvey and Reid (1997) found children with ADHD scored lower on the Test of Gross Motor Development (TGMD) (a test that measures basic fundamental motor skills such as throwing and catching and running and jumping) when compared to peers without ADHD. Kadesjo and Gillberg (1998) and Peik, Pitcher, and Hay (1999) found 50% of children with ADHD they studied had developmental coordination disorder (DCD), a significant impairment in general motor coordination and control. Yan and Thomas (2002), found children with ADHD took more time and were less accurate and more variable completing a rapid arm movement task compared to children without ADHD. Finally, Beyer (1999) found boys with ADHD 7 to 12 years of age performed significantly poorer in fine motor and motor coordination timed tests compared to children with learning disabilities. Interestingly, there were no differences in balance and upper limb coordination tests. It is possible that children with ADHD do poorly in timed and accuracy tests (e.g., Beyer, 1999, and Yan & Thomas, 2002) because of difficulties with impulsivity (moving without thinking) and attention to exact movement requirements of the task. Similarly, tests that measure developmental coordination (Kadesjo & Gillberg, 1998; and Piek, et al., 1999) often require attending to a task and moving carefully, something that may be difficult for children with ADHD. It is less clear why some children with ADHD would have problems with fundamental motor patterns at seen in Harvey and Reid's study (2003).

Teaching and Coaching Strategies for Children with ADHD

Sherrill (2004) presented several suggestions for teaching children with ADHD. Since most of the problems associated with ADHD are behavioral rather than physical, the suggestions focus on managing the environment to help the child with ADHD focus.

Establish a Highly Structured Program

To prevent distractibility and to compensate for a short attention span, instructors should establish a routine and follow it as closely as possible. This routine should include a consistent entry routine (how children should enter the gym and where they should go and sit), a relatively set order of activities, a consistent place to received instructions, and even personal space markers such as poly spots and carpet squares (perhaps just for the child with ADHD). Once a routine is established it is important to explain rules and consequences and remind the child often of these rules and consequences. In some cases a special behavior management plan might need to be established just for the child with disabilities. Whether class-wide rules or a specific behavior plan, it is important for the instructor to follow the plan as designed. While the child may not enjoy having to sit out or have a piece of equipment taken away for a few minutes, he will appreciate the consistency. It also is important to provide positive reinforcement when the child is doing what he is supposed to be doing.

Reduce Wait Time and Have Clear Start/Stop Signals

Children with ADHD cannot sit and focus for long periods of time. A simple way to help them focus on directions in is to reduce how long a child sits and listens to directions, For example, rather than explaining in detail what to do at five different stations, provide a quick demonstration at each station and then post more detailed directions and different challenges at each station. Then children can be assigned to stations and start the activity. Peers can or the instructor can help those students who do not understand what to do. Similarly, keep transition times to a minimum, and have clear stop commands. For example, a nice auditory cue is music playing while children work at a station. When the music is turned off, that is a cue to stop, sit and listen for instructions. Peers can add an extra verbal reminder to the child with ADHD to help him know to stop. Finally, the instructor can position him/herself close to the child and provide a pre-cue to let the child know that it will be time to stop in 30 seconds.

Reduce Environmental Space

Children with ADHD often cannot handle large open spaces or spaces without any clear boundaries. Therefore, it is important to delimit large spaces by adding partitions and floor markers. Special emphasis should be given to boundaries and how to make these boundaries visually clear to the child. Cones, tape markings, and ropes are good boundary markers, while gym mats can turn into an attractive nuisance (i.e., the child may find the mats attractive to jump on).

Eliminate Irrelevant Auditory and Visual Stimuli

A child with ADHD will be easily distracted by extraneous things in the gym, so it is important to maintain neat, uncluttered, well-ordered gym. As noted above, create partitions to keep children from looking at other stations or equipment, and try to avoid setting up equipment until needed. When giving instructions try and stand so that children see only you and not other distractors in environment. For example, if you are outside giving instructions, position yourself so the children have their back to other children playing on the playground.

Enhance Stimulus Value of Instructional Materials

To help children with ADHD focus on the targeted task, use brightly colored objects and markers such as balls and targets. Color coding activities can help as well such as throwing red balls to a red target. When possible, use auditory equipment (balls with bells) to provide further motivation to the child. Finally use mirrors so that children can look at themselves when performing an activity. In all of these cases enhanced stimulation will help the child focus.

Children with Autism

Autism is part of the larger cluster of disabilities known as pervasive developmental disorder (PDD). PDDs comprise a spectrum of similar disorders that affect communication, behaviors, and social skills. The term spectrum connotes a range in the severity of the characteristics from relatively mild (children with Asperger syndrome) to severe (children with Rett disorder). There is a spectrum within the classification of autism with some children having relatively mild communication, behavioral, and social deficits while others may display more severe deficits. Whether mild or severe, the deficits and unique behaviors that characterize autism are not typical for the child's developmental age. Table 3 presents the diagnostics criteria for autistic disorder from the American Psychiatric Association (APA, 2000).

Communication deficits are one of the characteristics of autism. In the most severe cases children with autism may have no speech or even an ability to communicate using sign language, but often these children learn to point to things they want, take a parents hand and lead them to an item, or use a picture board and point to pictures showing wanted items. In other cases children with autism learn to speak but at an inappropriate level (e.g., whisper or too loud for the context) or in inappropriate ways (Powers, 1989; Towbin, 2001). For example, some children with autism may repeat certain words that create an interesting sound or interesting feeling in their mouth. In other cases, children echo what was asked. To illustrate, when asked, "How are you, John?" the child repeats the question, "How are you, John?" In addition to expressive language deficits, children with autism also have a difficult time understanding verbal language. In very severe cases, parents reported they thought their child was deaf because their child was completely unresponsive to any speech or sounds. In mild cases, a child with autism may not understand multiple directions when give verbally or may not understand abstract, pretend, or sarcastic speech (Powers, 1989; Towbin, 2001). For example, a physical educator tells the class to pretend the gym floor is water and carpet squares are islands. He then tells the class to jump from one "island" to another without falling into the water. The child with autism may start to cry worried he may actually get wet or even drown.

Table 2. Diagnostic Criteria for Attention Deficit (ADHD)*

A. Either (1) or (2):

(1) Inattention: at least 6 of the following symptoms of inattention have persisted for at least 6 months to a degree that is maladaptive and inconsistent to a developmental level:

   a. Often fails to give close attention to details or makes careless mistakes in schoolwork, work, or other activities;

   b. Often has difficulty sustaining attention in tasks or play activities:

   c. Often does not seem to listen to what is being said to him/her;

   d. Often does not follow thru on instructions and fails to finish schoolwork, chores, or duties in the workplace (not due to oppositional behavior or failure to understand instructions).

   e. Often has difficulties organizing tasks and activities;

   f. Often avoids or strongly dislikes tasks (such as schoolwork or homework) that require sustained mental effort;

   g. Often loses things necessary for tasks or activities (e.g., school assignments, pencils, books, tools, or toys);

   h. Is often easily distracted by extraneous stimuli;

   i. Often forgetful in daily activities

(2) Hyperactivity-Impulsivity: at least 4 of the following symptoms of hyperactivity-impulsivity have persisted for at least 6 months to a degree that is maladaptive and inconsistent with developmental level:

   Hyperactivity:

a. Often fidgets with hands or feet or squirms in seat;

b. Leaves seat in classroom or in other situations in which remaining seated is
    expected;

c. Often runs about or climbs excessively in situations where it is inappropriate (in
    adolescents or adults, may be limited to subjective feelings of restlessness);

d. Often has difficulty playing or engaging in leisure activities quietly.

    Impulsivity:

a. Often blurts out answers to questions before the questions have been completed;

b. Often has difficulty waiting in lines or waiting turn in games or group situations.

B. Onset no later than age 7.

C. Symptoms must be present in 2 or more situations (e.g., at school, work, and at
    home).

D. The disturbance causes clinically significant distress or impairment in social,
    academic, or occupational functioning.

E. Does not occur exclusively during the course of PDD, Schizophrenia, or other
    Psychotic Disorder, and is not better accounted for my Mood, Anxiety,
    Dissociative, or Personality Disorder.

- American Psychological Association (APA) (2000). *Diagnostic and
  statistical manual of mental disorders* (4th ed, TR). Washington, DC:
  Author.

Table 3. Diagnostic Criteria for Autistic Disorder*

A. A total of six (or more) items from (1), (2), and (3), with at least two from (1), and on each from (2) and (3):

(1) qualitative impairment in social interaction, as manifested by at least two of the following:

    a. Marked impairment in the use of multiple nonverbal behaviors such as eye-to-eye gaze, facial expression, body postures, and gestures to regulate social interactions.

    b. Failure to develop peer relationships appropriate to developmental level.

    c. A lack of spontaneous seeking to share enjoyment, interests, or achievements with other people (e.g., by a lack of showing, bringing, or pointing out objects of interest).

    d. Lack of social or emotional reciprocity.

(2) Qualitative impairments in communication as manifested by at least one of the following:

    a. Delay in, or total lack of, the developmental of spoken language (not accompanied by an attempt to compensate through alternative modes of communication such as gestures or mime).

    b. In individuals with adequate speech, marked impairment in the ability to initiate or sustain a conversation with others.

    c. Stereotyped and repetitive use of language or idiosyncratic language.

> d. Lack of varied, spontaneous make-believe play or social imitative play appropriate to developmental level.
>
> (3) Restricted repetitive and stereotyped patterns of behavior, interests, and activities as manifested by at least one of the following:
>
> a. Encompassing preoccupation with one or more stereotyped and restricted patterns of interest that is abnormal either in intensity or focus.
>
> b. Apparently inflexible adherence to specific, nonfunctional routines or rituals.
>
> c. Stereotyped and repetitive motor mannerisms (e.g., hand or finger flapping or twisting, or complex whole-body movements).
>
> d. Persistent preoccupation with parts of objects.
>
> B. Delays or abnormal functioning in at least one of the following areas, with onset prior to age 3 years: (1) social interactions, (2) language as used in social communication, or (3) symbolic or imaginative play.
>
> C. The disturbance is not better accounted for by Rett's Disorder or Childhood Disintegrative Disorder.

American Psychological Association (APA) (2000). *Diagnostic and statistical manual of mental disorders* (4th ed, TR). Washington, DC.

Social deficits are another characteristic of children with autism and perhaps the one most associated with autism. Children with autism have a very difficult time interacting appropriately including making eye contact with others, playing with others, sharing toys, and seeking to be with others. Children with autism often do not seem interested in being with, interacting with, and enjoying others company (Mundy & Sigman, 1989; Powers, 1989; Towbin, 2001). However, limited social interactions do not mean children with autism do want to interact with parents and peers. Unfortunately, these children often lack communication and behavioral skills necessary to initiate and sustain contact. In addition, it is important to note that children with autism do not always want to be alone and may enjoy cuddling- up with or hugging a parent or sibling.

Unique behaviors are the final major characteristic associated with autism. In many cases unique and odd behaviors is the first thing that differentiates children with autism from their peers. As with other characteristics associated with autism, behaviors can range from mild mannerisms such as rocking or shaking hands to more severe behaviors including self-abuse, tantrums, and aggression. Many feel the more severe behaviors are associated with limited communication skills. In other words, a child becomes frustrated when he cannot tells someone what he wants or does not understand what to do. In addition, children with autism like routines and "sameness," and sudden changes in routines can lead to unwanted behaviors. Another unique behavioral characteristic associated with autism is inappropriate play with toys and objects. For example, a child with autism might repeatedly spin the wheels on a toy car rather than playing with the car like same-age peers. Similarly, a child may line up objects in a certain way but never actually play with the objects. A final behavioral idiosyncrasy associated with autism is sensitivity to sensory stimulations. Some children with autism might be sensitive to touch, others might be sensitive to sounds, and still others may be sensitive to light and visual stimulation. In severe cases children may wear ear phones to block out extraneous sounds in the environment while other children may not like to wear certain clothes or like being touched (Block, Block, & Halliday, 2006; Powers, 1989; Towbin, 2001).

Motor delays are usually considered a common characteristic of autism (Reid & Collier, 2002), but some feel that children with autism do not have any true motor delays or deficits and can demonstrate some fairly advanced, unique motor skills (e.g., Sigman & Capps, 1997). For example, it is not uncommon for parents to comment anecdotally that their child displays excellent balance and climbing skills (can easily traverse even advanced playground structures), can run, gallop, even skip when in an open field, and can manipulate small and complex objects easily. Unfortunately, these same well coordinated and athletic looking children do not do well when given formal motor tests. For example, Slavoff (1997) found all of the 13 pre-K through 3rd grade children she tested using the gross-motor section of the Peabody Developmental Motor Scales (PDMS) scored significantly below their peers. The gross motor section of the PDMS measures motor development using quantitative measures of balance (e.g., standing on one foot, walking a balance beam), locomotion (run, jump, gallop), and object manipulation (catching a tossed ball). Similarly, Berkeley, Zittel, Pitney, and Nichols (2001) found seventy-five percent of their sample of children with high functioning autism ages 6-8 scored at a level that that was significantly delayed compared to peers on the Test of Gross Motor Development (TGMD). The TGMD tests qualitative aspects of locomotor (e.g., run, gallop) and object control (e.g., throw, catch) skills. Finally, Manjiviona and Prior (1995) found that two-thirds of their sample of high functioning children with autism ages 7-17 performed at a delayed level on the Test of Motor Impairment-Henderson Revision (TOMI). The TOMI evaluates motor abilities in children such manual dexterity (sorting objects), ball skills (catching a ball), and balance (walking on a beam, standing on one foot).

While all three studies clearly showed children with autism having significant motor delays, it still is unclear whether these delays are purely motor in nature or due to lack of motivation, attention, and understanding the task. For example, all three tests used in the study measures jumping either qualitatively (TGMD) or quantitatively (PDMS, TOMI). To score well in a jumping test one needs to forcefully swing arms back and then forward and forcefully bend then extend legs. While most children with autism can jump very easily, children with autism tend to not move forcefully (at least not on command). Whether due to lack of motivation or not understanding exactly what to do, the result is children with autism would not score well on jumping items. Similarly, some items on the TOMI are timed (e.g., sort objects or stringing bead as quickly as possible) and some items on the TGMD and PDMS (e.g., running) require a child to move quickly. Again, whether a lack of interest, short attention span, or some other reason, most children with autism do not do well when asked to move quickly, and as a result may not score well on these types of items.

Teaching and Coaching Strategies for Children with Autism

Children with autism require unique teaching strategies that help take advantage of their strengths while accommodating their unique behaviors and learning deficits. There are many strategies that can be employed to help children with autism be more successful in physical education.

Setting up the Environment
The first general strategy focuses on setting up the environment that takes advantage of the child's visual strengths (many children with autism respond much better to visual rather than verbal cues). Setting up a visual environment also prevents behavior outbursts which often occur when a child is confused with the environment or what to do. Specific strategies for setting up the environment include organizing the physical layout so that it clearly explains to the child where to go and what to do (e.g., poly spots to sit on when the child enters the gym, pictures on stations to show the child what to do, and equipment set up in such a way that the child clearly understand what to do with the equipment. Establishing a clear routine with a visual schedule also is helpful for children with autism. The visual schedule explains via pictures everything the child will do in physical education (e.g., stretches, run laps, ride stationary bike, throw to target, kick to target, stretch, and leave the gym). Related to the visual schedule is establishing a routine and having a clear ending to the class. Children with autism often have difficulties with transition from one place to another and from one activity to another. A routine can be as simple as always sitting down on a poly spot when entering the gym followed by a review of the visual schedule followed by stretching as a group. It also is important to have clear, consistent closure to session to help the child understand physical education is over and it is time to move to another activity (Blubaugh & Kohlmann, 2006; Groft-Jones & Block, 2006).

Communication
How to present information is critical for children with autism. As noted, above many children with autism respond better to visual cues rather than verbal cues. However, children with autism can respond to verbal cues under certain conditions (Sigman & Capps, 1997). First, get the child's attention and try and get eye-contact with the child. Any child who is not focused on the instructor's verbal cues will do poorly, so it is imperative to get the child's attention. Asking the child to follow simple directions you know the child can do such as touching body parts often breaks a child away from a daydreaming state to a state of focus. Once the child is attending to the instructor, use very simple verbal directions. For example, rather than saying "watch me as I throw the ball, and pay particular attention to how I step with my opposite foot," say "watch me" (then demonstrate the throwing exaggerating the stepping motion), followed by "you do it." Similarly, avoid verbal jargon that might confuse the child with autism. For example, saying "gallop like a horse" might confuse a child who

does not know how a horse gallops or who does not understand how he (the child with two legs) can gallop like a horse with four legs. Finally, as noted above use alternative forms of communication including pictures, gestures, signs language, and environmental cues. For example, an instructor might demonstrate a proper kick in soccer, and he also shows a child a picture of a player kicking a soccer ball. Then the instructor puts a red footprint next the ball to show the child where to step (environmental cue). He also places a red piece of tape on the child's left foot. Now the child is told to step on the red spot with the red show and kick the ball. Simplifying cues and instruction often allows children with autism to respond to verbal cues, but pairing verbal cues with visual cues is probably the best solution (Groft-Jones & Block, 2006).

Prevent Challenging Behaviors

Communication and social deficits often result in children with autism getting confused with their environment and what to do. This confusing can lead to behavioral outbursts directed at teachers, peers or even back towards the child him/herself (known as self-abusive behaviors). Teachers and coaches should be aware of challenging behaviors and try to avoid situations that lead to these behaviors. Many of the suggestions above (e.g., visual schedules, routines, keeping communication simple) are a good start to preventing behavior problems. It also is important to let the child know that he/she is doing the activity or skill correctly. That is why it is important to provide a lot of positive reinforcement to the child when he/she does do the activity correctly (or even attempts to activity). For example, if you ask a child run and he attempts to run by doing a fast walk, the instructor would still reinforce the child ("good running Johnny, let's try again lifting our feet higher off the ground. Watch me run …. Now you do it."). Positive reinforcement includes finding a powerful reinforce the child wants to earn by following directions. This reinforce might start out with food and gradually fade to bouncing on a therapy ball or riding a scooter. Children with autism also need to be taught and then reinforced on appropriate behaviors and appropriate play and use of equipment. For example, a child might turn a scooter board over and just play with the wheels. The instructor would go to the student, turn the scooter back over, and show him how to ride the scooter. When the child does ride the scooter the teacher would provide praise and perhaps a treat for playing appropriately, reinforcing appropriate behaviors. Despite best efforts to prevent behavioral outburst, children with autism may get frustrated with an activity or may get over stimulated with sensory input (environment is too loud or the lights are too bright for the child). Dealing with challenging behaviors when they do occur should first eliminate the cause of the problem (e.g., turn down the music or place earphones on the child' ears to muffle the sound), remove the child from the activity or setting if possible, and having a calming activity for the child such as lying on a matt or rolling on a therapy ball. Often gently removing the child from the environment and allowing the child to do a calming activity will quickly end the behavior problem (MacDonald, Jones, and Istone, 2006).

Children with Visual Impairments

The term visual impairment is a global term describing someone who has a significant visual loss that cannot be adequately corrected by glasses (Holbrook, 2006). Vision and visual impairment are measured two ways: visual acuity and field of vision. V*isual acuity* measures how clearly one can see from a standard distance. Visual acuity is measured using the Snellen chart which contains letters of the alphabet arranged by line with each line decreasing in size. For younger children the Lighthouse Flash Card Test is used with pictures or shapes substituting for letters). To test vision the subject stands 20' (6.1 meters) away from the chart. The bottom line represents 20/20 vision and the single letter on the top represents 20/200 vision. A person with normal visual acuity (20/20 vision) can read all the lines on the chart including the bottom line (Miller & Menacker, 2007). Legal blindness is defined as 20/200 vision even with corrective glasses, so a person who is legally blind would be able to read only the top letter from 20'. Put another way, a person with 20/200 vision sees at 20' what a person with normal vision sees at 200' (Holbrook, 2006; Miller & Menacker, 2007). Those with more severe visual impairments would not be able to even read the top letter.

Field of vision measures the total area that can be seen without moving the eyes or head. To test visual field the subject sits still focusing on forward on a spot on the wall. Objects are then slowly moved from behind the subject into the subject's visual field. The subject tells the examiner the object can be seen, and the examiner records the visual field. Young children can sit in a parent's lap and do this test with a favorite object or toy slowly brought into the child's visual field. A normal visual field is 160-170 degrees, and a visual impairment is considered a visual field of 20 degrees or less in the better eye. Some people have both visual acuity and visual field losses, while others just have one or the other (Holbrook, 2006; Miller & Menacker, 2007). Table 4 provides a definition of various levels of visual impairment based on visual acuity.

Visual impairment describes a functional loss of vision. Various eye disorders can result to a visual impairment. Some of the more common types of eye disorders include can include retinal degeneration, albinism, cataracts, glaucoma, muscular problems that result in visual disturbances (e.g., strabismus, nystagmus), corneal disorders, diabetic retinopathy, congenital disorders (cortical blindness), and infection. These disorders can cause partial or complete visual loss (NICHCY, 2004) (see Holbrook, 2006, for more detailed descriptions).

Most children with a visual impairment do not have intellectual or physical disabilities (although some can have multiple disabilities). However, visual loss can have a significant effect on overall development. The effect of visual loss on a child's development depends on many factors including the type of disorder and severity of loss, age at which the condition appears, and overall functioning level of the child (NICHCY, 2004). Of particular importance for normal development is whether a child is born with a visual impairment (congenital) or acquires a visual loss later in childhood (acquired) (Holbrook, 2006; NICHCY, 2004). Social development is a particularly delayed in children born with visual impairments. Early social development is dependent on visual observation including preverbal communication (e.g., gesturing, understanding non-verbal cues) and social reciprocity (taking turns and social imitation). These delays are most notable in children with visual impairments of 20/500 or greater. However, these delays are usually overcome as the child develops (Miller & Menacker, 2007).

Table 4. Classification of Visual Impairment Based on Visual Acuity*

Acuity	Visual Impairment	Functional Description
20/70	*Partial sighted*	Some type of visual problem has resulted in a need for special education
20/70-20/200	*Low vision*	isual impairment, not necessarily limited to distance vision. Low vision applies to all individuals with sight who are unable to read the newspaper at a normal viewing distance, even with the aid of eyeglasses or contact lenses. They use a combination of vision and other senses to learn, although they may require adaptations in lighting or the size of print, and, sometimes, Braille;
20/200	*Legally blind*	also includes a visual field of 20 degrees or less. Can see from 20' what a sighted person can see from 200' Will require Braille or books on tape.
5/200-10/200	*Motion perception*	sees 5-10'what a sighted person can see at 200'. Can detect movement from 3-5' away but cannot say what is moving.
3/200	*Light perception*	Can detect a strong light at a distance of 3' but unable to detect movement at 3' from eye.
0	*Total blindness*	Inability to recognize a strong light straight into eye.

* modified from Lieberman, L.J. (2005). Visual impairments. In J.P. Winnick (ed.). *Adapted physical education and sport* (4th ed.). (pp. 205-219). Champaign, IL: Human Kinetics., and National Dissemination Center for Children with Disabilities (NICHCY) (2004). *Visual Impairments – Fact Sheet 13*. Retrieved November 22, 2008m from http://old.nichcy.org/pubs/factshe/fs13txt.htm.

Table 5. Classification of Hearing Impairment Based on Decibel Level*

Level of Hearing Loss	Decibel Level Loss	Sound Equivalent
Typical or Stand	less than 20dB	
Mild	20-40dB	Cannot hear a whispered
conversation in a quiet atmosphere at close range.		
Moderate	40-60dB	Atmosphere at close range.
Severe	60-90dB	Cannot hear speech; may only hear
loud noises such as a vacuum cleaner or lawn mower at close range.		
Profound	90dB+	Cannot hear speech; may only hear
		extremely loud noises such as a
chain saw or the vibrating component of a loud sound.		

* Alexander Graham Bell Association for the Deaf and Hard of Hearing (AGBell) (2008). Hearing Loss
    Chart. Retrieved November 23, 2008, from http://www.agbell.org/DesktopDefault.aspx?
    p=Hearing_Loss_Chart.

Motor Delays

Motor delays are often found in children with visual impairments. Motor delays are not neurologically or motor related but rather due to lack of the ability to observe others. A child who is born with a visual impairment or acquires a visual impairment very early in childhood has little reason to explore interesting objects in the environment. This results in missed opportunities and experiences that effect motor development and learning. Lack of exploration may continue until learning becomes motivated or until intervention begins (Fraiberg, 1977). In addition, a child may actually fear movement, and parents often are concerned their child may get injured which further limits motor exploration and normal rough and tumble play (Lieberman, 2005; Miller & Menacker, 2007). Early locomotor patterns are most affected by visual loss including crawling, creeping, cruising, and walking with delays of 4-6 months, while stationary patterns such as sitting show only a 1-2 month delay (Fraiberg, 1977; Hatton, Bailey, & Burchinal, 1997). Children with visual impairments eventually catch up and develop these and other locomotor skills. However, it is common for children with visual impairments to have a unique walking pattern noted by a slow, shuffling gait with a wide base of support. Again, this is due to not being able to see where one is going rather than any neurological delays (Lieberman, 2005).

Other motor problems associated with children with visual impairments include postural deviations and hypotonia. Hypotonia is low muscle tone which is a direct byproduct of limited movement. Postural problems are related to hypotonia and an inability to observe normal postures. Both of these conditions usually correct themselves as a child begins early intervention and becomes more active. However, children with visual impairments tend have muscle tone and overall physical fitness delays well into childhood and adolescence (Lieberman & McHugh, 2001); Winnick & Short, 1986). Balance also may be a problem in children with visual impairments, and again these delays are related to lack of movement experiences and practice. In addition, balance is aided by focusing on a reference point which is obviously not available to children with visual impairments (Lieberman, 2005). Finally, children with congenital visual impairments tend to take longer to learn object control skills such as throwing and kicking, and often never develop a smooth, integrated pattern when performing these skills. For example, it is more difficult to learn all the components of an overhand throw when a child has never seen what a skillful throw looks or receives visual feedback. On the other hand, children who have already acquired object control skills before losing their vision should not have any of these problems with object control skills.

Teaching and Coaching Strategies for Children with Visual Impairments

Teaching strategies for children with visual impairments focus on how to present information using other means other than vision (Drane & Block, 2006; Lieberman, 2005). Demonstration will only be useful for children with visual impairments of 20/200 or better, and you will want to place the child as close to you as possible for the demonstration. Verbal explanations will be more important for children with visual impairments, and these verbal cues need to be very specific. Providing a verbal cue for throwing such as "put your arm over here" is too general for a child with a visual impairment. A more appropriate cue would be "when throwing bring your arm back so that your hand is behind your ear and your elbow is pointing towards the target." Physical guidance also will be an important teaching tool with the teacher or coach manipulating the child through the correct pattern. Pairing physical guidance with verbal cue words is a good strategy with gradual fading of physical guidance. For example, putting a child into side orientation to the target for the throw can be paired with the cue words "side orientation." After placing the child into side orientation for several trials, the teacher can fad this physical guidance and verbally cue the child with "side orientation." A final tool for communicating how to move to a child with a visual impairment is *tactile modeling* (Lieberman, 2005). Tactile modeling is when you (the teacher) do the movement with the child holding on to you to feel how you move. As you move your arm for the throw, the child places one hand on your elbow and one on your wrist to get a feel for how the movement is performed. Tactile modeling tends to be better for smaller motor skills or components of larger movement skills.

It also is important to enhance targets and boundaries with brighter colors, tactile cues, and sound devices (Lieberman 2005). Children with low vision will appreciate bright contrasts such as yellow tape over a blue floor as well as bright orange cones contrasting a white wall. Placing tape over a rope on the floor provides a raised, tactile surface that makes it easier for a child with a visual impairment to locate a space and to know when he/she is crossing a boundary. Finally, sound devices can be used to help a child with a visual impairment locate targets and equipment. This can be as easy as placing a bell into a ball or putting a portable radio under a target. Peers also can clap to help a child locate a target. Equipment with electronic beepers such as beepers in balls and cones can be purchased.

The type of activity is also important to consider when working with children with visual impairments. *Closed motor skills* are consistent and predictable with stationary target and generally set movements. Throwing to a set target, kicking to a set target, bowling, hitting a golf ball, and archery are good examples of closed skills. *Open motor skills* are those that have variables that change often and thus are unpredictable. Hitting a tennis ball or playing a game of volleyball, soccer or basketball, are examples of open motor skills. Clearly closed motor skills will be easier to teach and will allow more success and independence in children with visual impairments compared to open motor skills (Lieberman, 2005). However, open motor skills and activities can be adjusted to make them closed for the child with a visual impairment. For example, in a volleyball game a peer can catch the ball for a child with a visual impairment, hand it the child, and then let the child do his/her standard serve to a teammate. Similarly, a child can receive a free pass in basketball, and the pass has to be a bounce pass from 10' away followed by the child allowed free pass to teammate who claps to cue the child where to pass.

Finally, safety should be a concern when planning the physical education and sport environment for children with visual impairments. The teacher or coach needs to think from the perspective of the child to analyze the environment for safety concerns. For example, volleyball standards or gym mats stored in the corner of the gym might be a hazard for a child with a visual impairment. Similarly, setting up equipment or stations before children enter the gym can cause an injury. Some equipment cannot be moved, and the best resolution is walking the child through the gym or play environment pointing out permanent objects. On days when equipment is set up ahead of time, make sure the entry way is clear for the child. In addition, explain to the child where equipment is placed around the gym. A clock analogy is often easy for a child with a visual impairment to understand. For example, with the child facing a particular direction the teacher can say "station 1 with cones for dribbling is at 9 o'clock, station 2 has cones and balls on the floor where you will pass with a partner is at 11 o'clock, the shooting station with various size targets on the wall and balls on the floor is at 1 o'clock, and throw-ins with a partner will be a station 4, and I have cones and balls on the floor ready at that station." Peers can provide these extra cues and can be used to guide the child into the gym as well as from activity to activity.

SUMMARY AND CONCLUSIONS

As discussed above, lifespan motor development or performance is an important area of overall human development. Motor skill development and its associated changes in the cognitive and affective domains have a number of theoretical and practical implications. The knowledge of age-related but not age-dependent motor development is a foundation for physical education programs in school, sport programs outside school, and the clinical applications. The studies of "normal" motor development can yield critical information for understanding of "abnormal" motor development and generate important assessment tools or rehabilitation approaches for motor disorders for people of various ages. Age-related changes in physical and motor development are useful for ordinary and special populations in tracking normal development or delay in people of different ages and motor capacities, as well in identifying individuals who have special needs. The course of motor development should be offered to teachers, coaches, recreational leaders, and parents.

REFERENCES

Adolph, K.E., Vereijken, B., & Denny, M.A. (1998). Learning to crawl. *Child Development. 69*(5), 1299-1312.

Alexander Graham Bell Association for the Deaf and Hard of Hearing (AGBell) (2008). *About Hearing Loss.* Retrieved November 23, 2008, from http://www.agbell.org/ DesktopDefault.aspx?p=About_Hearing_Loss

American Psychological Association (APA) (2000). *Diagnostic and statistical manual of mental disorders* (4th ed, TR). Washington, DC.

Angle, B. (2007, September). Winning the "game" against learning disabilities. *Coach and Athletic Director*. Retrieved November 10, 2008, from http://findarticles.com/p/articles/ mi_m0FIH/is_/ai_n27379279

Berkeley, S.L., Zittel, L.L., Pitney, L.V., & Nichols, S.E. (2001). Locomotor and object control skills of children diagnosed with autism. *Adapted Physical Activity Quarterly. 16*, 403-414.

Beyer, R. (1999). Motor proficiency of boys with attention deficit/hyperactivity disorder and boys with learning disabilities. *Adapted Physical Activity Quarterly. 16*, 403-414.

Block, M.E. (2007). *A teachers' guide to including students with disabilities in general physical education* (3rd ed.). Baltimore: Paul H. Brookes.

Block, M.E. (1991). Motor development in children with Down syndrome: A review of the literature. *Adapted Physical Activity Quarterly. 8*, 179-209.

Block, M.E., Block, V.E., & Halliday, P. (2006). What is autism? *Teaching Elementary Physical Education. 17*(6), 7-11.

Blubaugh, N., & Kohlmann, J. (2006). TEACCH model for children with autism. *Teaching Elementary Physical Education. 17*(6), 16-19.

Bredekamp, S., & Copple, C. (1997). Developmentally appropriate practices in early childhood programs. Washington, D.C.: National Association for the Education of Young Children.

Clark, J.E., & Metcalfe, J.S. (2002). The mountain of motor development: A metaphor. In J.E. Clark and J. Humphrey (Eds.), *Motor development: Research and reviews*. Reston, VA: NASPE Publications.

Clark, J.E., & Whittal, J. (1989). What is motor development: The lessons of history. *Quest. 41*, 183-202.

DiRocco, P. J., Clark, J. E., & Phillips, S.J. (1987). Jumping coordination patterns of mildly mentally retarded children. *Adapted Physical Activity quarterly. 4,* 178-191.

Drane, D., & Block, M.E. (2006). *Accessible golf.* Champaign, IL: Human Kinetics.

Frankenburg, W.K., Dodds, J.B., Fandal, A.W., Kazuk, E., & Cohrs, M. (1992). The Denver II: A major revision and restandardization of the Denver Developmental Screening Test. *Pediatrics. 89,* 91-97.

Fraiberg, S, (1977). *Insights from the blind: Comparative studies of blind and sighted infants.* New York: Perseus Books Group.

Gallahue, D.L., & Ozmun, J.C. (2006). Understanding motor development: Infants, children, adolescents, adults. New York: McGrwa-Hill.

Glanzman, M.M, & Blum, N.J. (2007). Attention Deficits and Hyperactivity. In M.L. Batshaw, L Pellegrino, & N.J. Roizen (Ed.), *When your child has a disability* (6th ed.) (pp. 345-366). Baltimore: Paul H. Brookes.

Groft-Jones, M., & Block, M.E. (2006). Strategies for teaching children with autism in physical education. *Teaching Elementary Physical Education. 17*(6), 25-28.

Harvey, W.J., & Reid, G. (2003). Attention deficit/hyperactivity disorder: A review of research on movement skill performance and physical fitness. *Adapted Physical Activity Quarterly. 20*, 1-25.

Harvey, W.J., & Reid, G. (1997). Motor performance of children with attention deficit/hyperactivity disorder: A preliminary investigation. *Adapted Physical Activity Quarterly. 14*, 189-202.

Hatton, D.D., Bailey, D.B., & Burchinal, J.R. (1997). Developmental growth curves of preschool children with visual impairments. *Child Development. 68*, 788—806.

Herer, G.R., Knightly, C.A., & Steinberg, A.G. (2007). Hearing: Sounds and silence. In M.L. Batshaw, L. Pellegrino, & N.J. Roizen (Ed.), *When your child has a disability* (6th ed.) (pp. 157-183). Baltimore: Paul H. Brookes.

Holbrook, M.C. (Ed.). (2006). *Children with visual impairments: A parents' guide (2nd ed.).* Bethesda, MD: WoodbineKadesjo, B., & Gillberg, C. (1998). Attention deficits and clumsiness in Swedish 7-year-old children. *Developmental Medicine and Child Neurology. 40*, 796-804.

Individuals with Disabilities Education Improvement Act (IDEA) of 2004. 20 U.S.C.

Kadesjo, B., & Gillberg, C. (1998). Attention deficits and clumsiness in Swedish 7-year-old children. *Developmental Medicine and Child Neurology. 40*, 796-804.

Krebs, P.L. (2005). Intellectual Disabilities. In J.P. Winnick (Ed.), Adapted and physical education and sport (4th ed.) (pp. 133-153). Champaign, IL: Human Kinetics.

Lavay, B.W. (2005). Specific learning disabilities. In J.P. Winnick (Ed.), *Adapted physical education and sport.* (4th ed.) (pp. 189-204).

LDOnline. *What is a learning disability?* Retrieved November 10, 2008, from http://www.ldonline.org/ldbasics/whatisld.

Lieberman, L.J. (2005). Deafness and Deaf blindness. In J.P. Winnick (ed.). *Adapted physical education and sport* (4th ed.). (pp. 221-234). Champaign, IL: Human Kinetics.

Lieberman, L.J., Volding, L., & Winnick, J.P. (2004). A comparison of the motor development of Deaf children of Deaf parents and hearing parents. *American Annals for the Deaf,* July.

Lieberman, L.J. (2005). Visual impairments. In J.P. Winnick (ed.). *Adapted physical education and sport.* (4th ed.). (pp. 205-219). Champaign, IL: Human Kinetics.

Lieberman, L.J., & McHugh, B.E. (2001). Health-related fitness for children with visual impairments and blindness. *Journal of Visual Impairment and Blindness. 95*(5), 272-286.

Luckasson, R.A., Schalock, R.L., Spitalnik, D.M., Spreat, S., Tassé, M., Snell M.E., Coulter, D.L., Borthwick-Duffy, S.A., Alya Reeve, A., Buntinx, W.H.E., & Ellis, M.C. (2002). *Mental retardation: definition, classification, and systems of supports.* (10th ed.). Washington, DC: American Association of Intellectual and Developmental Disabilities.

MacDonald, C., Jones, K., & Istone, M. (2006). Positive behavioral support. *Teaching Elementary Physical Education. 17*(6), 20-24.

Malina, R.M., Bouchard, C., & Bar-Or, O. (2004). *Growth, maturation, and physical activity.* (2nd ed). Champaign, IL: Human Kinetics.

Manjiviona, J., & Prior, M. (1995). Comparison of Asperger syndrome and high functioning autistic children on a test of motor impairment. *Journal of Autism and Developmental Disorders. 25*, 23-39.

Miller, M.M., & Menacker, S.J. (2007). Vision: Our window to the World. In M.L. Batshaw, L. Pellegrino, & N.J. Roizen (Ed.). *When your child has a disability.* (6th ed.) (pp. 137-155). Baltimore: Paul H. Brookes.

Miyahara, M. (1994). Subtypes of students with learning disabilities based on gross motor function. *Adapted Physical Activity Quarterly. 11*, 368-382.

Moffitt, T.E. (1990). Juvenile delinquency and attention deficit disorder: Boys developmental trajectories from age 3 to age 15. *Child Development. 61*, 893-910.

Mundy, P., & Sigman, M. (1989). Specifying the social impairment in autism. In G. Dawson (Ed.), *Autism – Nature, diagnosis, and treatment.* (pp. 34-41). New York: Guilford Press.

National Dissemination Center for Children with Disabilities (NICHCY) (2004). *Deafness and Hearing Loss: Fact sheet No. 3.* Retrieved November 22, 2008 from http://www.nichcy.org/InformationResources/Documents/NICHCY%20PUBS/fs3.pdf

National Information Center for Children and Youth with Disabilities (NICHCY). (2001, December). *NICHCY Fact sheet #19: Attention deficit/hyperactivity disorder.* Washington, DC.

Payne, V.G., & Isaacs, L.D. (2008). *Human motor development: A lifespan approach.* New York: McGraw Hill.

Piek, J.P. (2006). *Infant motor development.* Champaign, IL: Human kinetics.

Piek, J.P., Pitcher, T.M., & Hay, D.A. (1999). Motor coordination and kinesthesis in boys with attention deficit-hyperactivity disorder. *Developmental Medicine and Child Neurology. 41*, 159-165.

Powers, M.D. (1989), What is autism? In M.D. Powers (Eds.), *Children with autism: A parent's guide.* (pp. 1-29). Bethesda, MD: Woodbine House.

Pueschel, S.M. (2000). *A parent's guide to Down syndrome: Toward a brighter future.* Baltimore: Paul H. Brookes.

Rarick, G. L. (1980). Cognitive-motor relationships in the growing years. *Research Quarterly for Exercise and Sport. 51*, 174-192.

Reid, G., & Collier, D. (2002). Motor behavior and the autism spectrum disorders – introduction. *Palaestra. 18*, 20-27, 44.

Roberton, M.A. (1983). Changing motor patterns during childhood. In J. Thomas (Ed.), *Motor development during childhood and adolescence.* Minneapolis: Burgess.

Roberton, M.A. & Halverson, L.E. (1984). *Developing children: Their changing movement.* Philadelphia: Lea & Febiger.

Schalock, R.L. Luckasson, R.A., Shogren K.A., Borthwick-Duffy, S., Bradley, V., Buntinx, W.H.E., Coulter, D.L., Craig, E.M., Gomez, S.C., Lachapelle, Y., Reeve, A., Snell, M.E., Spreat, S., Tasse´, M.J., Thompson, J.R., Verdugo, M.A., Wehmeyer, M.L., & Yeager M.H. (2007). The Renaming of *Mental Retardation*: Understanding the change to the term *Intellectual Disability. Intellectual and Developmental Disabilities. 45*, 116–124.

Seefeldt, V. & Haubenstricker, J. (1982). Patterns, phases, or stages: An analytical model for the study of developmental movement. In J.A.S Kelso & J.E. Clark (Eds.), *The development of movement control and coordination.* New York: Wiley.

Seefeldt, V, Reuschlein, P., & Vogel, P. (1972). *Sequencing motor skills within the physical education curriculum.* Paper presented at the American Association for Health, Physical Education, and Recreation. Houston, TX.

Shapiro, B. (2001). Specific learning disabilities. In M.L. Batshaw (Ed.), *When your child has a disability* (revised) (pp. 373-390). Baltimore: Paul H. Brookes.

Sherrill, C. (2004). *Adapted Physical Activity, Recreation and Sport* (6th ed.). New York: McGraw Hill.

Sigman, M., & Capps, L. (1997). *Children with autism: A developmental perspective:* Cambridge, MA: Harvard University Press.

Slavoff, G. (1997). *Motor development in children with autism.* Unpublished doctoral dissertation. University of Virginia, Charlottesville.

Stewart, D., & Kluwin, T.N. (2002). *Teaching deaf and hard-of-hearing students: Content, strategies, and curriculum.* Needham Heights, MA: Allyn & Bacon.

Szapacs, C. (2006). Applied behavioral analysis *(ABA., Teaching Elementary Physical Education. 17*(6), 12-15.

Thomas, J.R. (1997). Motor behavior. In J.D Massengale and R.A. Swanson (Eds.), *The history of exercise and sport science.* IL: Human Kinetics.

Thomas, J. R., Yan, J. H., & Stelmach, G. E. (2000). Movement characteristics change as a function of practice in children and adults. *Journal of Experimental Child Psychology. 75,* 228-244.

Towbin, K.E. (2001). Autism spectrum disorders. In M.L. Batshaw (Ed.), *When your child has a disability.* (revised ed.) (pp. 341-353). Baltimore: Paul H. Brookes.

Wall, A. E. T. (2004). The developmental skill-learning gap hypothesis: Implications for children with movement difficulties. *Adapted Physical Activity Quarterly. 21,* 197-218.

Werry, J.S., Elkind, G.S., Reeves, J.C. (1987). Attention deficit, conduct, oppositional, and anxiety disorders in children. III. *Journal of Abnormal and Child Psychology. 15,* 409-428.

Winders, P.C. (1997). *Gross motor skills in children with Down syndrome: A guide for parents and professionals.* Bethesda, MD: Woodbine House.

Winnick, J., & Short, F. (1986). The influence on physical fitness test performance. *Journal of Visual Impairment and Blindness. 80,* 729-731.

Woolrich, D.L. (1994). *Attention deficit hyperactivity disorder.* Baltimore: Paul H. Brookes.

Yan, J.H., & Thomas, J.R. (2002). Arm movement control: Differences between children with and without attention deficit/hyperactivity disorder. *Research Quarterly for Exercise and Sport. 73,* 10-18.

Yan, J. H., Thomas, J. R. Stelmach, G. E., & Thomas, K. T. (2000). Developmental features of rapid aiming arm movements across the lifespan. *Journal of Motor Behavior. 32,* 121-140.

Yun, J., & Ulrich, D.A., (1997). Perceived and actual physical competence in children with mild mental retardation. *Adapted Physical Activity Quarterly. 14,* 285-297.

Zafeiriou, D.I. (2004). Primitive reflexes and postural reactions in the neural developmental examination. *Pediatric Neurology, 31*(1), 1-8.

Zelazo, P. D., Craik, F. I. M., & Booth, L. (2004). Executive function across the life span. *Acta Psychologica. 115*, 167-184.

Zelazo, N.A., Zelazo, P., Cohen, K.M., & Zelazo, P.D. (1993). Specificity of practice effects on elementary neuromotor patterns. *Developmental Psychology. 29*(4), 686-691.

Zhang, J. (2005). A quantitative analysis of motor developmental delays by adolescents with mild mental retardation. *Palaestra. 21*(1), 7-8.

In: Handbook of Motor Skills
Editor: Lucian T. Pelligrino

ISBN: 978-1-60741-811-5
© 2009 Nova Science Publishers, Inc.

Chapter 2

DEVELOPMENTAL COORDINATION DISORDER IN CHILDREN AND ADOLESCENTS

Andreas D. Flouris[*]

Institute of Human Performance and Rehabilitation, Centre for Research
and Technology Thessaly. 32 Siggrou Street. Trikala, GR42100, Greece

ABSTRACT

Developmental Coordination Disorder (DCD) is a term used to describe a condition of motor incoordination found in children. Prevalence estimates for DCD obtained internationally indicate that about 6 to 10% of the school-aged population may be affected. Despite the high prevalence rates, a systematic review of the literature reveals that data have been mainly reported for north America and northern Europe. Recent evidence shows that DCD has a significant physiological impact on children's health and well-being. Specifically, it has been found that children with DCD are at increased risk for developing coronary artery disease at a later age. This has been attributed to the fact that children with DCD systematically avoid being active. Thus participation in physical activity has been suggested as a significant mediator in the relationship between clumsiness and coronary artery disease. These findings underline the necessity to identify individuals with DCD early in life, in order to prevent many of the secondary problems that may arise in later years. The factor contributing the most to the scarcity of DCD data is the challenge of screening/identification of children with this disorder. To date, no gold-standard has been universally recognized. Furthermore, widely accepted screening methods such as the Bruininks Oseretsky Test of Motor Proficiency, or the Movement Assessment Battery for Children, are neither practical nor cost-effective. A solution to this problem may be found in the Children's Self-Perceptions of Adequacy in and Predilection for Physical Activity (CSAPPA) scale. However, further investigation of the validity and precision of the CSAPPA scale in different populations is required.

---

[*] e-mail: aflouris[at]cereteth.gr

INTRODUCTION

Poor motor coordination in children has been recognized as a developmental problem since the beginning of the 20th century [1]. Withdrawal or exclusion from play, sports, and games significantly affects children's social interaction, skill practice, fitness, health, and – ultimately – quality of life [2]. Ergo, considerable concern has been expressed for the children whose deprived motoric abilities put them at risk for withdrawal or exclusion from physical activity [3].

As early as 1937 children with coordination difficulties have been described as 'clumsy', 'awkward', or 'having movement difficulties' [1]. The introduction of the term 'Developmental Coordination Disorder' (DCD) in the Manual for Mental Disorders of the American Psychiatric Association [4] has increased awareness on this condition, forming criteria which distinguish DCD as a separate disorder from similar conditions such as apraxia or developmental dyspraxia [3, 5, 6].

In addition to the motoric difficulties apparent in children with DCD, the development in later childhood and adolescence of distress, heightened anxiety, low self-esteem, and secondary social, academic and behavioural problems has been frequently documented [7, 8]. Results from longitudinal studies report strong associations between DCD and later learning difficulties, school failure and psychological problems [9, 10].

Concurrently, research conducted during the past decade has provided evidence to suggest significant physiological outcomes of DCD on children's health and well-being [11-19]. Specifically, it has been found that children with DCD are at increased risk for developing coronary artery disease (CAD) at a later age [11, 12, 18-21]. This has been attributed to the fact that children with DCD systematically avoid being active [12, 15, 18, 20, 22]. Thus participation in physical activity has been suggested as a significant mediator in the relationship between clumsiness and CAD. These findings underline the necessity to identify individuals with DCD early in life, in an effort to prevent many of the secondary problems that may arise in later years [7, 23, 24].

Prevalence estimates for DCD obtained internationally indicate that about 6 to 10% of the school-aged population may be affected [4, 25-28]. Despite the high prevalence rates, a systematic review of the literature reveals that research data have been mainly reported for north America [4, 17] and northern Europe [29, 30]. Limited information can also be found for some parts of Asia [28, 31], and Australia [32]. However, the explicit impact of DCD on children's' motoric, psycho-social, and academic cosmos suggests the further investigation of this condition in other counties.

One of the factors contributing to the scarce research data on DCD is the challenge of screening/identification of children with this disorder. To date, no gold-standard test has been universally recognized. Furthermore, widely accepted screening methods such as the Bruininks Oseretsky Test of Motor Proficiency (BOTMP) [33], or the Movement Assessment Battery for Children (mABC) [34], are neither practical nor cost-effective. These tests, conducted only by a trained individual, require a minimum of 30 minutes to be conducted, and cost approximately $50 to $100 per child. Furthermore, since testing can be performed only on individual-student basis, the ability to conduct mass screening over short time periods is not feasible. As a result, schools and other organizations often object to time consuming screenings due to interference with daily academic requirements. This limits the potential for research and the degree to which intervention programs can be made available to children with DCD.

A solution to this problem may be found in the Children's Self-Perceptions of Adequacy in and Predilection for Physical Activity (CSAPPA) scale [35]. The CSAPPA is a paper-pencil group-administered instrument, which has been introduced as a cost-effective and practical proxy of the short form of the BOTMP test (BOTMP-SF) in screening for DCD [17, 36]. The use of CSAPPA scale is advantageous in that it allows for mass screening with minimum budget in very short periods of time. Thereafter, the BOTMP-SF or other comprehensive tests can be administered solely to the children diagnosed by CSAPPA to be at risk for DCD.

A REVIEW ON DEVELOPMENTAL COORDINATION DISORDER

Developmental coordination disorder is a term used to describe the unaccountable failure of some children to acquire age-appropriate motor skills. These skills are not generally as dependent on formal education as, for example, mathematics, reading, or music. A significant portion of the actions that people perform in every-day life have been acquired informally, and are able to be performed with no close attention. Under normal conditions, people become aware of the complexity in various movements only when deprived of ability (e.g. fastening buttons with very cold fingers). A relevant example is provided by a child who is unable to complete even the most fundamental motor tasks without help. Being challenged to use utensils, fasten buttons, or ride a bike to school may seem insignificant to a certain extent, but such deficiencies may have significant impact on the educational development of children, their psycho-social, and academic cosmos.

Historical Review

The phenomenon of clumsiness has received considerable attention over the years and a number of studies have investigated its nature. Historically, amidst the earliest were the investigations performed by Dimock [37], Orton [1], and Espenschade [38]. These authors mainly examined the development of motor performance in children and adolescents across time. Research on clumsiness remained focused on motor development and growth during the '60s with Schnabel [39] and Winter [40] forming theories regarding a "temporary regression in motor performance of males between the ages of 11 and 17".

It was at that time when the first theoretical models were developed, attempting to explain the role of the nervous system in motor development [41]. The theoretical basis of these early models was based on a hierarchy of motor control. According to this notion, motor planning and executing is performed by higher centers, without external or internal feedback from lower centers of the central nervous system (CNS). During the last two decades, the coordination of movement has become the object of systematic experimental enquiry. The more recently proposed models, suggest an interaction of increased complexity among various levels of the CNS, but research results have been markedly contradictory [42]. Nevertheless, it was unanimously agreed that due to the conglomerate of the reported symptoms without any known pathophysiology, children's motor deficiencies needed to be classified as a separate disorder.

Terminology

Although the debate regarding the most suitable term for a disorder may seem entirely of 'academic' concern, exact terminology may have significant theoretical and practical implications. In research settings, ambiguous terminology may generate complexity in defining and comparing different samples. In real-life scenarios, definitions of a specific condition by different societies may or may not present with special privileges and/or services. These issues have been addressed frequently in the scientific literature of motor deficiency [43, 44].

Ergo, it is not surprising to find that contemporary reviews focused on the terminology of the condition examined herein have found that it represents a significant problem [45, 46]. The variance in terminology appears to be considerably systematic, depending mainly on country and profession [3, 6, 47]. Health professionals in Sweden have utilized the label 'Disorder of Attention and Motor Performance' [48]. The same condition is labeled 'Dyspaxia' in Italy [49], and 'Minimal Neurological Disfunction' in Australia [50]. In contrast, the classification scheme employed by the World Health Organization incorporates the label 'Specific Developmental Disorder of Motor Function' [51]. In Canada, The Netherlands, and USA different terms have been employed depending on the profession. However, insurance companies in these countries generally acknowledge the term 'Developmental Coordination Disorder' [DCD [4]], deeming compensation only when its specific criteria are met. This definition and its criteria are further discussed in the following section.

Definition of DCD

The 1994 International Consensus Conference on Children and Clumsiness introduced the term "Developmental Coordination Disorder" (DCD) to describe the condition of children with motor incoordination [4]. Four criteria are incorporated in this term. Two criteria are inclusive (i.e. satisfaction of the criteria is imperative if the diagnosis is to be assigned), while the remaining two criteria are exclusive (satisfaction of the criteria results in rejecting the diagnosis). The four DSM-IV diagnostic criteria for DCD are:

a. Performance in daily activities that require motor coordination is substantially below that expected given the person's chronological age and measured intelligence quotient (IQ). This may be manifested by marked delays in achieving motor milestones (e.g. walking, crawling, sitting), dropping things, "clumsiness, poor performance in sports, or poor handwriting.
b. The disturbance in Criterion A significantly interferes with academic achievement or activities of daily living.

c. The disturbance is not due to a general medical condition (e.g. cerebral palsy, hemiplegia, or muscular dystrophy) and does not meet the criteria for a Pervasive Developmental disorder.

d. If mental retardation is present the motor difficulties are in excess of those usually associated with it.

Nevertheless, some authors have argued that the use of these criteria does not ensure the specificity required to differentiate DCD from various classic medical models [52]. In acquired movement disorders such as Parkinson's disease, the underlying symptomatology includes positive features such as resting tremor and 'cogwheel' rigidity, which, although present in patients, are absent in healthy individuals. Furthermore, the same disease incorporates negative features such as abnormal movement slowness, where the patient lacks the movement speed available by the healthy individual [52]. In contrast, no distinct pathology can be identified in the features indicated in manual of psychiatric disorders for DCD [4]. These features can be considered abnormal only in a statistical sense.

Nevertheless, positive features are not only apparent in acquired disorders. The symptoms of obsession and stereotyped action in autism, and the hyperactivity of attention deficit hyperactivity disorder (ADHD) individuals both appear to have distinct positive facets. A distinct positive aspect characterizing DCD is the awkward or influent style of performance. However, although the latter is evident, it is difficult to assess and/or quantify with objectivity. This lack of fixed positive features results in a diagnosis based on norm-referenced test items that yield continuous measurements of performance for which statistically determined cut-off points can be developed [52].

If the symptomatology of DCD does not represent a distinctive set of pathologic features, it can still be questioned whether they form a consistent pattern. Similar to schizophrenia, the etiology of DCD is unknown. Nevertheless, the symptoms of schizophrenia appear to be formed into two distinct clusters [52]. Within the germane literature, a number of studies have attempted to recognized subtypes of DCD [53-55]. However, there is still no complete evidence suggesting that motor features of DCD form cohesive and/or contrasting clusters.

The problem in defining DCD mainly arises from the lack of convincing evidence that DCD is clearly distinguishable from the features of other developmental disorders. The notion of a separate syndrome entails that the disorder constitutes a discrete clinical entity. Ergo, one may reasonably question whether coordination deficits represent a separate syndrome, or merely a symptom. Studies examining the occurrence of co-morbidity report that over two thirds (68%) (figure 2.1.) of children exhibiting coordination difficulties are diagnosed with multiple disorders [56]. Hence, it seems important to briefly discuss whether the motor deficits apparent in children are indeed similar in nature and degree or whether these deficits are significantly re-shaped when combined with another disorder.

DCD and Frequent Co-Morbidities

Recent studies [56, 57] have suggested that children who experience difficulties in reading (i.e. dyslexic) will, more than often, present with attentional problems (i.e. ADHD) and difficulties in acquiring the movement skills that are required at home and at school (i.e. DCD). It appears that, although often one feature will be more evident, it is not a completely isolated problem. This generates the question whether the nature and symptomatology of each individual disorder is affected by the presence of another. Moreover, it has been suggested that many of these syndromes are, in fact, variable manifestations of a single, underlying etiology [56]. Were this to be true, understanding the exact nature of this co-morbidity effect would increase knowledge in differentiating between various developmental disorders. Theories concerning the nature and origins of DCD and other developmental disorders are discussed in a subsequent section.

Prevalence

Clumsiness is a common condition of childhood, usually identified in children between six and 12 years of age. It was previously believed that coordination deficits occurred in 10 to 19% of school-aged children [58, 59]. Using the more precise definition of DCD with the incorporated criteria [4], the current prevalence is estimated to be between six and 10% of all school-aged children [4, 5, 31, 49, 52, 60, 61]. It further appears that DCD is more apparent in boys than girls with ratios ranging from 2:1 [62] to 4:1 [30]. Furthermore, a higher occurrence of DCD has been found in children with a history of prenatal or perinatal difficulties [5].

All the aforementioned characteristics of this disorder have been derived from studies performed in a small number of developed countries. Current knowledge on DCD is, essentially, based on populations from Australia [61], Canada [17], Singapore [60], Japan [6], Sweden [30], The Netherlands [63], UK [64], and USA [65]. Despite the high prevalence rates of DCD [129,000 children may suffer in Canada alone [17]], research in this area has not been repeated in other countries. As a result, research findings have arisen consistently from the same populations for the last 30 years. This may be reflected on the current knowledge of this disorder generating considerable bias on views regarding its origins, identification, and treatment.

Signs and Symptoms

A systematic review of the relevant literature shows that researchers from various disciplines have endeavored to understand the nature of the condition. However, there continues to be considerable controversy concerning the etiology of DCD, mostly due to the heterogeneous nature of the motor difficulties [5, 65, 66].

In summary, research has shown that children with DCD have difficulties with movement and spatial organization [67]. Descriptions of the multitude of problems that children with DCD experience at school include: messy, slow handwriting and immature drawing (figure 2.2); difficulty in coping with classroom tasks including cloakroom, lunchroom, and bathroom routines; difficulty in acquiring the necessary motor skills for participation in gym class; difficulty in relating to peers and participating on the playground; reduced participation in structured and unstructured physical activities; distress, heightened anxiety and low self-esteem [7, 17, 52, 68-70].

The majority of referrals for children with DCD are made by teachers on the basis of secondary academic problems, such as handwriting (figure 2.2) and difficulty with written work or task completion. Thus, it may appear that the learning problems are eventually addressed within the school system. As suggested, however, if a child's problems are present primarily outside the classroom, children may suffer socially and emotionally but are rarely referred for assessment and intervention [7, 15]. Motor difficulties are extremely obvious to a child's peer group. These individuals may be labeled by their peers and excluded from group play. It seems reasonable that these factors may contribute significantly to the social and emotional problems that are commonly observed in these children.

Indeed, teenagers with DCD have reported that their clumsiness: a) prevented them from participating in, and learning many sports, b) contributed to negative feelings about themselves, and c) resulted in less self-confidence with respect to physical and social skills [71, 72]. This reluctance to practice motor skills, a generally reduced motivation to participate in physical activities, and low perceived competence in the physical domain has been frequently noted in the literature [7, 35, 73, 74].

Children with DCD also experience feelings of inferiority [75], and of being less well-liked by peers [76]. High rates of behavioral problems, emotional problems, difficulties in school adjustment, and other social problems have also been reported in the literature [30, 77, 78]. Adolescents with DCD are likely to withdraw from physical activities that involve social interaction and to have fewer physical hobbies [72]. Furthermore, recent studies proposed that 9 to 13 year-olds with DCD are at high risk for developing coronary artery disease (CAD) at a later age [14, 15]. This has been attributed to the aforementioned withdrawal or exclusion from physical activity. It also appears that DCD exhibits several risk factors reported for CAD and type II diabetes, such as low birth weight [79, 80] and obesity [81]. The wide range of dysfunctions of children with DCD have been recently [65] grouped into three areas: gross motor, fine motor, and psychosocial.

Gross Motor Deficits

The majority of children with DCD experience soft neurological signs such as hypotonia, primitive reflexes persistence, and/or immature balance responses that influence gross motor development [82, 83]. Furthermore, awkward running pattern, falling, dropping of items, and difficulty in imitating body positions are frequently identified [84]. It is because of these problems in gross motor development that children with DCD perform poorly in sporting events [6]. The latter has been attributed in part to delayed reaction and movement time [58], to decreased muscle force generation [84], low levels of total anaerobic output, relative peak power, as well as absolute and relative mean power output [85, 86]. However, it seems that the cause and effect relationship in some of these factors is markedly complex.

Fine Motor Deficits

Problems with handwriting or drawing have been frequently reported as the first identifiable sign of fine motor deficits in children with DCD. Moreover, difficulty in planning and executing other fine motor skills (i.e. gripping, dressing) have been often reported [87-89].

Psychosocial Deficits

Unfortunately the problems of children with DCD are not limited in fine and gross motor areas, but extend to psychosocial problems at school. These children often demonstrate learning disabilities and reading deficits [82, 84]. They demonstrate increased prevalence for lower intelligence [82, 84] although, according to the DSM-IV criteria for DCD, low IQ is not a contributing factor [4]. Furthermore, children with DCD may generate disturbance in the class more often than their peers [90], they have a tendency of being the 'class-clown', and they demonstrate less socially desirable means of obtaining recognition and friends [84].

Etiology

Researchers from various disciplines have attempted to explain the nature of DCD. However, there is no convincing data to support any theory to date. Considerable controversy exists regarding the etiology of this condition, mostly due to the heterogeneous nature of motor deficits [66]. Until 10 years ago, research was focused in establishing theoretical models to explain the role of the nervous system in motor development. For the last 10 years, the focus has been progressively shifted towards the neurochemical level. Thus, research endeavors on the origins of DCD can be presented as 'Early Theoretical Models' and 'Current Biophysical Approaches'.

Early Theoretical Models
Numerous scientific results suggest that motor coordination problems of children with DCD are the result of sensory processing problems [91-94]. However, the specific nature of this sensory problem has been debated. Some have argued that the motor coordination problems are the result of a multi-sensory problem [91-94], while others have argued that they are the result of a uni-sensory problem [70, 95, 96].

Multi-Sensory Deficit Theories
Several authors have suggested that DCD results from problems in inter-sensory perception or sensory integration [91-94]. However, the exact relationship between sensory integration and motor coordination is poorly understood [76, 97]. In 1972, Ayers proposed a theoretical explanation of the relationship between sensory input and motor problems in children – the Sensory Integration Theory [91]. According to this theory, the inability to simultaneously integrate information from a number of sensory modalities is the cause of learning difficulties and motor impairment. Ayres suggested that 'one of the most important organizers of sensory information is movement; therefore, a lack of interaction with the physical environment impedes learning. When a child meets environmental demands through emitting an appropriate motor response, an adaptive response is made. The adaptive response serves to help organize the nervous system. Children with sensory integrative dysfunction will often demonstrate poorly planned, stereotyped, or unsuccessful movements as they interact with their environment [91, 92].'

Uni-Sensory Deficit Theories
An alternative explanation for motor coordination problems in children with DCD is that where causality is represented by a dysfunction in a single sense (i.e. are of uni-sensory origin) [70, 96]. The processing of information from a single sense, rather than the ability to simultaneously integrate various sensory information, is what differentiates a uni-sensory theory from a multi-sensoty theory. Several scientists supported the uni-sensory theory including Hulme and colleagues [98], Laszlo and Bairstow [70, 96], and van der Meulen and colleagues [95]. In general, results from numerous studies suggest that the processing of

information from a single sense (such as vision) may have an important role in motor coordination problems of children with DCD [98-101]. However, findings have not been consistent and further research is required in order to specify exactly how uni-sensory integration affects the motor coordination of children with DCD.

Current Biophysical Approaches

Progress in science, technology, and medicine during the last two decades has significantly aided research on DCD. Several theories hold that the etiology of DCD is a component of the cascade of cerebral palsy [82, 90]. Other reports in the literature suggest that DCD is a result from prenatal, perinatal, or neonatal insult [5]. Hadders-Algra [102, 103], who proposed that DCD is a result of neuronal damage at the cellular level in the neurotransmitter or receptor systems. This was based on evidence suggesting that cerebral palsy often results from prenatal damage that is impossible to identify by current diagnostic techniques. Ergo, the motor deficits experienced by children with DCD should not emanate from damage to specific groups of neurons or brain regions, but from abnormalities in neurotransmitter or receptor systems.

Indeed, while no studies have examined germane neurochemical agents in relation to DCD, opinions were raised recently [89, 104] suggesting a close resemblance of this condition with various neurophysiological disorders. A recent finding of increased left-handedness among DCD-children [105] provides further evidence to support such views, suggesting that the DCD-predisposing factors may be biophysical in nature. Causal theories of hand preference in humans range from purely learned behavior, to neurochemical variations during the prenatal stage, and to solely genetics. The increased left-handedness among children with DCD is congruent with the higher prevalence of DCD in males; the chemical causative agent of left-handedness being male-hormone-linked [106]. This further mirrors the increased prevalence of left-handedness in developmental disorders, as well as increased language disorders in males [106]. Nevertheless, the association of handedness and DCD has received limited attention in the literature.

The crossing of pathways that lead to the transmission of proprioceptive information has been widely recognized, as well as the mediating role of corpus callosum in the transmission of information between the two cerebral hemispheres. Children with DCD exhibit right hemisphere insufficiency (lesion/disconnection), frequently accompanied by a dysfunctional corpus callosum [107]. According to leading neurophysiological theories, these abnormalities are also responsible for the occurrence of left-handedness [106]. Injury to the developing cortex appears to result in reorganization of both the cortical architecture and the pattern of connectivity. Enlargements in certain brain regions may result, disrupting the biochemical environment of the fetus which, in turn, results in specific cerebral abnormalities such as left-handedness [106].

A common neurochemical basis to the causative agents of various developmental disorders has been a long-standing belief [106]. The general role of neurochemical factors in regulating human behavior is well accepted, based on both animal and human clinical models [108]. Prominent neuropsychological disorders (e.g. autism, ADHD, dyslexia, depression, phenylketonuria) that dramatically affect cognitive and social competence are mainly attributable to neurochemical imbalances [108]. Moreover, many other eminent disorders such as Alzheimer's disease, Huntington's disease, and Parkinson's disease present neuroanatomical lesions that are accompanied by neurochemical deficits [108].

Neurotransmitters such as dopamine are critically involved in exploratory, motor, and other 'extra personal' functions that are localized in the left hemisphere. Other principal monoamines such as serotonin and norepinephrine are very important in 'peripersonal' visuomanual behavior localized in the right hemisphere [108]. Aberrant dopaminergic activity is a major contributing factor in most prominent disorders with psychological or neurological symptoms including Alzheimer's disease, attention-deficit disorder, autism, and schizophrenia [108]. Various symptoms of DCD [17, 45] may well be explained by reductions in brain dopamine activity, which has been associated with changes in motor and cognitive functions such as handwriting, language, motor planning, and spatial organization [108, 109].

In conclusion, it appears that contemporary evidence on various developmental disorders may be used as guidelines in exploring the origins of DCD. Nevertheless, there is no scientific evidence to support such views hitherto. Research in the specific causative agents of DCD suggested the influence of the cerebellum and basal ganglia [110]. Children with DCD from several studies closely resemble those obtained for patients with lesions of the posterior parietal cortex, patients with ADHD, cerebral palsy, or Parkinson's disease [89, 102, 103]. The most salient evidence to support these contemporary biophysical approaches is the pathophysiological similarities of DCD with developmental disorders in terms of risk factors: low birth weight, exposure to specific pharmacological agents and/or toxins during pregnancy and lactation [111] as well as the recent finding of increased left-handedness among DCD-children [105]. These are further discussed in the following section.

Risk Factors

Reports in the literature have defined several risk factors for DCD. Short gestation, low birth weight, and male gender were among the most pronounced risk factors [112]. However, as in all characteristics of DCD, significant complexity continues to exist in the literature. Even the incidence rates differentiate from one study to the other, according to the diagnostic criteria and the assessment methods. Both familial and prenatal risk factors are reported [113, 114], as well as environmental and social risk factors [113, 115].

Recent findings suggest that exposure to a range of toxicants during pregnancy and lactation, such as alcohol and smoking, are related to DCD symptoms [111]. Moreover, studies examining the effect of specific pharmacological treatments suggest that several drugs may have a significant impact to the infants' brain function and motor behavior [111].

Results from other studies raise the possibility that abnormalities in the processing of efference copy signals could underlie motor impairment in the majority of children with DCD. Such an abnormality may provide a parsimonious explanation for the abnormal performance found on a variety of tasks in DCD where children are required to utilize internal representations of motor acts (e.g. remembering movements, remembering drawings, localizing an unseen finger) [89, 116, 117].

Prognosis

In the past, parents were advised not to worry about their child's clumsiness because the child would 'grow out' of the problem [118]. However, research findings on DCD during the past decade suggest that children do not 'grow out' of clumsiness and that, with no intervention, there will be no improvement [84, 88, 118-120].

Specifically, in the study by Losse [118], 17 children with DCD were tested at 6 years of age, and were re-tested 10 years later. Results indicated that motor deficits continued to exist at 16 years of age. In another study [121] 818 children with DCD were evaluated twice for reading comprehension at 7 and 10 years of age. The authors found a significant positive relationship in poor reading comprehension for children with DCD in the two measurements.

Finally, a follow-up study at 22 years of age was performed on 55 individuals who at the age of 7 had either DCD, AHDH, or both [24]. Children with DCD and those with comorbidity demonstrated lower scores at both measurements, while at the age of 22 were found to have more criminal offences, greater preponderance for substance abuse or other psychiatric disorders, and lower levels of schooling [24].

These findings underline the necessity for early identification of individuals with DCD, in an effort to prevent many of the secondary problems that may arise in later years [7, 23, 24]. The following section represents a review of tests widely accepted as valid and reliable diagnostic instruments of DCD.

Diagnosis and Screening

The identification of DCD requires a comprehensive assessment that includes a valid and reliable evaluation of the child's motor skills, as measured by standardized tests. In addition, the assessment needs to include observations of how the child interacts with his/her environment and the quality of the child's movement. The careful evaluation of multiple sources of information is especially important in the field of DCD because there is no 'gold standard', that can be used alone to confidently identify the condition.

In screening for DCD, the majority of the investigators use a two-step process to identify children who are suspected of having the condition. This two-step process usually includes initial screening for indicators of movement incompetence followed by a confirmatory motor test [95]. Typical procedures involve the teachers' or parents' identification of a child as one whose motor performance falls below the expected of age-related peers, whose motor development lags behind intellectual development, or whose motor behavior appears clumsy [70]. These indicators are not necessarily markers of interference in the activities of daily living, but rather are predictors of motor incoordination. Below is the description for the most widely used screening instruments for DCD.

The Bruininks Oseretsky Test of Motor Proficiency

One of the most popular measures used by North America's therapists and other professionals to assess motor skills is the Bruininks Oseretsky Test of Motor Proficiency (BOTMP) [122]. The BOTMP is designed to assess both gross and fine motor skills, containing 46 items intended for children from 4.5 to 14.5 years of age, and has been previously validated for elementary school-aged children [122]. Feinberg and Bruininks [123] found multiple correlations of approximately 0.60 between preliminary versions of subtests from the BOTMP and scores on peer status and self-esteem measures, with sub-tests of gross motor performance producing the highest correlations.

In the original study, however, the reported factor analysis identified five factors, one of which (general motor development) accounted for 70% of the variance [122]. No fine motor factors were identified, which led Hattie and Edwards [124] to question whether the distinction between gross and fine motor items was justified. These authors also raised concerns about: a) the grouping of the items into subtests, b) the pattern of loading subtests into the gross and fine motor areas, c) the existence of sex differences on many items, d) the low item consistency, and e) variable test-retest reliability, especially in girls [124]. They concluded that 'the test has little value in providing dependable scores and any decisions based on the test are suspect'.

Other investigators have also questioned the validity and reliability of the BOTMP. Burton and Miller [125] stated that 'the most impressive aspect of the BOTMP is its great and sustained popularity throughout the United States and Canada', something that, according to these authors, is not justified. They report the major problems of this test being the large confidence intervals within which the true score may lie and its focus on motor abilities rather than motor skills. A recent study by Wilson and others [126] who examined the reliability of the BOTMP reported that correlations between scores given by two tests were significant but the percentage of disagreement between tests was markedly high. Nevertheless, the BOTMP continues to represent one of the most valid and reliable diagnostic instruments for DCD.

The Movement Assessment Battery for Children

An alternative test used frequently outside of North America to assess motor skills in children is the Movement Assessment Battery for Children (mABC) [127]. The primary focus of the mABC is to objectively assess, identify, and describe movement difficulties in children. However, it is believed that there has not been adequate investigation of either the reliability or validity of the mABC [125]. Nevertheless, this test may be useful for screening, planning intervention, and clinical exploration. Although the reliability and validity of the mABC have not been adequately established, studies of the Test of Motor Impairment (TOMI) [128], the predecessor of the mABC indicate that it is reliable and useful in identifying children with motor problems. Significantly higher impairment score have been found for children with learning disabilities and for low birthweight children [127].

Agreement between Tests

The identification of DCD requires a comprehensive assessment that includes a valid and reliable evaluation of the child's motor skills. Adapted physical activity professionals must be aware of differences between the two aforementioned screening instruments in terms of validity and practicality, in order to select the diagnosing tool that is most suitable for different settings. However, validation processes in the area of DCD are markedly complex since there is a lack of a gold standard diagnosing tool. Ergo, the validity of generally accepted methods as well as novel screening tools that are introduced is questionable.

Due to the lack of gold standard, agreement among the two most widely accepted diagnostic tests is of considerable value. Several studies in the literature have addressed this issue, investigating whether the BOTMP and the mABC consistently identify the same children as displaying motor difficulties. Riggen and colleagues [129] compared the last revision of the TOMI (which with minor revisions became the mABC) to the BOTMP using a sample of preschool children. They found that overall agreement between impaired and non-impaired status was 88% (kappa = 0.71). In all the cases in which there was a disagreement regarding impairment, the TOMI identified the child as displaying motor impairments whereas the BOTMP did not.

In a different study, Henderson and Sugden [127] found only a moderate correlation between the impairment score of the mABC and performance score of the BOTMP (r= -0.53). Wilson [117] reported that the overall agreement between the mABC and the BOTMP was only 40% in a sample of 43 children with attention and/or reading problems. Again, approximately 50% of the sample who scored within normal limits on the BOTMP had an impairment score on the mABC. Many of the children identified by the mABC tended to have attention disorders as well. When both the BOTMP and mABC identified children with motor problems, they tended to have attention and/or reading disorders, indicating more extensive developmental problems. In general, reports in the literature suggest an overall agreement of approximately 80% between the two tests.

However, the validity of both diagnosing instruments has been questioned repeatedly. Tests that identify individual differences in the performance of specific gross motor tasks often assess performance areas such as locomotor skills, balance, and ball skills that do not reflect the daily play activity of children [130]. Ball tasks, for instance, appear with regularity in these and other assessment instruments, though the extent to which ball tasks are routinely used by females in daily activities may be questionable. Hopping, stork stand, and walking backwards are also common test items, but the extent to which ineptitude in these particular tasks is associated with an inability to take part in activities of daily living has not been documented. In other words, while current tests may identify children with motor difficulties, complementary assessments of interference in everyday or culturally normal activities are essential to ensure that proper decisions are made about individual children [130].

Major practical limitations for both the BOTMP and the mABC include the high cost (approximately $150 CAD), inefficient amount of time (approximately 45 minutes) as well as a trained researcher required to administer each test. As a result, schools often object to time consuming screenings due to interference with daily academic requirements. This limits the potential for research and the degree to which intervention programs can be made available to children with DCD. In response to these limitations Hay [35] introduced the Children's' Self-Perception of Adequacy in and Predilection for Physical Activity (CSAPPA) scale. This test is discussed in detail in the following section.

The Children's' Self-Perception of Adequacy in and Predilection for Physical Activity Scale

The CSAPPA scale [35] is a 20-item questionnaire designed for children 9-16 years of age. Its purpose is to measure children's self perceptions of their adequacy in performing, and their desire to participate in physical activities, utilizing a structured alternative choice format to present descriptions of physical activities. Initially, the objective of the test was to detect children at risk for hypoactivity [35], and was introduced for the first time as a proxy for BOTMP-SF in a later study [17]. The CSAPPA scale requires approximately 20 minutes to be completed and has a marginal cost. Results from preliminary validation studies reported increased sensitivity, specificity, and precision of this test as a proxy for the BOTMP-SF in DCD screening [16, 17]. Nevertheless, the CSAPPA scale remains a newly designed test that requires further investigation in order to be established as a valid screening tool for diagnosing DCD. Published work pertaining to this test is scrutinized in the following section.

Systematic Literature Review of Diagnostic Studies for the CSAPPA Scale

"Evidence-based medicine" refers to a specific approach to the practice of clinical epidemiology [131]. The main objective of this approach has been to help researchers and clinicians base their diagnostic decisions on appropriate evidence from the health care literature. In order to satisfy the main objective of this study, a systematic literature review was conducted of all studies on the CSAPPA scale published in peer-reviewed journals from 1992 (i.e. year when the CSAPPA was introduced) to 2003. Using these criteria, eight articles were selected. The appendix provides a complete chart of the individual studies with explicit details regarding the reference standard, blinding, patient spectrum, settings, tactics, the reproducibility and utility of the test, as well as the diagnostic outcome.

Criteria for Study Evaluation

The selected articles were evaluated on a 7-point rating scale [131] based on seven specific methodological criteria:

1. Was there a comparison with the diagnosis of a gold standard for this disorder?
2. Was the comparison with the diagnosis of the gold standard independent and blind?
3. Has the diagnostic test been evaluated in a patient sample that included an appropriate spectrum of mild and severe, treated, and untreated, disease, plus individuals with different but commonly confused disorders?
4. Was the setting for this evaluation, as well as the filter through which study patients passed, adequately described?
5. Have the tactics for carrying out the test been described in sufficient detail to permit their exact replication?
6. Has the reproducibility of the test result (precision) been determined?
7. Was the "utility" of the test determined?

A systematic review designed to evaluate the scientific methods of the selected articles validating the efficacy of the CSAPPA scale as a proxy for the BOTMP in the diagnosis of DCD can be found in the Appendix.

Comparison with an Acceptable "Gold Standard"

As was mentioned previously, there is no "gold standard" diagnostic test for DCD in the traditional sense. A solution that has been suggested in such scenarios is to select one or more consequences of the target disorder and make these the gold standard [131]. These logical consequences often are called constructs. Ergo, in subsequent chapters the reader will frequently come upon the term "construct validity". Motor performance below the 15th percentile in the BOTMP-SF has been unanimously accepted as the closest measure to a gold-standard diagnosis for DCD. Hence, for the purposes of this systematic literature review, the BOTMP-SF will be accepted as the reference standard diagnostic tool. Four of the eight

(50%) articles reviewed incorporated an appropriate reference standard in diagnosing DCD. Initially, the objective of the CSAPPA scale was to detect children at risk for hypoactivity [35], and was later introduced for the first time as a proxy for BOTMP-SF [17]. This may explain the fact that two studies were focused in long-term stability of the CSAPPA scale [132, 133], while the remaining two articles under review examined the agreement of CSAPPA scores with participation in physical activity and a questionnaire administered to the teachers [134, 135]. However, all articles published following the introduction of the CSAPPA as a proxy for BOTMP-SF [17] have incorporated the appropriate reference standard in diagnosing DCD [14, 16, 17].

Independent and Blind Comparison with Gold Standard

In establishing the accuracy of a diagnostic tool, a blind and independent assessment of the gold standard and the proxy under examination represents a vital criterion [131]. Neglecting to blind increases the opportunity for expectation bias, whereby the investigator is aware of the diagnostic outcome prior to conducting the examination. Despite the importance of a blinded trial to avoid screening expectation bias, the explicit statement of independent and blind comparison of the CSAPPA and BOTMP-SF can only be found in one of the articles examined [135]. However, this study did not examine the accuracy of the CSAPPA in diagnosing DCD. Instead, it was more focused on investigating the existence of gender bias in CSAPPA scores. In two articles the BOTMP-SF examiner was blinded from the CSAPPA results [17, 35]. However, validity was compromised since the BOTMP-SF in these studies was administered only to the children with the 5% higher and 5% lower CSAPPA scores. Specific procedures to avoid expectation bias were not mentioned in the remaining five articles.

Patient Spectrum

The diagnostic value of a test frequently resides in its ability to distinguish between the target disease and other similar conditions [131]. Due to the increased prevalence of co-morbidities in DCD (figure 2.1) [56, 57] this criterion is of increased importance. A large spectrum of patients including those suffering from frequent DCD co-morbidities such as dyslexia and ADHD is vital. All but one [133] the studies reviewed used large convenience samples of school children. The number of subjects measured in almost all studies promises a spectrum of subjects with various types of developmental disorders and/or DCD co-morbidities. Nevertheless, the ability of the CSAPPA scale to distinguish between DCD and frequent co-morbidities has not been specifically examined. It should be mentioned at this point, however, that none of the currently utilized diagnostic instruments for DCD is able to distinguish between DCD and frequent co-morbidities.

Evaluation Settings

Since a test's predictive value changes with the prevalence of the target disorder [131], an article must include information regarding the study site and subject selection criteria to permit a calculation of the tests predictive value in a different population. Five of the eight articles reviewed [16, 17, 35, 134, 135] provided explicit information with respect to the evaluation settings, as well as the criteria through which the study subjects passed. The remaining three papers [14, 132, 133] represented abstract publications. It seems reasonable that information regarding the evaluation settings were not included in the latter papers due to insufficient space allowed.

Test Tactics

When the conclusion of a study is that a diagnostic test is acceptable, the methods and procedures of administering the test and interpreting the results should be provided with explicit details. Five of the eight articles reviewed [16, 17, 35, 134, 135] provided explicit information with respect to the test tactics and interpretation. The remaining three papers [14, 132, 133] represented abstract publications. As previously mentioned, it is believed that information regarding the test tactics were not included in the latter publications due to insufficient space allowed.

Test Reproducibility (Precision)

Validity of a diagnostic test requires both the absence of systematic deviation from the truth (i.e. elimination of bias) and the presence of precision (i.e. the same test applied to the same, unchanged, patient must produce the same result). A comprehensive description of a diagnostic test must provide the potential users with information on reproducibility. Precision of CSAPPA scale was examined only in the first study which introduced the CSAPPA scale [35]. The precision of the test was reported significant at $p<0.001$. None of the remaining studies tested this attribute.

Test Utility

Utility is defined as a numerical estimate of the worth or value of a given outcome [136]. Possibly the most practical criterion for a diagnostic test is whether its use will benefit the patient significantly [131]. Typically, a number of questions addresses the value of a test. Is the disorder identified? Is the need for further investigation reduced? In addition, does its use bring reductions in cost and time? Utility is dependent on the practicality of the clinical test, diagnostic accuracy as well as concerns for costs and benefits [131]. Preliminary evidence concerning diagnostic utility for the CSAPPA scale suggests that the test is highly practical, inexpensive, and time efficient [16]. Furthermore, all studies reviewed incorporated various forms of descriptive evidence (e.g., sensitivity, specificity, positive and negative predictive values, false-positive and false-negative rates) or analytical statistics (McNemar chi-square, Kappa statistic, Pearson product moment correlation or Spearman rank correlation) to evaluate the accuracy and diagnostic utility of the CSAPPA scale. However, the positivity criterion for the CSAPPA scale has been frequently altered.

Summary of Systematic Literature Review

The majority of diagnostic articles reviewed herein failed to meet the standard criterion to accurately validate clinical tests. Overall, only the article which introduced the CSAPPA scale satisfied all criteria and received a perfect 7-point rating [35]. Two studies were given a 6- [17] and 5-point [16] rating, respectively. Two articles received a 4-point rating [134, 135] and the three abstract publications reviewed [14, 132, 133] received a 1-point rating for including an appropriate patient spectrum.

Treatment Approaches

The primary objective of all methods of intervention for children with DCD is to improve their motor skill and their ability to function in every-day life. Several interventions for children with DCD have been examined according to the underlying pathophysiology attributed to the disorder. Pless and Carlsson [137] in a meta-analysis examining the effects of a motor skill intervention on DCD suggested that a specific-skills approach may be effective strategy in enhancing motor skill development. Further, some research supports a shift towards a 'Top-Down approach' to interventions based on cognitive, problem-solving theories [138]. In contrast, certain neurophysiological theories suggest pharmacological treatments focusing on the neurotransmitter or receptor systems [102, 103]. However, no effective treatment for DCD has been found to date. Detailed information regarding the most widely known interventions can be found elsewhere [138].

CONCLUDING REMARKS

Research conducted during the past decade has provided evidence to suggest significant physiological outcomes of DCD on children's health and well-being [11-19]. Specifically, it has been found that children with DCD are at increased risk for developing coronary artery disease (CAD) at a later age [11, 12, 18-21]. This has been attributed to the fact that children with DCD systematically avoid being active [12, 15, 18, 20, 22]. Thus participation in physical activity has been suggested as a significant mediator in the relationship between clumsiness and CAD. These findings underline the necessity to identify individuals with DCD early in life, in an effort to prevent many of the secondary problems that may arise in later years [7, 23, 24].

Prevalence estimates for DCD obtained internationally indicate that about 6 to 10% of the school-aged population may be affected [4, 25-28]. Despite the high prevalence rates, a systematic review of the literature reveals that research data have been mainly reported for north America [4, 17] and northern Europe [29, 30]. Limited information can also be found for some parts of Asia [28, 31], and Australia [32]. However, the explicit impact of DCD on children's' motoric, psycho-social, and academic cosmos suggests the further investigation of this condition in other counties.

One of the factors contributing to the scarce research data on DCD is the challenge of screening/identification of children with this disorder. To date, no gold-standard test has been universally recognized. Furthermore, widely accepted screening methods such as the Bruininks Oseretsky Test of Motor Proficiency (BOTMP) [33], or the Movement Assessment Battery for Children (mABC) [34], are neither practical nor cost-effective. A solution to this problem may be found in the Children's Self-Perceptions of Adequacy in and Predilection for Physical Activity (CSAPPA) scale [35]. However, further investigation of the validity and precision of the CSAPPA scale in different populations is required. Concurrently, the therapeutic ramifications of identifying DCD children through the CSAPPA scale must be further explored, as variations in treatment outcomes are highly dependent on the method of identification.

APPENDIX

Table 1. Summary of Diagnostic Literature

Article	Clinical Tests	Reference Standard	Blind & Independent Comparison	Subject Spectrum	Detailed Settings & Tactics	Establish precision	Establish utility	Diagnostic Outcome
[35]	CSAPPA BOTMP-SF PQ TE	BOTMP-SF PQ TE	BOTMP-SF administered only to the highest and lowest scoring 5%. Examiner blinded	1149 school-children attending 4th through 8th grade	Yes	Test-retest correlation coefficients ranged from 0.84** to 0.90**	Yes	CSAPPA scale identified children at risk for hypoactivity. Significant gender difference in CSAPPA scores. No age effect in CSAPPA. Correlation coefficients between CSAPPA and BOTMP-SF ranged from 0.70* to 0.82*; between CSAPPA and PQ ranged from 0.27* to 0.76*; between CSAPPA and TE ranged from 0.50* to 0.67*. Test-retest correlation coefficients for CSAPPA scores were significant*
[132]†	CSAPPA	No	No mention	340 school-children attending 7th through 9th grade x 32 months	No	No	No	Gender differences in CSAPPA scores. Overall predictive accuracy: 78%. Overall specificity: 91%. The high specificity values allow a diagnosis of long term hypoactivity

Article	Clinical Tests	Reference Standard	Blind & Independent Comparison	Subject Spectrum	Detailed Settings & Tactics	Establish precision	Establish utility	Diagnostic Outcome
[133]†	CSAPPA HAES	No	No mention	36 of 85 children in grade 9 and 10 who 5 years ago completed the CSAPPA scale	No	No	No	Test-retest correlation coefficient of 0.79* in CSAPPA scores Correlation of 0.50* between CSAPPA and HAES CSAPPA scores in 9th and 10th grade lower* compared to 5 years ago
[135]	CSAPPA PQ TE	No	Yes	567 school-children attending 4th through 8th grade; 27 teachers	Yes	No	No	Gender differences in CSAPPA scores Low to moderate correlations between CSAPPA and TE Significantly stronger correlations between CSAPPA and TE in girls
[134]	CSAPPA PQ	No	No mention	284 school-children attending 7th through 9th grade x 3 years	Yes	No	Yes	Low CSAPPA scores predicted rejection of physical education class with accuracy ranging from 76 to 100%. None of the 15 males and 15 females with the lower CSAPPA scores selected physical education class High CSAPPA scores predicted selection of physical education class with accuracy ranging from 73 to 84%. Gender differences in CSAPPA scores were apparent.
[17]	CSAPPA BOTMP-SF PQ TE	BOTMP-SF	BOTMP-SF administered only to the highest and lowest scoring 5%. Examiner blinded.	492 school-children attending 4th through 8th grade	Yes	No	Yes	Significant gender differences in CSAPPA scores Significant correlation between CSAPPA and TE Correlation coefficient of 0.79* was found between CSAPPA and BOTMP-SF rank percentile.

Table 1. (Continued).

Article	Clinical Tests	Reference Standard	Blind & Independent Comparison	Subject Spectrum	Detailed Settings & Tactics	Establish precision	Establish utility	Diagnostic Outcome
[14] †	CSAPPA BOTMP-SF PQ 20mMST BIA	BOTMP-SF	No mention	209 children	No	No	No	Prevalence of DCD: 9% Positivity criterion for CSAPPA: >46 (S_E=83%; S_P=89%) Significant* Kappa agreement between CSAPPA and BOTMP-SF
Article	Clinical Tests	Reference Standard	Blind & Independent Comparison	Subject Spectrum	Detailed Settings & Tactics	Establish precision	Establish utility	Diagnostic Outcome
[16]	CSAPPA BOTMP-SF PQ 20mMST BIA	BOTMP-SF	No mention	492 school-children attending 4th through 8th grade	Yes	No	Yes	Male CSAPPA cutoff score: <47 (S_E=0.90; S_P=0.89). Female CSAPPA cutoff score: <53 (S_E=0.88; S_P=0.75). CSAPPA demonstrated significant Kappa agreement with BOTMP-SF in diagnosing DCD No gender differences in CSAPPA scores. DCD males had significantly lower CSAPPA scores and aerobic fitness compared to non-DCD males DCD females had significantly lower CSAPPA scores and aerobic fitness, and higher BMI.

Note: † : abstract publication; * : significant at p<0.01.

Key: CSAPPA= Children's Self Perception of Adequacy in and Predilection in Physical Activity Scale; BOTMP-SF=Bruininks-Oseretsky Test of Motor Proficiency; PQ=Participation in Physical Activity Questionnaire; TE=Teacher's Evaluation Questionnaire; 20mMST=20m Multistage Shuttle Run Test; BIA=Bioelectrical Impedance Analysis; HAES=Habitual Activity Estimation Scale; S_E=sensitivity; S_P=specificity.

REFERENCES

[1] Orton S. Reading, writing and speech problems in children. London: *Chapman & Hall*; 1937.

[2] Sallis JF, Patterson TL, Buono MJ, Nader PR. Relation of cardiovascular fitness and physical activity to cardiovascular disease risk factors in children and adults. *Am. J. Epidemiol.* 1988 May;127(5):933-41.

[3] Missiuna C, Polatajko H. Developmental dyspraxia by any other name: are they all just clumsy children? *Am. J. Occup. Ther.* 1995 Jul-Aug;49(7):619-27.

[4] DSM-IV. Category 315.4 Developmental Coordination Disorder. Diagnostic and Statistical Manual. 4th ed. Association AP, editor. Washington, DC: Author; 1994.

[5] Miyahara M, Mobs I. Developmental dyspraxia and developmental coordination disorder. *Neuropsychol. Rev.* 1995 Dec;5(4):245-68.

[6] Miyahara M, Register C. Perceptions of three terms to describe physical awkwardness in children. *Res. Dev. Disabil.* 2000 Sep-Oct;21(5):367-76.

[7] Denckla M. Developmental dyspraxia: The clumsy child. In: Levine M, Satz P, editors. Middle childhood: *Development and dysfunction.* Baltimore, M..D: University Park Press; 1984. p. 245-60.

[8] Laszlo JI, Bairstow PJ, Bartrip J, Rolfe VT. Clumsiness or perceptuo-motor dysfunction? In: Colley AM, Beech JR, editors. *Cognition and action in skilled behaviour.* Amsterdam: North-Holland; 1988. p. 293-310.

[9] Henderson SE. Motor development and minor handicap. In: Kalverboer AF, Hopkins B, Geuze RH, editors. Motor development in early and later childhood: *Longitudinal approaches.* Cambridge, UK: Cambridge University Press; 1993. p. 286-306.

[10] Cantell MH, Smyth MM, Ahonen TP. Clumsiness in adolescence: Educational, motor, and social outcomes of motor delay detected at 5 years. *Ad. Phys. Act. Quart.* 1994.

[11] Tsiotra GD, Flouris AD, Koutedakis Y, Faught BE, Nevill AM, Lane AM, et al. A comparison of developmental coordination disorder prevalence rates in Canadian and Greek children. *J. Adolesc. Health.* 2006 Jul;39(1):125-7.

[12] Faught BE, Hay JA, Cairney J, Flouris A. Increased risk for coronary vascular disease in children with developmental coordination disorder. *J. Adolesc. Health.* 2005 Nov;37(5):376-80.

[13] Flouris AD, Faught BE, Hay J, Cairney J. Exploring the origins of developmental disorders. *Dev. Med. Child Neurol.* 2005 Jul;47(7):436.

[14] Faught B, Hay J, Flouris A, Cairney J, Hawes R. Diagnosing Developmental Coordination Disorder using the CSAPPA Scale. *Can. J. Appl. Physiol.* 2002;27:S17.

[15] Hay J, Cairney J, Faught B, Flouris A. The Contribution of Clumsiness to Risk Factors of Coronary Vascular Disease in Children. *Revista Portuguesa de Ciências do Desporto.* 2003;3(2):127-9.

[16] Hay J, Hawes R, Faught B. Evaluation of a Screening Instrument for Developmental Coordination Disorder. *J. Ad. Health.* 2004;34:308-13.

[17] Hay J, Missiuna C. Motor proficiency in children reporting low levels of participation in physical activity. *Can. J. Occup. Ther.* 1998;65:64-71.

[18] Cairney J, Hay JA, Faught BE, Wade TJ, Corna L, Flouris A. Developmental coordination disorder, generalized self-efficacy toward physical activity, and participation in organized and free play activities. *J. Pediatr.* 2005 Oct;147(4):515-20.

[19] Cairney J, Hay JA, Faught BE, Flouris A, Klentrou P. Developmental coordination disorder and cardiorespiratory fitness in children. *Pediatr. Exerc. Sci.* 2007 Feb;19(1):20-8.

[20] Cairney J, Hay JA, Wade TJ, Faught BE, Flouris A. Developmental coordination disorder and aerobic fitness: is it all in their heads or is measurement still the problem? *Am. J. Hum. Biol.* 2006 Jan;18(1):66-70.

[21] Faught BE, Hay J, Flouris A, Cairney J, Hawes R. Diagnosing Developmental Coordination Disorder using the CSAPPA Scale. *Can. J. Appl. Physiol.* 2002;27:S17.

[22] Flouris AD, Faught BE, Hay J, Vandijk A. Modeling risk factors for coronary heart disease in children with developmental coordination disorder. *Ann. Epidemiol.* 2003 Sep;13(8):591.

[23] Henderson SE, editor. The natural history and long term consequences of clumsiness in children. *International Consensus Meeting on Children and Clumsiness.* 1994; London, Ontario.

[24] Rasmussen P, Gillberg C. Natural outcome of ADHD with developmental coordination disorder at age 22 years: a controlled, longitudinal, community-based study. *J. Am. Acad. Child Adolesc. Psychiatry.* 2000;39:1424-31.

[25] Gubbay SS. Clumsy children in normal schools. Med J Aust. 1975 Feb 22;1(8):233-6.

[26] Henderson SE, Hall D. Concomitants of clumsiness in young schoolchildren. *Dev. Med. Child Neurol.* 1982 Aug;24(4):448-60.

[27] Iloeje SO. Developmental apraxia among Nigerian children in Enugu, Nigeria. *Dev. Med. Child Neurol.* 1987 Aug;29(4):502-7.

[28] Wright HC, Sugden DA, Ng R, Tan J. Identification of children with movement problems in Singapore: Usefulness of the Movement ABC Checklist. *Ad. Phys. Activ. Quart.* 1994;11:150-7.

[29] Van Dellen T, Vaessen W, Schoemaker MM. Clumsiness: definition and selection of subjects. In: Kalvelboer AF, editor. *Developmental Biopsychology, Experimental and Observational Studies in Children at Risk. Ann. Arbour.* MI: University of Michigan Press; 1990. p. 135-52.

[30] Kadesjo B, Gillberg C. Developmental coordination disorder in Swedish 7-year-old children. *J. Am. Acad. Child Adolesc. Psychiatry.* 1999 Jul;38(7):820-8.

[31] Nomura K, Hashimoto O. [Developmental coordination disorder]. *Ryoikibetsu Shokogun Shirizu.* 2003(39):509-12.

[32] Piek JP, Edwards K. The identification of children with developmental coordination disorder by class and physical education. *Br. J. Educ. Psych.* 1997;67:55-67.

[33] Bruininks RH. Bruininks-Oseretsky Test of Motor Proficiency. Circle Pines, MN: *American Guidance Service.* 1978.

[34] Henderson SE, Sugden DA. Movement assessment battery for children. Kent: *The Psychological Corporation.* 1992.

[35] Hay J. Adequacy in and predilection for physical activity in children. *Clin. J. Sports Med.* 1992;2:192-201.

[36] Hay J, Hawes R, Faught BE. Evaluation of a Screening Instrument for Developmental Coordination Disorder. *J. Ad. Health.* 2003;23:article in press.

[37] Dimock HS. A research in adolescence I. Pubescence and physical growth. *Child Dev.* 1935;6:177-95.

[38] Espenschade A. Motor performance in adoleschence: Including the study of relationships with measures of physical growth and maturity. *Monoghraphs of the Society for Research in Child Development.* 1940;5(1).

[39] Schnabel G. Zur bewegungscoordination in der Pubessenz. Theorie und Praxis der Körperkultur: *Wissenschaftliches Organ des Staatliches Komitee für Körperkultur und Sport der Deutschen Demokratischen Republik.* 1961;11/12:1070-9.

[40] Winter R. Zur entwicklung der laufbewegungen bei knaben und mädchen in schulalter. Theorie und Praxis der Körperkultur: *Wissenschaftliches Organ des Staatliches Komitee für Körperkultur und Sport der Deutschen Demokratischen Republik.* 1964;13:754-8.

[41] Heriza C. Motor development: traditional and contemporary theories. *Contermporary Management of Motor Control Problems: Proceedings of the II STEP Conference. Alexandria, Va: Foundation of Physical Therapy;* 1991. p. 99-126.

[42] Edelman GM. Neural Darwinism: selection and reentrant signaling in higher brain function. *Neuron.* 1993 Feb;10(2):115-25.

[43] Bax M. Specific learning disorders/neurodevelopmental disorders. *Dev. Med. Child Neurol.* 1999 Mar;41(3):147.

[44] Hart H. Terminology to benefit children. *Dev. Med. Child Neurol.* 1999 Oct;41(10):651.

[45] Polatajko H. Developmental Coordination Disorder (DCD) alias the clumsy child. In: Whitmore K, Hart H, Willems GW, editors. A neurodevelopmental approach to specific learning disorders: *The clinical nature of the problem.* London: MacKeith Press; 1998. p. 119-33.

[46] Henderson SE, Barnett A. The classification of specific motor coordination disorders: Some problems to be solved. *Human Mov. Sci.* 1998;17:449-70.

[47] Peters J, Barnett A, Henderson SE. Clumsiness, dyspraxia and developmental coordination disorder: How do health and educational professional in the UK define the terms? *Child, Care, Health and Development.* 2001;27:399-413.

[48] Gillberg C. Deficits in attention, motor control and perception and other syndromes attributed to minimal brain dysfunction. In: Aicardi J, editor. *Diseases of the nervous system in childhood.* Oxford: Blackwell; 1992. p. 1321-37.

[49] Zoia S. Normal and impaired motor skills development [PhD thesis]. Trieste: University of Trieste; 1999.

[50] Henderson SE, Henderson L. Toward an Understanding of Developmental Coordination Disorder. *Ad. Phys. Act. Quart.* 2002;19:12-31.

[51] WHO S-MI. The ICS-10 Classification of Mental and Behavioural disorders. Geneva: *World Health Organization;* 1992.

[52] Henderson S, Henderson L. Toward an Understanding of Developmental Coordination Disorder. *Ad. Phys. Act. Quart.* 2002;19:12-31.

[53] Dewey D, Kaplan BJ. Subtyping of developmental motor deficits. *Dev. Neurophysiol.* 1994;10:265-84.

[54] Hoare D. Subtypes of developmental coordination disorder. *Ad. Phys. Act. Quart.* 1994;11:158-69.

[55] Macnab J, Miller L, Polatajko H. The search for sub-types of DCD:Is cluster analysis teh answer? *Human Mov. Sci.* 2001;20:49-72.

[56] Kaplan B, Wilson B, Dewey D, Crawford S. DCD may not be a discrete disorder. *Human Mov. Sci.* 1998;17:471-90.

[57] Miller L, Missiuna C, Macnab J, Malloy-Miller T, Polatajko H. Clinical description of children with developmental coordination disorder. *Can. J. Occup. Ther.* 2001 Feb;68(1):5-15.

[58] Henderson L, Rose P, Henderson S. Reaction time and movement time in children with a Developmental Coordination Disorder. *J. Child Psychol. Psychiatry.* 1992 Jul;33(5):895-905.

[59] Smyth TR. Impaired motor skill (clumsiness) in otherwise normal children: a review. *Child, Care, Health and Development.* 1992;18:283-300.

[60] Wright H, Sugden D, Ng R, Tan J. Identification of children with movement problems in Singapore: Usefulness of the Movement ABC Checklist. *Ad. Phys. Activ. Quart.* 1994;11:150-7.

[61] Piek J, Edwards K. The identification of children with developmental coordination disorder by class and physical education. *Br. J. Educ. Psych.* 1997;67:55-67.

[62] Sugden DA, Chambers ME. Intervention approaches and children with developmental coordination disorder. *Pediatr. Rehabil.* 1998;2:139-47.

[63] Smits-Engelsman B, Henderson S, Michels C. The assessment of children with Developmental Coordination Disorders in the Netherlands: The relationship between the Movement Assessment Battery for Children and the Körperkoordinations Test für Kinder. *Human Mov. Sci.* 1998;17:699-709.

[64] Peters J, Barnett A, Henderson S. Clumsiness, dyspraxia and developmental coordination disorder: How do health and educational professional in the UK define the terms? *Child, Care, Health and Development.* 2001;27:399-413.

[65] Barnhart R, Davenport M, Epps S, Nordquist V. Developmental coordination disorder. *Phys. Ther.* 2003 Aug;83(8):722-31.

[66] Henderson S. Motor development and minor handicap. In: Kalverboer AF, Hopkins B, Geuze RH, editors. Motor development in early and later childhood: Longitudinal approaches. Cambridge, UK: Cambridge University Press; 1993. p. 286-306.

[67] Polatajko H, Fox A, Missiuna C. An international consensus on children with developmental coordination disorder. *Can. J. Occup. Ther.* 1995;62:3-6.

[68] Cermak S. Developmental dyspraxia. In: Roy EA, editor. Neuropsychological studies of apraxia and related disorders. Amsterdam: Elsevier; 1985. p. 225-48.

[69] McKinlay H. Children with motor difficulties: Not so much a syndrome - a way of life. *Physiotherapy.* 1987;73:635-7.

[70] Laszlo J, Bairstow P, Bartrip J, Rolfe V. Clumsiness or perceptuo-motor dysfunction? In: Colley AM, Beech JR, editors. Cognition and action in skilled behaviour. Amsterdam: North-Holland; 1988. p. 293-310.

[71] Schoemaker M, Kalvelboer A. Treatment of clumsy children. In: Kalvelboer AF, editor. Developmental Biopsychology: Experimental and Observational Studies in Children at Risk. *Ann. Arbor:* University of Michigan Press; 1990. p. 241-56.

[72] Hellgren L, Gillberg C, Beganholm A, Gillberg C. Children with deficits in attention, motor control and perception (DAMP) almost grown up: Psychiatric and personality disorders at age 16 yars. *J. Child Psychol. Psychiatry.* 1994;35:1255-71.

[73] Cadman D. Issues in the evaluation of screening programs: Guidelines and results. (Research Report 92-2). Hamilton, ON: Neurodevelopmental Clinical Research Unit.; 1992.

[74] Henderson S, editor. The natural history and long term consequences of clumsiness in children. International Consensus Meeting on Children and Clumsiness; 1994; London, Ontario.

[75] Gordon N, McKinlay I. Helping Clumsy Children. New York: Churchill Livingston; 1980.

[76] Gubbay S. Clumsy children in normal schools. *Med. J. Aust.* 1975 Feb 22;1(8):233-6.

[77] Cantell M, Smyth M, Ahonen T. Clumsiness in adolescence: Educational, motor, and social outcomes of motor delay detected at 5 years. *Ad. Phys. Act. Quart.* 1994.

[78] Gueze R. Longitudinal and Cross-Sectional Approaches in Experimental Studies in Motor Development. Cambridge, England: Cambridge University Press; 1993.

[79] Ong KK, Dunger DB. Perinatal growth failure: the road to obesity, insulin resistance and cardiovascular disease in adults. *Best Pract. Res. Clin. Endocrinol. Metab.* 2002 Jun;16(2):191-207.

[80] Leeson CP, Kattenhorn M, Morley R, Lucas A, Deanfield JE. Impact of low birth weight and cardiovascular risk factors on endothelial function in early adult life. *Circulation.* 2001 Mar 6;103(9):1264-8.

[81] Ijzerman RG, Stehouwer CD, de Geus EJ, van Weissenbruch MM, Delemarre-van de Waal HA, Boomsma DI. The association between low birth weight and high levels of cholesterol is not due to an increased cholesterol synthesis or absorption: analysis in twins. *Pediatr. Res.* 2002 Dec;52(6):868-72.

[82] Dewey D, Wilson B. Developmental coordination disorder: what is it? *Phys. Occup. Ther. Pediatr.* 2001;20:5-27.

[83] Schoemaker M, Hijlkema M, Kalverboer A. Physiotherapy for clumsy children: an evaluation study. *Dev. Med. Child Neurol.* 1994 Feb;36(2):143-55.

[84] Smyth T. Impaired motor skill (clumsiness) in otherwise normal children: a review. *Child, Care, Health and Development.* 1992;18:283-300.

[85] O'Beirne C, Larkin D, Cable T. Coordination problems and anaerobic performance in children. *Ad. Phys. Act. Quart.* 1994;11:141-9.

[86] Larkin D, Hoare D. Out of step. Coordinatind kids' movement. Nedlands, Western Australia: Active Life Foundation; 1991.

[87] Smits-Engelsman B, Niemeijer A, van Galen G. Fine motor deficiencies in children diagnosed as DCD based on poor grapho-motor ability. *Hum. Mov. Sci.* 2001;20:161-82.

[88] Schoemaker M, van der Wees M, Flapper B. Perceptual skills of children with developmental coordination disorder. *Hum. Mov. Sci.* 2001;20:111-33.

[89] Wilson P, Maruff P, Ives S, Currie J. Abnormalities of motor and praxis imagery in children with DCD. *Hum. Mov. Sci.* 2001 Mar;20(1-2):135-59.

[90] Waterson T. Managing the clumsy and non-reading child. *Practitioner.* 1999;243:675-7.

[91] Ayres A. Sensory integration and learning disorders. Los Angeles: *Western Psychological Services;* 1972.

[92] Ayres A. Sensory integration and the child. Los Angeles: *Western Psychological Services*; 1980.

[93] Walk R, Pick H. Intersensory perception and sensory integration. New York: Plenum; 1981.

[94] Fisher A, Nurray E, Bundy A. Sensory integration: *Theory and practice.* Philadelphia: E.F. Davis; 1991.

[95] van der Meulen J, Denier van der Gon J, Gielen C, Gooskens R, Willemse J. Visuomotor performance of normal and clumsy children. II: Arm-tracking with and without visual feedback. *Dev. Med. Child Neurol.* 1991 Feb;33(2):118-29.

[96] Laszlo J, Bairstow P. Kinaesthesis: Its measurement, training and relationship to motor control. *Q. J. Exp. Psychol. A Hum. Exp. Psychol.* 1983;35A:411-21.

[97] Polatajko H, Kaplan B, Wilson B. Sensory integration treatment for children with learning disabilities: Its status 20 years later. *Occup. Ther. J. Res.* 1992;12:323-41.

[98] Hulme C, Biggerstaff A, Moran G, McKinlay I. Visual, kinaesthetic and cross-modal judgements of length by normal and clumsy children. *Dev. Med. Child Neurol.* 1982;24:461-71.

[99] Lord R, Hulme C. Visual perception and drawing ability in clumsy and normal children. *Br. J. Dev. Psych.* 1982;6:1-9.

[100] Lord R, Hulme C. Perceptual judgements of normal and clumsy children. *Dev. Med. Child Neurol.* 1987a;29:250-7.

[101] Lord R, Hulme C. Kinaesthetic sensitivity of normal and clumsy children. *Dev. Med. Child Neurol.* 1987b;29:720-5.

[102] Hadders-Algra M. The neuronal group selection theory: promising principles for understanding and treating developmental motor disorders. *Dev. Med. Child Neurol.* 2000 Oct;42(10):707-15.

[103] Hadders-Algra M. Early brain damage and the development of motor behavior in children: clues for therapeutic intervention? *Neural. Plast.* 2001;8(1-2):31-49.

[104] Flouris AD, Faught BE, Hay J, Cairney J. Exploring the origins of developmental disorders. *Developmental Medicine and Child Neurology.* 2005 Jul;47(7):436.

[105] Flouris A, Faught B, Hay J, Vandijk A. Modeling risk factors for coronary heart disease in children with developmental coordination disorder. *Ann. Epidemiol.* 2003 Sep;13(8):591.

[106] Geschwind N, Galaburda A. Cerebral lateralization. Biological mechanisms, associations, and pathology: I. A hypothesis and a program for research. *Arch. Neurol.* 1985 May;42(5):428-59.

[107] Sigmundsson H, Ingvaldsen R, Whiting H. Inter- and intrasensory modality matching in children with hand-eye coordination problems: exploring the developmental lag hypothesis. *Dev. Med. Child Neurol.* 1997 Dec;39(12):790-6.

[108] Previc F. Dopamine and the origins of human intelligence. *Brain Cogn.* 1999 Dec;41(3):299-350.

[109] Volkow N, Gur R, Wang G, Fowler J, Fowler J. Association between decline in brain dopamine acticity with age and cognitive and motor impairment in healthy individuals. *Am. J. Psych.* 1998;155:344-58.

[110] Lundry-Ekman L, Ivry R, Keele S, Woollacott M. Timing and force control deficits in clumsy children. *J. Cogn. Neurosc.* 1991;3:367-76.

[111] Jacobson S, Chiodo L, Sokol R, Jacobson J. Validity of maternal report of prenatal alcohol, cocaine, and smoking in relation to neurobehavioral outcome. *Pediatrics.* 2002 May;109(5):815-25.

[112] Salokorpi T, Rautio T, Sajaniemi N, Serenious-Sirve S, Tuomi H, von Wendt L. Neuropogical development up to the age of four years of extremely low birthweight infants born in Southern Finland in 1991-1994. *Acta Paed.* 2001;90:218-21.

[113] Gillberg C, Rasmussen P. Perceptual, motor and attentional deficits in seven-year-old children: background factors. *Dev. Med. Child Neurol.* 1982;24:750-2.

[114] Hadders-Algra M, Touwen B. Body measurements, neurological and behavioural development in six-year-old children born preterm and/or small-for-gestation-age. *Early Hum. Dev.* 1990;22:1-13.

[115] Fawler C, Besnier S, Forcada M, Buclin T, Calame A. Influence of perinatal, developmental and environmental factors on cognitive abilities of preterm children without major impairments at 5 years. *Early Hum. Dev.* 1995;43:151-64.

[116] Drwyer C, McKenzie B. Visual memory impairment in clumsy children. *Ad. Phys. Act. Quart.* 1994;11:179-89.

[117] Wilson B, McKenzie B. Information processing deficits associated with Developmental Coordination Disorder: A meta-analysis of research findings. *J. Child Psychol. Psychiatry.* 1998;39:829-40.

[118] Losse A, Henderson S, Elliman D, Hall D, Knight E, Jongmans M. Clumsiness in children--do they grow out of it? A 10-year follow-up study. *Dev. Med. Child Neurol.* 1991 Jan;33(1):55-68.

[119] Coleman R, Piek J, Livesey D. A longitudinal study of motor ability and kinaesthetic acuity in young children at risk of developmental coordination disorder. *Hum. Mov. Sci.* 2001 Mar;20(1-2):95-110.

[120] Sugden D, Chambers M. Intervention approaches and children with developmental coordination disorder. *Pediatr. Rehabil.* 1998;2:139-47.

[121] Kadesjo B, Gillberg C. The comorbidity of ADHD in the general population of Swedish school-age children. *J. Child Psychol. Psychiatry.* 2001;42:487-92.

[122] Bruininks R. Bruininks-Oseretsky Test of Motor Proficiency. Circle Pines, MN: *American Guidance Service;* 1978.

[123] Feinberg F, Bruininks R. Motor Performance as correlates of peers status and self-esteem in elementary school children. *Circle Pines,* MN: American Guidance Service; 1975.

[124] Hattie J., Edwards H. A review of the Bruininks-Oseretsky Test of Motor Proficiency. *Br. J. Educ. Psych.* 1987;57:104-13.

[125] Burton A, Miller D. Movement skill assessment. Champaign, IL: *Human Kinetics;* 1998.

[126] Wilson B, Kaplan B, Crawford S, Campbell A, Dewey D. Reliability and validity of a parent questionnaire on childhood motor skills. *Am. J. Occup. Ther.* 2000;54:484-93.

[127] Henderson S, Sugden D. Movement assessment battery for children. Kent*: The Psychological Corporation;* 1992.

[128] Scott D, Moyes F, Henderson S. The Test of Motor Impairment-Henderson Revision. San Antonio, TX: *The Pscyhological Corporation;* 1984.

[129] Riggen K, Ulrich D, Ozmun J. Reliability and concurrent validity of a test of motor impairment-Henderson revision. *Ad. Phys. Act. Quart.* 1990;7:249-58.

[130] Butcher J. Development of a playground skill test. *Per. Mot. Skills.* 1991;72:259-66.

[131] Sackett D, Haynes R, Guyatt G, Tugwell P. *Clinical Epidemiology: A Basic Science for Clinical Medicine.* Toronto: Litte, Brown and Company; 1991.

[132] Hay J. Predictive validity of the CSAPPA scale, a lingitudinal investigation. *Ped. Exerc. Sci.* 1993;5:427.

[133] Hay J. The stability of children's self-perceptions regarding activity: a 5-year follow-up. *Ped. Exerc. Sci.* 1995;7:217.

[134] Hay J. Predicting the selection of pysical education class in grade ten from self-perceptions reported in grades seven, eight, and nine. *Brock. Education.* 1996;6:59-69.

[135] Hay J, Donnelly P. Sorting out the boys from the girls: teacher and student perceptions of student physical ability. *Avante.* 1996;2:36-52.

[136] Knapp RG, Miller MC. Clinical Epidemiology and Biostatistics. Philadelphia: Williams and Wilkins; 1992.

[137] Pless M, Carlsson M. Effects of motor skill intervention on developmental coordination disorder: A meta-analysis. *Ad. Phys. Act. Quart.* 2000;17:281 - 401.

[138] Mandich A, Polatajko H, Macnab J, Miller L. Treatment of children with Developmental Coordination Disorder: what is the evidence? *Phys. Occup. Ther. Pediatr.* 2001;20(2-3):51-68.

In: Handbook of Motor Skills
Editor: Lucian T. Pelligrino

ISBN: 978-1-60741-811-5
© 2009 Nova Science Publishers, Inc.

Chapter 3

THE PROFILE OF AQUATIC MOTOR SKILLS FOR ABLE-BODIED AND SWIMMERS WITH AN IMPAIRMENT

Ludovic Seifert[*1], *Daniel Daly*[2],
Brendan Burkett[3] *and Didier Chollet*[1]

[1] Centre d'Etude des Transformations des Activités Physiques et Sportives (CETAPS), EA 3832, Faculty of Sports Sciences, University of Rouen, France.
[2] Faculty of Kinesiology and Rehabilitation Sciences, Katholieke Universiteit Leuven, Belgium
[3] Centre for Healthy Activities, Sport and Exercise (CHASE), University of the Sunshine Coast, Australia.

ABSTRACT

Motor skills in an aquatic environment are typically defined with stroking parameters, in conjunction with the kinematic, kinetic and coordination profile of the swimmer. The collection and analysis of this data has followed the traditional processes of video and/or motion analysis of the entire body, followed by quantification of motor skill of specific body segments, such as the upper limbs. A similar process of analysis can be applied for able-bodied swimmers as well as swimmers with an impairment - with some variations. For example, if the swimmer does not have the use of their arms through disease or amputation the motor skill variable of arm stroke rate is not relevant. This chapter reviews motor skill development for both able-bodied and for swimmers with an impairment. By understanding the skill characteristics of both groups the unique process of aquatic motor skill development can be better understood. This profile is presented based on the established theories on aquatic motor skills, and is followed by practical examples based on data collected at elite competitions (Olympic and Paralympic Games) and motor skill profiles of unskilled swimmers.

* Corresponding author: Ludovic Seifert; CETAPS, Faculté des Sciences du Sport, Boulevard Siegfried, Université de Rouen, 76821 Mont-Saint-Aignan, France; Tel: +33 232 10 77 84; Fax : +33 232 10 77 95; E-mail : ludovic.seifert@univ-rouen.fr

Keywords: swimming, motor control, biomechanics, disability.

1. INTRODUCTION

Swimming performance is typically defined by the fundamental biomechanical parameters of velocity, stroke rate, stroke length and stroke index (Costill et al., 1985; Hay et al., 2002; Pendergast et al., 2006); active drag, power output and propelling efficiency (Pendergast et al. 2005; Toussaint & Truijens, 2005; Toussaint et al., 2000); as well as by hand kinematics and kinetics during underwater phases (Schleihauf, 1979; Schleihauf et al., 1988). Swimming performance has also been examined from the standpoint of energetic characteristics, including lactate production and degradation, oxygen consumption and the heart rate variability (di Prampero et al., 2008; Lavoie & Montpetit, 1986; Ogita, 2006; Pelayo et al., 2007; Toussaint & Hollander, 1994). Previous to 2000 little attention was given to motor organization (Pelayo et al., 2007; Seifert & Chollet, 2008). To achieve a certain velocity, the swimmer adopts an individual ratio between stroke rate and stroke length (Craig & Pendergast, 1979; Craig et al., 1979, 1985; Hay, 2002), concomitant with an individual inter-limb coordination (Seifert & Chollet, 2009). For example, in front crawl swimming two common cases are observed for a given velocity. Firstly using a high stroke rate induces a superposition coordination mode where the right arm propulsion overlaps the left arm propulsion. In this case the swimmer favors propulsive continuity. Secondly, using a high stroke length induces a catch-up coordination mode. In this case, the swimmer favors a high force peak and consequently a long glide time. This last strategy corresponds to adopting a streamline body position, i.e. with one arm stretched forward while the second arm applies a large impulse. These two cases suggested that stroking parameters (velocity, stroke rate and stroke length) influence the inter-limb coordination. As commonly observed in other cyclic tasks (in bimanual coordination, see Kelso, 1995; in postural regulation, see Bardy et al., 2002; in walking-running transition, see Diedrich & Warren, 1995) these stroking parameters in swimming can be manipulated by the scientists, coaches and teachers. This review therefore incorporates the findings on inter-limb coordination and stroking parameters in a motor control approach, to analyze aquatic skill development in relation to population (able-bodied and swimmers with impairment).

2. STROKING PARAMETERS

Cyclic activities such as swimming, walking, running, cycling, kayaking, rowing, crosscountry skiing follow the general laws that govern locomotion. According to Hay (2002), cyclic locomotion is defined as the motion of a body from one place to another produced by the repetition of a basic sequence (or cycle) of body movements. In swimming, cyclic locomotion is characterized by the alternation of propulsive and resistive impulses. Therefore, the goal for the swimmer is: 1) to maximize the propulsive impulses, 2) to minimize the resistive impulses, and 3) to coordinate the propulsive and resistive impulses of each segment in an optimum manner. This review has specifically focused on how inter-arm coordination is related to this goal in front crawl swimming. There are three indirect indicators that enable a cyclic motor skill to be assessed: 1) the cycle rate, called "stroke rate" in swimming, which is the number of strokes per unit of time (stroke.min[-1]) or Hertz (Hz); 2) the cycle length, called "stroke length" in swimming, which is the distance the body travels during one arm stroke (from the entry in the water of the hand at the first cycle to the entry in the water of the hand at the second cycle) and is measured in meters per stroke (m.stroke[-1]); and 3) the velocity, which is the product of stroke rate and stroke length. Thus, swimmers with high aquatic motor skills are able firstly to select the best ratio between stroke rate and stroke length to sustain a given velocity over a given distance (time); and secondly either increase stroke rate, or stroke length, without detriment to the other variable in a new combination to produce a higher velocity.

2.1. Stroking Parameters and Inter-Arm Coordination

The inter-arm coordination in front crawl can not be understood without considering the performance criteria velocity, stroke length, stroke rate and stroke index. In fact, the inter-arm coordination was found to evolve from the swimming velocity (in accordance with aquatic resistance), the stroke length and the freely chosen stroke rate. Notably stroke rate appeared to be the main parameter influencing inter-arm coordination (r = 0.54, Chollet et al., 2000; r = 0.71, Millet et al., 2002; r = 0.76, Seifert et al., 2004a). A stepwise regression showed that the best predictors of coordination changes are stroke rate (r^2 = 35.9 %), stroke length (r^2 = 21.2 %), and swimming velocity (r^2 = 20.7 %) (Seifert et al., 2007b). Furthermore the inter-arm coordination switched from a catch-up to a superposition mode at a velocity ~ 1.8 m.s[-1] and/or at a stroke rate ~ 50 stroke.min[-1], suggesting that the manipulation of these parameters would result in coordination changes (Alberty et al., 2008; Potdevin et al., 2003, 2006; Seifert et al. 2007b; Swaine & Reilly, 1983). Through five conditions of stroke rate, Swaine and Reilly (1983) showed that the best performance at 400 yards was achieved using the preferred stroke rate. During a time to exhaustion swam at 100 % of the 400 m race velocity, Alberty et al. (2008) found that performance decreased when stroke rate was controlled (the mean stroke rate was imposed by a metronome) when compared to the swimmer's freely chosen stroke rate. However, no changes in inter-arm coordination occurred. On the other hand, through three sessions of three 150 m trials (slow, moderate and fast pace), Chollet et al. (1996a) showed that for non-expert swimmers (335 s for 400 m front crawl) the energy cost (heart rate and post-swim blood lactate values) was slightly lower when swimmers concentrated on maintaining a prescribed stroke rate, rather than one that felt intuitively correct. In expert swimmers, pace monitoring appears to be an effective means for determining the individual's optimal stable ratio between stroke rate and stroke length; and from this to establish the corresponding inter-arm coordination. For example, Potdevin et al. (2006) imposed five 25 m maximum swims where five conditions of stroke rate were imposed (35, 40, 45, 50 and 55 stroke.min[-1]). They observed that both expert and non-expert swimmers switched from catch-up to superposition coordination mode at a stroke rate close to 50 stroke.min[-1]. In 63.4 % of the expert swimmers, the inter-arm coordination switched at a stroke rate close to 50-55 stroke.min[-1]. The inter-arm coordination of 45 % of the non-experts switched at a stroke rate close to 45-50 stroke.min[-1]. Velocity pacing and stroke rate monitoring appears to influence performance and/or inter-arm coordination, suggesting that these control parameters can be used to develop aquatic motor skills.

2.2. Changes of Stroke Rate and Stroke Length with Velocity

As swimming velocity increases from the 200 m to the 100 m event, the stroke rate also increases (Arellano et al., 1994; Chollet et al., 1996b; Craig et al., 1985; Pai et al., 1984; Pelayo et al., 1996). In contrast the stroke length is either similar (Chollet et al., 1996b) or shorter (Arellano et al., 1994; Craig et al., 1985; Pai et al., 1984; Pelayo et al., 1996). During five race distances stroke length was shown to increase for both males and females from the 50 m to the 200 m race, and to decrease from the 200 m to the 1500 m race. The cause of this change was thought to be the fact that swimmers develop greater propulsive power per stroke in the 200 m race (Pelayo et al., 1996). According to the study on stroking parameters by Pelayo et al. (1996), the inter-arm coordination shifted from a catch-up mode, at long and mid-distance pace, to a superposition coordination mode when sprinting. The transition occurred at the critical 200 m pace as the swimmer moved toward the preferred sprint coordination mode (Seifert et al., 2004b).

The stroke rate / velocity, and stroke length / velocity relationship has been found to follow a quadratic regression in swimming (Craig & Pendergast 1979, Craig et al. 1979, 1985; Seifert & Chollet, 2009; Figure 1), and more recently in twelve forms of human locomotion (Hay, 2002). These findings support the idea of an individual optimal stroke rate and stroke length for each race pace. The distance of the races was also shown to have a higher effect on the stroke rate against velocity curve. Notably when swimming above the lactate threshold, velocity increase is due only to an increase in stroke rate, while the stroke length progressively decreases (Dekerle et al., 2005; Fernandes et al., 2006; Keskinen & Komi, 1988). As shown in section 3, these changes of stroke rate and stroke length with velocity are followed by those of inter-arm coordination with velocity (Figs. 2 and 8) (Seifert & Chollet 2009).

1A

$$SR = 78.39v^2 - 219.16v + 186.15$$

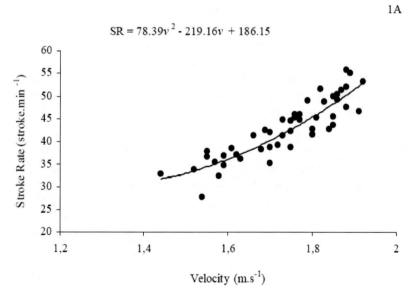

Figure 1. (Continues)

1B

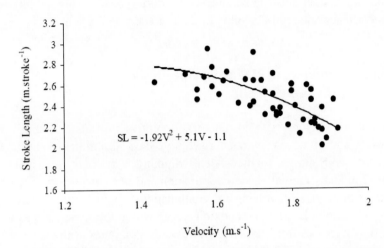

$$SL = -1.92V^2 + 5.1V - 1.1$$

Figure 1. Changes of stroking parameters in relation to swimming velocity: 1A: Stroke rate (SR) – velocity (v) curve; 1B: Stroke length (SL) – velocity (v) curve established from three trials per swimmer at four paces (N=12 elite) (adapted from Seifert & Chollet, 2009).

2.3. Stroking Parameters as Regards Skill Level

Craig and Pendergast (1979) showed that expert swimmers had a greater maximal stroke length and could maintain this longer stroke length as the stroke rate increased, resulting in a higher velocity. For a given race pace, the swimming velocity was found to positively correlate to stroke length, this last parameter being the most discriminant of skill level. Indeed, the faster performances in the 100 m men's event in the 1984 Olympic Games, as compared to the values in the 1976 Games, was attributed to increased stroke length and decreased stroke rate (Craig et al., 1985). Based on this finding Costill et al. (1985) proposed a stroke index (product of stroke length and swimming velocity) which was found to be higher in expert swimmers. In the 100 m event the higher velocity of expert swimmers was related to a greater stroke length, when compared to lower performers (Chollet et al., 1997; Seifert et al., 2005, 2007a).

Moreover, from studying stroke rate every 5 s in 100 m and 200 m events (in a 50 m pool) Sidney et al. (1999) concluded that stroke rate evolution is also quite stable in experts, except at the start of the event. Conversely Letzelter and Freitag (1983) found in a 25 m pool a "zigzag" stroke rate pattern during the four laps of the 100 m. Furthermore Haljand (2002) established six main models for stroke rate strategies during a race: 1) increasing stroke rate throughout the race; 2) decreasing stroke rate; 3) no change of stroke rate; 4) a U-pattern, i.e. decreasing then increasing; 5) a inverted U-pattern, i.e. increasing then decreasing; and 6) zigzag pattern, i.e. decreasing, increasing, decreasing. Studying the 100 m events in a 25 m pool for international and national swimmers, Kjendlie et al. (2006) showed that the top three performers used a U-pattern, while the finalists decreased their stroke rate throughout the race. In the 200 m events (in a 50 m pool) the elite swimmers of the Athens 2004 Olympic semi-finals exhibited greater stroke length and velocity, and had a similar stroke rate but a smaller stroke rate variability than the French national 2004 Championship semi-finalists

(Hellard et al., 2008). As with other sport skill activities the greater the aquatic motor skill level, the more stable their stroking parameters are during a race. This stability is transferred into higher consistency and reproducibility of their motor organization.

2.4. Stroking Parameters as Regards Able-Bodied and Swimmers with Impairment

Competition for persons with locomotor disabilities is organized under a functional classification system in which swimmers with various disabilities compete against one another in one of ten S classes for freestyle. Swimming is the only sport that combines the conditions of limb loss, cerebral palsy (coordination and movement restrictions), spinal cord injury (weakness or paralysis involving any combination of limbs) and other disabilities (such as Dwarfism, major joint restriction conditions) both within the same class as well as across classes. Function decreases from class S10 downward. Swimmers with visual impairment are divided into three classes - S11, S12, and S13 based on visual acuity, visual field, and light perception and one class (S14) is organized for those with intellectual disability presently outside the Paralympic Games. This functional system has been used during the previous five Paralympics Games (held immediately following the Olympics at the same venue) and is subject to continued evaluation.

Swimmers with a locomotor disability competing at Paralympic level have been found to exhibit some similar patterns of stroke rate and race velocity patterns (Daly et al., 2003), whilst other components such as start, turn and finish times differ, when compared to the higher swimming velocity of Olympic swimmers (Daly et al., 2001). Using cluster analysis Daly et al. (2003) in fact found that with minor exceptions Paralympic 100 m finalists (long course) in nine classes of men and women, employed similar race velocity, as well as stroke length and stoke rate patterns despite the wide range of end times from 54 s for the best men to 163 s for women in the least functional classes. Mid-pool velocity decreased by around 3.5 % per section over the race with a slightly higher decrease of 5.9 % following the turn. Stroke rate decreased by 6 % at the beginning of the race and then by 1.5 % over the remaining sections and stroke length first increased by 2 % then to decrease by 3 % per remaining section.

Disabilities, such as visual impairment or blindness have been found to not influence the race strategy in this 100 m race when compared to Olympic swimmers (Burkett et al., 2003; Malone et al., 2001). When comparing the Olympic and Visually Impaired swimmers at the Sydney 2000 Games, within the four clean swimming sections of the 100 m event there were no significant differences in stroke rate between the Olympic or Paralympic swimmers. Despite the difference in average swimming velocity, as the stroke rate was not normalized for time, this suggests that a very similar race strategy is adopted by both the Olympic and Paralympic swimmers. This result of similar race patterns between Olympic and Paralympic swimmers have been found in other studies (Daly et al., 2001, 2003). As shown in Table 1 there was no significant difference between class 12 & 13 swimmers (they have different levels of impairment, where as class 11 are total blind). This similarity raises the controversial question should these two classes be combined, which has been raised in other research (Burkett et al., 2003; Malone et al., 2001). All this shows that for the visually impaired swimmers in this current study the ability to "see" the opposition swimmer and racing them may not be as important as employing a suitable race strategy. Optimal individual performance is the main goal. This all also indicates that the 100 m race is relatively simple in that in the long course event apparently only one strategy is used by a wide variety of swimmers who nevertheless have sufficient race experience.

Table 1. Means and standard deviations values of race variables in Male Olympic and Paralympic finalists with a visual impairment in the 100 m Freestyle at the Sydney 2000 Games

	Olympic	S13	S12	S11	
Number of subjects	72	13	25	16	Difference
Time (s)	48.94 (0.40)	58.81 (1.34)	58.61 (1.06)	63.02 (2.06)	11>(12=13)>Oly
Start (%)	12.12 (0.26)	12.17 (0.28)	12.29 (0.37)	12.01 (0.33)	
Turn (%)	14.68 (0.30)	14.59 (0.30)	14.69 (0.19)	15.07 (0.38)	11>(12=Oly=13)
Finish (%)	5.09 (0.11)	5.16 (0.24)	5.08 (0.26)	5.32 (0.27)	
Start (m.s^{-1})	2.53 (0.06)	2.13 (0.06)	2.08 (0.05)	1.98 (0.04)	Oly>(13=12)>11
Turn (m.s^{-1})	2.09 (0.04)	1.78 (0.06)	1.74 (0.01)	1.58 (0.02)	Oly>(13=12)>11
Finish (m.s^{-1})	2.01 (0.05)	1.68 (0.06)	1.68 (0.09)	1.50 (0.03)	Oly>(12=13)>11
Race segment (%)					
1 (15 m – 25 m)	9.74 (0.19)	9.79 (0.27)	9.83 (0.15)	9.04 (0.22)	(12=13=Oly)>11
2 (25 m – 42.5 m)	17.66 (0.13)	17.68 (0.31)	17.90 (0.36)	17.43 (0.50)	
3 (57.5 m – 75 m)	18.41 (0.28)	18.34 (0.22)	18.60 (0.30)	18.33 (0.43)	
4 (75 m – 95 m)	22.10 (0.20)	22.21 (0.52)	21.88 (0.30)	22.17 (0.58)	
Race segment (m.s^{-1})					
1 (15 m – 25 m)	2.10 (0.05)	1.77 (0.07)	1.74 (0.04)	1.69 (0.05)	Oly>(13=(12=)>1
2 (25 m – 42.5 m)	2.02 (0.02)	1.71 (0.05)	1.67 (0.02)	1.60 (0.05)	Oly>13>12>11
3 (57.5 m – 75 m)	1.94 (0.03)	1.65 (0.05)	1.61 (0.05)	1.52 (0.05)	Oly>(13=12)>11
4 (75 m – 95 m)	1.85 (0.03)	1.56 (0.05)	1.56 (0.04)	1.43 (0.06)	Oly>(12=13)>11
Stroke Rate (stroke.min^{-1})					
1 (15 m – 25 m)	55.55 (3.3)	52.62 (5.23)	53.65 (2.94)	54.68 (6.88)	
2 (25 m – 42.5 m)	51.47 (3.0)	49.00 (4.68)	49.34 (3.86)	50.51 (6.86)	
3 (57.5m – 75 m)	50.80 (2.7)	49.33 (5.89)	47.41 (2.48)	50.06 (6.27)	
4 (75 m – 95 m)	50.40 (4.0)	47.70 (5.04)	48.68 (4.52)	49.51 (5.69)	
Stroke Length (m.stroke^{-1})					
1 (15 m – 25 m)	2.31 (0.11)	2.02 (0.17)	1.94 (0.09)	1.87 (0.22)	Oly>(13=12=11)
2 (25 m – 42.5 m)	2.36 (0.14)	2.11 (0.18)	2.03 (0.15)	1.92 (0.22)	Oly>(13=12=11)
3 (57.5 m – 75 m)	2.29 (0.13)	2.03 (0.18)	2.04 (0.16)	1.84 (0.20)	Oly>(13=12=11)
4 (75 m – 95 m)	2.21 (0.17)	1.98 (0.17)	1.93 (0.20)	1.75 (0.19)	Oly>(13=12=11)

% =race section time/predicted section time (based on section percentage of total race distance); Class differences are listed from highest to lowest value from left to right. Symbols indicate that one class or group of classes had a significantly greater (>) value than a second or that the difference was not significant (=). Turn time measured as 7.5m from the wall.

Compared to able-bodied or Olympic swimming, Paralympic swimming has a shorter history of competition, with the first Olympic Games held in 1896, and the first Paralympic Games in 1960. This difference in evolution has resulted in differences in aquatic motor skills. This difference is best demonstrated by the variability of swimming performance within and between national and international competitions. In an Olympic year, potential Olympic medal swimmers need to improve their motor skill performance by ~1 % within competitions, and ~1 % within the year leading up to the Olympics (Pyne et al., 2004). Additional enhancements of ~0.4 % between competitions would substantially increase a swimmer's chance of a medal (Pyne et al., 2004).

In a recent study, 724 official finals times were analyzed for 120 male and 122 female Paralympic swimmers in the 100 m freestyle event at fifteen national and international competitions between 2004 and 2006 (Fulton et al., 2009). Separate analyses were performed for males and females in each of four Paralympic subgroups: S2-S4, S5-S7, S8-S10 (most through least physically impaired), and S11-S13 (most through least visually impaired). Mixed modeling of log-transformed times, with adjustment for mean competition times, was used to estimate variability and progression. Within-swimmer race-to-race variability expressed as a coefficient of variation, ranged from 1.2 % (male S5-S7) to 3.7 % (male S2-S4). Swimming performance progressed by ~0.5 %·y^{-1} for males and females. Typical variation in mean performance time between competitions was ~1 % after adjustment for the ability of the athletes in each competition, and the Paralympic Games was the fastest competition. Thus, taking into account variability, progression and level of competition, Paralympic swimmers who want a substantial increase in their medal prospects should aim for an annual improvement of at least 1-2 %, which is higher than the current 1 % for Olympic swimmers.

Other studies to compare the stroking parameters of Paralympic swimmers have been conducted over a four year period, analyzing thirteen competitions including the Paralympic Games, World Championships, and several national championships (Fulton et al., 2009). In total, 442 races of 100 m heat (225 performances) and finals (217 performances) were profiled. Correlation analysis for 100 m freestyle results are displayed in Table 2. On average start time correlated the highest with race time showing near perfect correlations for classes S7 (r = 0.90), S8 (r = 0.97) and S10 (r = 0.90). Turn time correlations were very high and consistent for all classes (r = 0.78 to 0.89) and finish time was consistently the lowest of the three race times for all classes showing moderate to high correlations (r = 0.30 for class 8 to r = 0.67 for class S10). This is somewhat in contrast to the findings of Daly et al., (2001) for Atlanta Paralympic heat swims where start time was not found to be as important (r = 0.6 and lower for classes S7 and above). The findings for turning and finished did coincide. When comparing the final race time with the stroke parameters for the different Paralympic classes several relationships were found, such as small correlations for stroke rate in the class S7 and S10 swimmers (r = -0.05 to -0.27), indicating that stroke rate may not be as important as stroke length for these swimmers. Stroke rate correlations for classes S8 and S9 were high to very high (r = -0.51 to -0.78) indicating that high stroke rate may be optimal for these classes. Classes S8 and S9 showed very small correlations for stroke length (r < -0.13) with class S9 displaying zero correlation for fourth 25 m stroke length. These results further highlight the importance of high stroke rate for S8 and S9 swimmers. Class S7 showed moderate correlations (r = -0.78 to -0.88) and class S10 very high correlations (r = -0.42 to -0.50) for stroke length. Classes S8 and S9 displayed small correlations (r = 0.09 to 0.23) for first and second stroke count while class S7 showed moderate stroke count correlations (r = 0.88 and 0.84) and class S10, high stroke correlations (r = 0.51 and 0.47) in relation to final time.

Correlation analysis results showed strong relationships between 25 m segment times and velocity to final race time in all events for each of the four classes represented. These results suggest that, as expected, a high velocity in any 25 m segment of a 100 m swimming performance is beneficial for optimal final time. These correlations suggest that S7-S10 swimmers do not possess the same skill level for start, turn, and finish time and suggest that different strategies are evident between Paralympic swimming classes. Recognizing differences in strategies between classes is important and may be the key to optimizing performance for Paralympic swimming. The majority of results for stroke parameters between the classes suggest that, in accordance with research in able-bodied swimming, focusing on stroke length is important for achieving optimal race time. These results suggests that swimmers should concentrate on using a long stroke and taking fewer strokes per lap for 100 m events to achieve optimal race time.

Table 2. Correlation analysis with associated lower and upper (90 %) confidence limits for performance elements to final race time in 100 m freestyle event for classes S7-S10 between two World Championship events

Freestyle Measure	S7	S8	S9	S10
Start Time	0.90	0.97	0.68	0.90
	(0.81-0.95)	(0.95-0.98)	(0.53-0.79)	(0.84-0.93)
Turn Time	0.80	0.89	0.78	0.84
	(0.64-0.89)	(0.83-0.93)	(0.66-0.86)	(0.76-0.90)
Finish Time	0.58	0.30	0.47	0.67
	(0.31-0.76)	(0.08-0.50)	(0.26-0.64)	(0.52-0.78)
1st 25 Time	0.93	0.98	0.87	0.96
	(0.86-0.96)	(0.97-0.99)	(0.79-0.92)	(0.94-0.98)
4th 25 Time	0.89	0.90	0.94	0.96
	(0.80-0.94)	(0.85-0.94)	(0.91-0.96)	(0.94-0.98)
1st 25 Velocity	-0.88	-0.96	-0.89	-0.77
	(-0.78--0.94)	(-0.94--0.98)	(-0.82--0.93)	(-0.65--0.85)
4th 25 Velocity	-0.93	-0.94	-0.92	-0.96
	(-0.87--0.96)	(-0.91--0.96)	(-0.87--0.95)	(-0.94--0.98)
1st 25 Stroke Rate	-0.05	-0.58	-0.61	-0.09
	(0.28--0.37)	(-0.40--0.71)	(-0.44--0.74)	(0.41--0.31)
4th 25 Stroke Rate	-0.27	-0.59	-0.78	-0.25
	(0.05--0.55)	(-0.41--0.72)	(-0.67--0.86)	(-0.02--0.45)
1st 25 Stroke Length	-0.88	-0.12	-0.05	-0.47
	(-0.79--0.94)	(0.11--0.34)	(0.19--0.28)	(-0.27--0.63)
4th 25 Stroke Length	-0.78	0.01	0.00	-0.42
	(-0.61--0.88)	(0.23--0.22)	(0.24--0.24)	(-0.21--0.59)
1st 50 Stroke Count	0.88	0.23	0.21	0.51
	(0.78-0.94)	(0.01-0.44)	(-0.03-0.43)	(0.32-0.66)
2nd 50 Stroke Count	0.84	0.09	0.12	0.47
	(0.71-0.91)	(-0.14-0.32)	(-0.12-0.35)	(0.28-0.63)

Table 3. Summary of race comparison for swimming Class 9

	Worlds final (2002)	Canada final (2003)	Grand Prix (2004)	Paralympic Athens heat (2004)	Paralympic Athens final (2004)	Common-wealth Games (2006)	Worlds final (2006)
Key times							
Total time (s)	63.97	62.78	59.64	58.77	58.15	57.41	56.67
Start Time (s)	7.81	7.85	7.31	6.70	7.17	6.86	6.89
25m Time (s)	13.94	13.88	13.29	12.60	12.67	12.58	12.57
Finish Time (s)	3.42	3.37	3.01	3.48	3.28	3.24	3.11
Start, Turns, Finish (s)	17.14	17.06	16.00	15.94	15.89	15.40	15.08
Free Swim Time (s)	46.83	45.72	43.64	42.83	42.26	42.01	41.59
Splits							
50m (s)	30.50	30.54	29.20	28.53	28.34	28.21	27.87
100m (s)	63.78	62.63	59.64	58.77	58.15	57.41	56.67
50m times							
1st 50m	30.51	30.54	29.20	28.53	28.34	28.21	27.87
2nd 50m	33.28	32.09	30.44	30.24	29.81	29.20	28.80
Turns							
Turn 1 (s)	5.91	5.84	5.68	5.76	5.44	5.30	5.08
Stroke count							
Lap 1	56	58	52	48	52	50	52
Lap 2	64	64	58	56	60	54	56
Averages							
Velocity (m.s^{-1})	1.49	1.53	1.60	1.63	1.65	1.65	1.68
Stroke Rate (stroke.min^{-1})	63.8	65.5	62.7	60.6	64.9	61.4	64.6
Stroke length (m.stroke^{-1})	1.43	1.42	1.54	1.63	1.54	1.61	1.57

Turn time measured as 5 m from wall.

Using competition analysis data from all 100 m freestyle finalists at the Sydney Paralympic Games, Daly at al. (2003) calculated correlations between stroke rate and length and mid-pool velocity as well as for within race and between race (heat and finals) changes in these parameters. They found that races were won or lost by better maintaining velocity in the second half of each 50 m race lap and that differences in velocity between swimmers were more related to stroke length than stroke rate. Within-race velocity changes were more related to changes in stroke rate. Stroke rate changes were also responsible for velocity changes between qualifying heats and finals in the first part of races while stroke length was responsible for better velocity maintenance at the end of races.

Other longitudinal based studies have tracked the performance of individual swimmers from their inaugural international competition as a 14 year old, through to their Paralympic and World record performances four years later (Burkett & Mellifont, 2008). This progression can provide an insight into the differences in skill level and subsequent motor skills in swimming. As seen in Table 3 the individual swimmer's performance improved ten percent from the final appearance performance at the 2002 World Championships, to the medal performance at the 2004 Paralympic Games, and an additional 2.6 percent to set the world record performance at the 2006 World Championships. More importantly this data identifies the details that contribute to this, such as stroke rate and length, segmental velocity, start and turn times etc... The key areas of improvement for this swimmer were to improve turn and finish times, and to evenly pace the race, knowing that high and stable values of the stroking parameters reveal high motor skills (Chollet et al., 1997; Hellard et al., 2008; Letzelter & Freitag, 1983; Seifert et al., 2005, 2007a).

Finally Osborough et al. (2009b) examined the relationships between velocity, stroke length and stroke rate for competitive single-arm amputee front crawl swimmers and assessed their relationships with anthropometric characteristics. Thirteen highly-trained swimmers were filmed during seven increasingly faster 25 m front crawl trials. Increases in velocity (above 75 % of maximal velocity) were achieved by a 5 % increase in stroke rate which coincided with a 2 % decrease in stroke length. At maximal velocity, inter-swimmer correlations showed that stroke rate was significantly related to velocity ($r = 0.72$) whereas stroke length was not.

Moderate but non-significant correlations suggested that faster swimmers did not necessarily use longer and slower strokes to swim at a common sub-maximal velocity when compared to their slower counterparts. No correlations existed between stroke length and any anthropometric characteristics, instead bi-acromial breadth, shoulder girth and upper-arm length all significantly correlated with the stroke rate used at maximal velocity. These findings imply that as a consequence of being deprived of an important propelling limb, at fast velocity, stroke rate is more important than stroke length in influencing the performance outcome of highly-trained front crawl swimmers with a single-arm amputation.

3. INTER-LIMB COORDINATION

Inter-limb coordination for the two different swimming strokes, namely the alternating strokes of front crawl and backstroke, and the simultaneous strokes of butterfly and breaststroke need to be considered separately. In the alternate strokes propulsion is mainly achieved by the arms rather than by the legs. In front crawl, the arms contributed ~85-90% of the propulsion, and consequently the legs are responsible for ~10-15% (Deschodt et al., 1999; Keskinen & Komi, 1992). For the simultaneous strokes, and particularly in breaststroke, the legs contribute 40-60% of the propulsion. Therefore, the analysis of the inter-limb coordination in the alternate strokes focused on the inter-arm coupling, while the arm-leg coupling has been investigated in the simultaneous strokes. The front crawl was regularly used for the freestyle races because it's the less regulated, the more optimal (as regards velocity / energetic cost ratio) and actually the most popular swimming stroke in competition for able-bodied and swimmers with impairment. This is also reflected in the volume of published literature. Our review has therefore been limited to the development of aquatic motor skills in front crawl (for further details in the other strokes, see Seifert & Chollet, 2008).

3.1. Arm Stroke Phase Organization and Inter-Arm Coupling

Knowing that aquatic resistance during swimming propulsion, also called "active drag" (D), varies with velocity (v) (equation 1), the challenge in swimming is to overcome aquatic resistance to achieve high swimming velocity:

$$D = K \bullet v^2 \qquad \qquad \text{(equation 1)}$$

where K is a constant of proportionality depending on body size and shape: K = 0.5 • Cx• Ap • rho, Cx is the hydrodynamic coefficient, Ap is the projected frontal area, and rho is the density of water.

To best overcome the aquatic resistance in front crawl swimmers must monitor their inter-arm coordination. This is best achieved by firstly organizing the transition between the underwater and above water phases of the cycle, and secondly the time devoted to propulsion and glide during the underwater part of the cycle. The time devoted to the above water arm recovery varies in relation to the stroke rate, changing from 0.44 to 0.65 s for a decrease in stroke rate from 58 to 41 strokes min^{-1} (Deschodt, 1996; Wilke, 1992). Therefore the relative time of the above water arm recovery corresponded to 25 to 45 % of the total cycle duration (Deschodt, 1996; Rouard & Billat, 1990; Seifert et al., 2004b; Vaday & Nemessury, 1971). However, the above water arm recovery duration varies less than the structure of the underwater part of the cycle. Indeed, during an intermittent graded velocity test (8 laps of 25 m), Seifert et al. (2004b) showed that the arm recovery duration changed only from 25.1 to 29.1 % of the total cycle duration for respective velocities of 1.43 to 1.93 m.s^{-1}. Conversely, the time devoted to the glide and catch phase, which corresponded to a downward hand sweep, varied from 37.8 % to 18.5 % of the total cycle duration for velocities of 1.43 to 1.93 m.s^{-1} respectively (Seifert et al., 2004b). In absolute duration, the value fluctuates between 0.5 s for a maximal 10m test (Maglischo et al., 1984) to 0.9 s for a maximal 400 yard test (Chatard et al., 1990). Similarly, the time devoted to the propulsion, during which the hand pulls and pushes the water (insweep and upsweep), changes greatly, varying from 39.1 % to 52.4 % of the total cycle duration for velocities of 1.43 to 1.93 m.s^{-1} respectively (Seifert et al., 2004b).

Moreover, the movement of one arm is not independent of that of the second arm, suggesting that while one arm propels, the second arm could glide, propel or recover. Monitoring of the time devoted to the different arm stroke phases (entry, glide and catch, propulsion, above water recovery) should be considered in terms of the inter-arm coordination. There are three theoretical modes of inter-arm coordination, namely catch-up, opposition and superposition mode (Maglischo, 2003). Based on the time gap between the start of the propulsion of one arm and the end of propulsion of the other arm, the index of coordination (IdC) quantifies the degree of continuity/discontinuity between the propulsive actions of the two arms (Chollet et al., 2000). Therefore, when IdC = 0 %, the mode is opposition, when IdC < 0 %, the mode is catch-up and when IdC > 0 %, the mode is superposition (for further details, see Chollet et al., 2000). However, from a functional point of view, it is reasonable to consider the opposition mode as -1 % < IdC < 1 %.

3.2. Inter-Arm Coordination as Regards the Aquatic Resistance

As suggested previously, increasing the time devoted to the propulsion of each arm is not sufficient; the swimmers must adapt the inter-arm coupling to overcome the aquatic resistance and achieve high velocity. Thus, when the velocity increased from 1.47 to 1.92 m.s^{-1}, the inter-arm coordination of elite males switches from a catch-up mode (IdC ~ -10±5 %) to a superposition mode (IdC ~ 3±6 %) (Seifert et al., 2007b). In fact, when the velocity increased above a critical value (~ 1.8 m.s^{-1}), only the superposition mode was observed (Seifert et al., 2007b). Kolmogorov et al. (1997) showed a particularly large increase in active drag and power near 1.8 m.s^{-1}, which would explain the transition in the arm coordination of elite males at this velocity step. Indeed, from 0.95 to 1.65 m.s^{-1}, active drag ranged from 15 to 50 N, and power ranged from 20 to 80 W, whereas from 1.8 to 2 m.s^{-1}, they ranged respectively from 90 to 120 N and from 150 and 230 W (Kolmogorov et al., 1997). As noted previously when moving at higher velocities (>1.5 m.s^{-1}) wave drag becomes even more important with wave drag accounting for up to 50% of total drag (Toussaint & Truijens, 2005). Using a similar process to calculate "hull velocity" for a ship, the hull velocity for a swimmer, with an arbitrary height of 2 m, is 1.77 m.s^{-1} (Toussaint & Truijens, 2005). This finding coincides with the large increase in active drag found above this critical velocity (>1.7-1.8 m.s^{-1}), as determined by the wave drag, the environmental constraints eliciting a superposition coordination of the arms. Recently, it was shown that the increase of velocity led to simultaneous changes in drag force, power out-put and index of coordination (Seifert et al., 2008). While swimming only with arms in the free swimming condition, the inter-arm coordination of front crawl national swimmers switched from catch-up mode (IdC < 0 %) to superposition mode (IdC > 0 %) when the velocity increased from 0.9 to 1.5-1.6 m.s^{-1} (maximal velocity) (Fig. 2) (Seifert et al., 2008). Using arms only on the Measuring Active Drag system (MAD), the same swimmers increased their drag force from 30 N to 100-110 N at maximal intensity, developing a mechanical power out-put (P_d) of ~200 W (Fig. 3) (Seifert et al., 2008), P_d being calculated following the equation 2.

$$P_d = D \cdot v \qquad \text{(equation 2) used to overcome aquatic resistance}$$

Therefore, a positive correlation (r = 0.70) and linear regression coefficient (r² = 0.49) were found between the inter-arm coordination and the active drag force (Fig. 4).

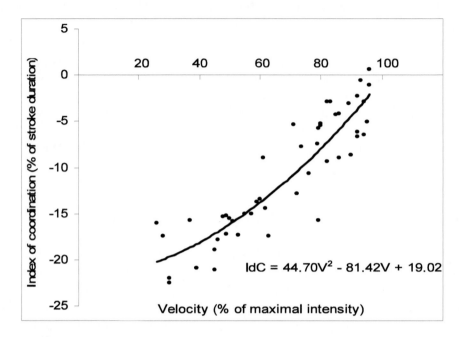

Figure 2. Relationship between index of coordination (IdC) and swimming velocity (*v*); adapted from Seifert et al. (2008).

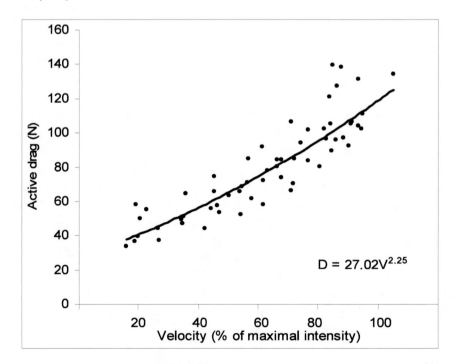

Figure 3. Relationship between active drag (D in Newton) and swimming velocity (*v*); adapted from Seifert et al. (2008).

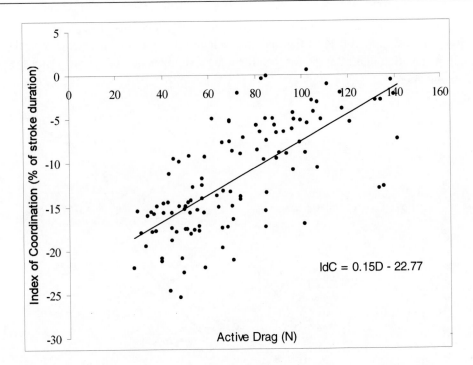

Figure 4. Relationship between index of coordination (IdC) and active drag (D in Newton).

3.3. Inter-Arm Coordination as Regards the Skill Level

The skill level or the capacity to overcome aquatic resistance reflects the motor skill needed to swim fast. Two cases should be distinguished, firstly swimmers over a similar race distance but with different velocities. For example, the maximal velocity of elite male swimmers was 1.92 m.s^{-1} in comparison to 1.78 m.s^{-1} for mid-level male swimmers, as shown in figure 5. Secondly, to swim at similar swimming velocity but different race distance pace, as shown in figure 4. For example the velocity of 1.7 m.s^{-1}, corresponded to the 200 m race pace for elite male, and to the 100 m race pace for mid-level male swimmers. This finding suggests that scientist, coaches and instructors should identify if the goal is to compare two populations in the same task (i.e. a similar race distance but at different velocity and with a difference of race time), or at an equivalent swimming velocity (i.e. similar aquatic resistance).

When swimming at their respective maximal velocities in front crawl, elite male swimmers used a superposition mode of coordination (IdC = 2.8±5.4%), while mid-level males swimmers exhibited catch-up coordination mode (IdC = -4.3±5.0%), as shown in figure 5. Conversely, at a similar velocity of 1.7 m.s^{-1}, the two groups of swimmers did not show any difference of coordination (IdC ~ -6±4.2%) (Seifert et al., 2007b). As elite male swimmers develop higher drag force and higher mechanical power output than mid-level swimmers, they could overcome higher aquatic resistance leading to the use of partially overlapping propulsive impulses (i.e. to increase the IdC). Figure 6 presents the changes in active drag force and mechanical power output when swimming with arms only, as measured on the MAD system. Also identified are the changes of inter-arm coordination when swimming arms only in the free swimming condition over eight laps of 25 m with increasing velocity (from 60 % to 100 % of the maximal velocity; with a maximal velocity in the free swimming condition of 1.52 m.s^{-1} for the elite male swimmers and of 1.44 m.s^{-1} for the mid-level swimmers).

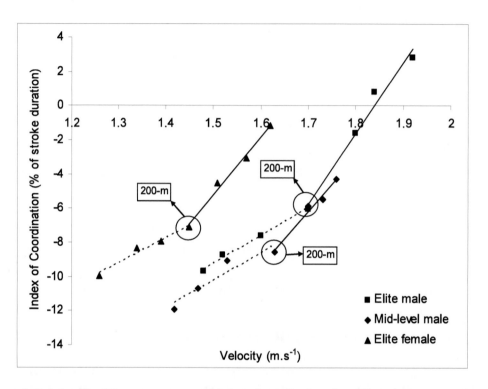

Figure 5. Relationships between race pace and index of coordination: dotted line: slow pace, continuous line: fast pace (adapted from Seifert et al., 2007b).

When swimming at their respective maximal velocities in front crawl, elite male swimmers used a superposition mode of coordination (IdC = 2.8±5.4%), while mid-level males swimmers exhibited catch-up coordination mode (IdC = -4.3±5.0%), as shown in figure 5. Conversely, at a similar velocity of 1.7 m.s^{-1}, the two groups of swimmers did not show any difference of coordination (IdC ~ -6±4.2%) (Seifert et al., 2007b). As elite male swimmers develop higher drag force and higher mechanical power output than mid-level swimmers, they could overcome higher aquatic resistance leading to the use of partially overlapping propulsive impulses (i.e. to increase the IdC). Figure 6 presents the changes in active drag force and mechanical power output when swimming with arms only, as measured on the MAD system. Also identified are the changes of inter-arm coordination when swimming arms only in the free swimming condition over eight laps of 25 m with increasing velocity (from 60 % to 100 % of the maximal velocity; with a maximal velocity in the free swimming condition of 1.52 m.s^{-1} for the elite male swimmers and of 1.44 m.s^{-1} for the mid-level swimmers).

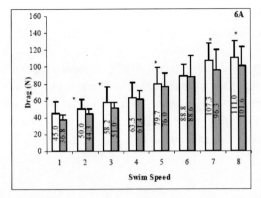
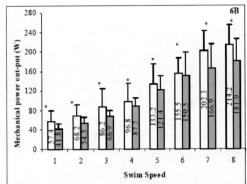

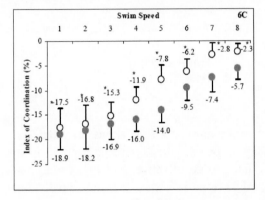

Figure 6. Difference of active drag force (6A), mechanical power output (6B) and index of coordination (6C) between elite male swimmers (white) and mid-level swimmers (grey) at 8 swimming velocitys (expressed in percentage of the maximal velocity).

The superposition coordination (positive value of IdC) was found not to be the cause of higher velocity, but the consequence of the high active drag that swimmers must overcome. Indeed, having a superposition coordination mode did not automatically lead to high velocity. For example, during a 100 m race, Seifert et al. (2007a) showed that elite men have a higher and more stable IdC (always in superposition mode) than the mid-level male swimmers. In fact, the increase in IdC for mid-level male swimmers in the second part of the 100 m resulted from a longer relative duration of the hand spent in the propulsion phase. However, this motor change was ineffective because, unlike in the elite male swimmers, stroke length continued to decrease both between and within 25 m laps. This suggests that the longer relative duration of the propulsion time of the mid-level male was related to their smaller hand velocity (Toussaint et al., 2006).

Similarly, high hand velocity did not guarantee effective propulsion and inter-arm coordination. For example if the hand slips through the water, the high hand velocity did not help in catching water. Therefore, the coordination value could not in itself explain the aquatic motor skills of the swimmers, but should be associated to the measurement of velocity, stroke length, stroke index, active drag, power out-put, propulsive efficiency, intra-cyclic velocity variation and some others parameters about efficiency.

3.4. Inter-Arm Coordination as Regards Froude
Efficiency and Intra-Cyclic Velocity Variation

To achieve high swimming velocity, the inter-arm coordination should be associated with effective propulsion. To generate propulsive force, the swimmer accelerated a mass of water. However, part of the total mechanical power output (P_o) is dissipated in the water as kinetic energy to accelerate the water past the body (P_k), while the remainder is used to overcome aquatic resistance (P_d), as shown in equation 3 (Toussaint et al., 2000; Toussaint & Truijens, 2005):

$$P_o = P_k + P_d \qquad\qquad\qquad\qquad\qquad\text{(equation 3)}$$

Knowing that P_o is greater than what is required to overcome aquatic resistance, the swimmers had to optimize P_d and to minimize P_k. The Froude efficiency (η_F) quantifies the useful power (equation 4) (Lighthill, 1975; Toussaint & Truijens, 2005):

$$\eta_F = P_d / P_o \qquad\qquad\qquad\qquad\qquad\text{(equation 4)}$$

As regards to the equations 3 and 4, the swimmers must accelerate a mass of water in an effective way. Therefore, if the tangential velocity of the swimmer's arm and hand leads to a high swimming velocity, his propulsion is assumed to be effective. Notably, Counsilman (1981) pointed out that high hand acceleration would result in high swimming velocity, only if the hand did not slip through the water. Thus, Martin et al. (1981) proposed a simple model, which was adapted by Zamparo et al. (2005) to assess the Froude efficiency (equation 5):

$$\eta_F = (v / (2\pi \cdot \text{SR} \cdot l)) \cdot (2 / \pi) \qquad\qquad\qquad\text{(equation 5)}$$

assuming that the arm is a rigid segment of length (l), rotating at constant angular velocity ($2\pi \cdot \text{SR}$).

Toussaint et al. (2006) found that η_F corresponded to the ratio between the swimming velocity (v) and the hand tangential velocity (u). As fatigue increased at 100 m race pace, Toussaint et al. (2006) showed that the propulsive force and the mechanical power output decreased, while v/u remained constant. This was demonstrated as the national swimmers both decreased their swimming velocity (from 1.69 m.s^{-1} in the first 25 m lap to 1.48 m.s^{-1} in the fourth lap), and their hand tangential velocity (from 2.14 m.s^{-1} in the first 25 m lap to 1.91 m.s^{-1} in the fourth lap). The two groups of swimmers presented in figure 5 showed a constant v/u, when v increased through the 8 x 25 m test set. The capacity of the elite and mid-level swimmers to overcome aquatic resistance is reflected by the higher propulsive force and mechanical power output, and by the adaptation of their inter-arm coordination during each lap of 25 m. Additionally v/u was greater for the elite swimmers ($v/u = 0.44\pm0.06$) than for the mid-level swimmers ($v/u = 0.36\pm0.03$). When comparing the mean of the eight laps of 25 m the elite swimmers produced a lower u than the mid-level swimmers ($u = 2.98\pm0.37$ m.s^{-1} vs. $u = 3.15\pm0.27$ m.s^{-1} respectively). These results suggest that the higher u of the mid-level swimmers caused them to slip through the water; while those of the elite swimmers enabled them to apply effective propulsive forces and achieve faster maximal v with their effective inter-arm coordination. Finally, the measurement of the hand tangential velocity and Froude efficiency in relation to inter-arm coordination permitted the examination of the effectiveness of aquatic motor skills.

The previous calculation of efficiency is acceptable but does not take into account the intra-cyclic velocity variation. In fact, the swimming velocity is not uniform as the application of propulsive forces in water leads to acceleration and deceleration within the cycle, i.e. to centre of gravity intra-cyclic velocity variation (Fujishima & Miyashita, 1999; Miller, 1975). Therefore, measure the efficiency, an estimation of energy wasted through intra-cyclic velocity variation is required (Miller, 1975). Generally, large intra-cyclic velocity variation leads to a loss of part of the mechanical power output. From a theoretical point of view, Nigg (1983) showed that a velocity change of 10 % within a stroke cycle resulted in an additional work demand of about 3 %, suggesting that the best solution to increase the capacity to produce propulsive force and to develop mechanical power output seems to be to reduce intra-cyclic velocity variation. As observed in figure 6, when velocity and active drag increased, elite front crawl swimmers seem to increase their propulsive continuity (i.e. increase in IdC), while their hip intra-cyclic velocity variation remained stable with a coefficient of variation close to 0.15 (Schnitzler et al., 2008; Seifert et al., 2008). This result suggests that elite swimmers have an effective motor adaptation to the aquatic resistance increase.

Mid-level swimmers also had low intra-cyclic velocity variation similar to (coefficient of variation close to 0.14) elite swimmers. While recreational swimmers showed greater intra-cyclic velocity variation with a coefficient of variation close to 0.18, increasing from 0.15 to 0.21 with swimming velocity. At the same time, the recreational swimmers did not change their inter-arm coordination, remaining in a catch-up mode (-3.6 % < IdC < -8.6 %), whereas their swimming velocity increased from 0.85 $m.s^{-1}$ to 1.40 $m.s^{-1}$. In summary, the quantification of the propulsive forces, the hand tangential velocity, the intra-cyclic velocity and of the inter-arm coordination should not be made since each parameter separately did not guarantee by itself effective aquatic motor skill.

3.5. Inter-Arm Coordination, Energetic Cost and Time Limit to Exhaustion

As previously found in human locomotion, notably in walking-running (Diedrich & Warren, 1995; Holt et al., 1991, 1995; Sparrow & Newell, 1998), the relationships between the inter-limb coordination and the energetic cost could also provide information on the effectiveness of the inter-limb coordination. In swimming, a pilot study assessed the relationships between the index of coordination (IdC) and the energetic cost through an intermittent incremental protocol of six to eight stages of 200 m, with increments of 0.05 $m.s^{-1}$ (Morais et al., 2008). Each increment was separated by a 30 sec rest interval until exhaustion (for further details, see Fernandes et al., 2003). The results showed an increase of propulsive continuity: the elite female front crawl swimmer switching from the catch-up coordination mode (IdC = -8.5 % for a VO_2max of 52. % at stage 1) and an energetic cost of 7.1 $J.Kg^{-1}.min^{-1}$, to the opposition coordination mode (IdC = -1.5 % for a VO_2max of 99.9% at stage eight) and an energetic cost of 13.9 $J.Kg^{-1}.min^{-1}$. This study found a strong correlation between IdC and energetic cost (r = 0.97) (Morais et al., 2008).

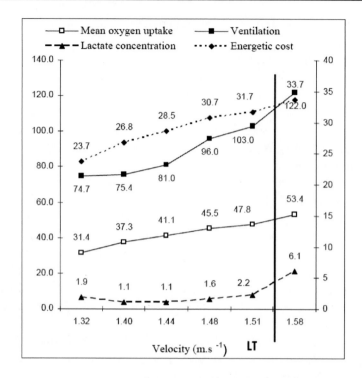

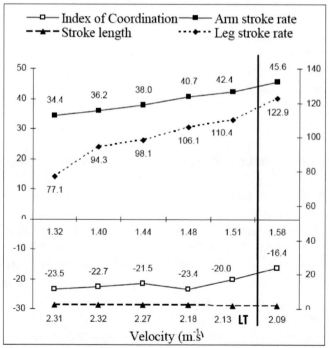

Figure 7. Physiological (7A) and stroking parameters and motor organization (7B) changes of the 2007 European 10 km open water swimming champion through six stages of 300 m with increasing velocity. LT: blood lactate threshold was 4.15 mmol.L^{-1}, with a LT of 78.6% of $_{max}$ and a vLT of 1.54 m.s^{-1}, representing 97.6% of v_{max}. Mean oxygen uptake in mL. kg^{-1}.min^{-1}, ventilation in L.min^{-1}, energetic cost in mL.min^{-1}.m^{-1}, arm and leg stroke rate in stroke.min^{-1}, stroke length in m.stroke^{-1}, index of coordination in % of a complete stroke duration.

In another study using an intermittent incremental protocol of six stages of 300 m until exhaustion the elite long distance swimmers also significantly increased their propulsive continuity (i.e. IdC increased) above their lactate threshold (LT) (Malenfant, 2007). In this protocol the stages were separated by 30 s rest with the first stage 30 s slower than the time required to swim 300 m at the adjusted 400 m pace. The swimming time was then reduced by 5 s for each consecutive 300 m. Because the swimmers, however, had never trained at high velocity (i.e. sprint intensity), their inter-arm coordination remained in catch-up mode (with very negative IdC ~ -20%) (see in figure 7 for an example from the European champion of the 10 km in 2007). In summary, above a certain ventilation, oxygen uptake, energetic cost and lactate production, some swimmers adapt their inter-arm coordination by switching from a catch-up to an opposition mode, or by reducing the degree of catch-up.

In the previous studies the change of coordination is not completely due to energy cost, as during the tests until exhaustion the velocity was also increased. Therefore coordination could be modified because of the increase of active drag. Thus, the use of time limit to exhaustion tests at a given velocity enabled the coordination changes to be examined, while still excluding the effect of velocity. Alberty et al. (2008) used a 400 m test at maximal intensity, knowing that the velocity achieved on this event is highly correlated to the maximal aerobic velocity. The authors then used time limit to exhaustion tests during which the swimming velocity corresponded to 95 %, 100 % and 110 % of mean velocity measured in the all-out 400 m. In the two first conditions, stroke length decreased while stroke rate and propulsive continuity increased through the test, the coordination switching from catch-up mode (IdC ~ -4 %) to opposition mode (IdC ~ -1 %) (Alberty et al., 2008). If the swimmers modified their stroke organization to maintain the imposed velocity, it did not guarantee better propulsion, because the distance covered at the velocity of 100 % of 400 m time varied from 400 m to 225 m (Alberty et al., 2008). As suggested by Seifert et al. (2007a), the higher degree of propulsive continuity could be reached by longer time spent in propulsion because the hand velocity decreased. Therefore, fatigue could lead either to a decrease in hand velocity and a increase in IdC, or to hand slip due to poor hand orientation and a decrease in IdC. Finally, the value of IdC by itself could not explain the effectiveness of propulsion and aquatic motor skills. Coaches, instructors and scientists should consider performance (velocity, stroke length, stroke index) in relation to the inter-limb coordination used by the swimmers.

3.6. Inter-Arm Coordination and the Inter-Individual Variation: Coordination Profiling and Swimmers with Impairment

When velocity increases, a similar adaptation of the inter-arm coordination (e.g. increase in IdC) is found (Chollet et al., 2000; Seifert & Chollet, 2009). However, when analyzing twelve elite front crawl sprint swimmers transiting from their slowest to their fastest velocity, the results showed inter-individual variation in the range of arm coordination and in velocity (Fig. 8; Seifert & Chollet, 2009).

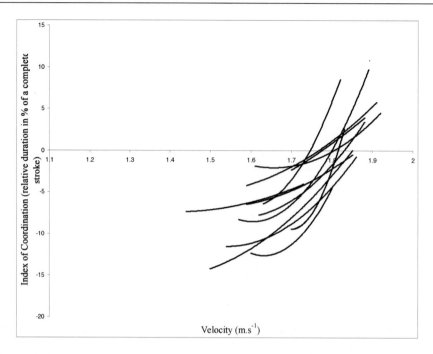

Figure 8. Quadratic regression between inter-arm coordination and velocity for twelve elite front crawl sprinters (adapted from Seifert & Chollet, 2009).

These results suggested four theoretical profiles (Fig. 9): 1) a small scale of velocity and coordination; 2) a small scale of velocity and a large scale of coordination; 3) a large scale of velocity and a small scale of coordination; 4) a large scale of velocity and coordination.

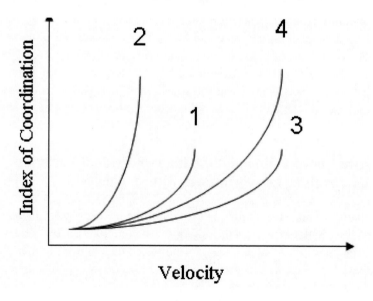

Figure 9. Four profiles of relationships between coordination and velocity.

The first profile corresponded to swimmers with little "motor flexibility" in coordination and velocity. These could be "ultra-specialists", training mostly in one way. For example, because they trained mostly for endurance triathlons (Hue et al., 2003) and long distance swimming (Malenfant, 2007) maintained their inter-arm coordination in catch-up mode with extremely negative values for IdC. The second profile corresponds to an ineffective large value for coordination, because high velocities cannot be attained. As pointed out by Seifert et al. (2007a), some unskilled swimmers switched to superposition mode (IdC > 0 %) because their hand spent more time in the propulsive phase, due to slow hand velocity, but therefore did not generate high force. The third profile corresponds to swimmers which less change in their coordination while reaching high velocity. These swimmers were focused on adaptation in the ratio between stroke rate and stroke length (see in figure 10 one swimmer of the French team which participated in the 4 x 100m at the Atlanta Olympic Games in 1996).

Finally for the fourth profile, the longer the coordination curve, the greater the swimmer's range of coordination; indicating motor flexibility in coordination. Indeed, the higher the maximal coordination, and the lower the minimal coordination of the curve, the more the swimmer is exploring human potential. To the coach, this indicates that these swimmers attain a range of velocities depending on the type of coordination mode: catch-up mode by using glide time, or superposition mode by overlapping the propulsive phases. Finally, the value of IdC does not indicate itself the aquatic motor skills of the swimmer, but should be related to the stroking parameters (velocity, stroke rate and stroke length).

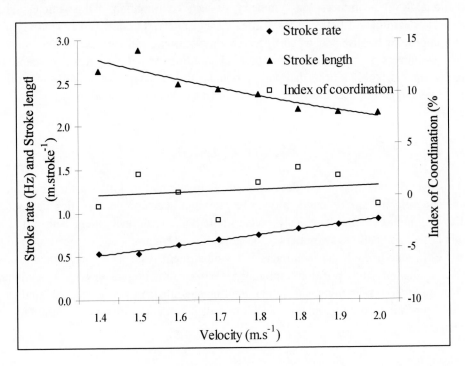

Figure 10. Change of stroke rate, stroke length and index of coordination in relation to seven stages of 25 m with increasing velocity.

Swimmers with locomotor disabilities, i.e. amputation, cerebral palsy, spinal cord injury may have a different aquatic motor control pattern due to their disability. For example a swimmer who is a single leg amputee will have a modified balance on the blocks prior to entering the pool and to maintain balance in the water their single leg kick may alternate from left to right, to counter the upper limb stroke. This natural compensation of a one-legged kick can change the motor skill of kicking and may also influence the inter-arm coordination. The neuro-muscular impairment that can be associated with cerebral palsy can also influence the aquatic motor skill, particularly as these athletes fatigue the asymmetry can be exaggerated. Similarly the loss of abdominal control and core stability associated with a spinal cord injury can also affect the aquatic motor control; this will depend on the location of the spinal lesion. These potentially smaller propulsive surfaces or an unbalanced capacity for propulsion, when compared to an able-bodied swimmers have been found to influence their inter-arm coordination (Satkunskiene et al., 2005) and consequently showed inter-individual variation that should be investigated to well understand aquatic motor skills. Three groups of swimmers are distinguished: swimmers using catch-up coordination (IdC varying from -30 % to 0 %), swimmers using normal superposition coordination mode (0 % < IdC < 10 %), swimmers using an exaggerated superposition mode usually not seen in able-bodied swimmers with IdC values ranging from 11 to 30 %. Satkunskiene et al. (2005) stated that even if swimmers with locomotor disabilities vary the coordination mode in relation to their degree of impairment, correct coordination is fundamental to front crawl swimming, just as in able-bodied swimmers.

More recently Osborough et al. (2009a) examined thirteen single arm amputee international level swimmers for symmetry of arm coordination. All swimmers showed asymmetric coordination between their affected and unaffected arm pulls. This asymmetry did not appear to be affected by an increase in swimming velocity up to maximum. The quickest swimmers possessed more symmetrical coordination between arms, compared to the slower swimmers. This suggests that pulling both arms through the water with similar timings might be beneficial for front crawl swimmers with a single arm amputation.

4. Conclusion

This overview deals with the development of aquatic motor skills showing how stroking parameters (velocity, stroke length and stroke rate) and inter-arm coordination in front crawl need to be monitored simultaneously both in able-bodied and swimmers with impairment. The goal of all competitive swimmers is the same, e.g. overcoming aquatic resistance to swim fastest. Both able-bodied and swimmers with impairment need to organize their body and limb coordination and position optimally. While the literature provides interesting information on how swimmers with impairment manage their race strategy, few studies point out the inter-limb coordination for this sample of swimmers. This is an important future research direction..

Acknowledgements

We thank Morgan Alberty and Ricardo Fernandes for the review of this paper and their instructive comments about inter-limb coordination and biomechanics in swimming.

REFERENCES

Alberty, M., Potdevin, F., Dekerle, J., Pelayo, P., Gorce, P. & Sidney, M. (2008). Changes in swimming technique during time to exhaustion at freely chosen and controlled stroke rates. *Journal of Sports Sciences.* 26, 11, 1191-1200.

Arellano, R., Brown, P., Cappaert, J. & Nelson, R.C. (1994). Analysis of 50, 100 and 200m freestyle swimmers at the 1992 Olympic Games. *Journal of Applied Biomechanics.* 10, 189-199.

Bardy, B.G., Oullier, O., Bootsma, R.J. & Stoffregen, T.A. (2002). Dynamics of human postural transitions. *Journal of Experimental Psychology: Human Perception and Performance.* 28, 499-514.

Burkett, B., Malone, L., & Daly, D. (2003). 100m race strategy comparison between Olympic and visually impaired Paralympic swimmers. *Journal of Science and Medicine in Sport.* Supplement. (6, 4), 80.

Burkett, B., & Mellifont, R. (2008). Sport Science and Coaching in Paralympic Swimming. *International Journal of Sports Science & Coaching.* 3, 1, 105-112.

Chatard, J.C., Collomp, C., Maglischo, E. & Maglischo, C. (1990). Swimming skill and stroking characteristics of front crawl swimmers. *International Journal of Sports Medicine.* 11, 2, 156-161.

Chollet, D., Chalies, S. & Chatard, J.C. (2000). A new index of coordination for the crawl: description and usefulness. *International Journal of Sports Medicine.* 21, 54-59.

Chollet, D., Moretto, P., Pelayo, P. & Sidney, M. (1996a). Energetic effects of velocity and stroke rate control in non-expert swimmers. In J.P. Troup, A.P. Hollander, D. Strasse, S.W. Trappe, J.M. Cappaert, & T.A. Trappe (Eds.), *Swimming Science* VII (pp. 172-176), London, E&FN Spon.

Chollet, D., Pelayo, P., Delaplace, C., Tourny, C. & Sidney, M. (1997). Stroking characteristic variations in the 100 m freestyle for male swimmers of different skill. *Perceptual and Motor Skills.* 85, 167-177.

Chollet, D., Pelayo, P., Tourny, C. & Sidney, M. (1996b). Comparative analysis of 100 m and 200 m events in the four strokes in top level swimmers. *Journal of Human Movement Studies.* 31, 25-37.

Costill, D.L., Kovaleski, J., Porter, D., Kirwan, J., Fielding, R. & King, D. (1985). Energy expenditure during front crawl swimming: Predicting success in middle-distance events. *International Journal of Sports Medicine.* 6, 266-270.

Counsilman J. (1981). Hand speed and acceleration. Swimming Technique, 18, 22-6.

Craig, A.B., Boomer, W.L., & Gibbons, J.F. (1979). Use of stroke rate, distance per stroke, and velocity relationships during training for competitive swimming. In J. Terauds & E.W. Bedingfield (Eds.) *Swimming Science.* III (pp. 65-274), Baltimore, University Park Press.

Craig, A.B. & Pendergast, DR. (1979). Relationships of stroke rate, distance per stroke, and velocity in competitive swimming. *Medicine and Science in Sports.* 11, 3, 278-283.

Craig, A.B., Skehan, P.L., Pawelczyk, J.A. & Boomer, W.L. (1985). Velocity, stroke rate, and distance per stroke during elite swimming competition. *Medicine and Science in Sports and Exercise.* 17, 6, 625-634.

Daly, D., Djobova, S., Malone, L., Vanlandewijck, Y. & Steadward, R. (2003). Swimming speed patterns and stroking variables in the Paralympic 100-m freestyle. . *Adapted Physical Activity Quarterly.* 20, 260-278.

Daly, D., Malone, L., Smith, D., Vanlandewijck, Y. & Steadward, R. (2001). The contribution of starting, turning, and finishing to total race performance in male Paralympic swimmers. *Adapted Physical Activity Quarterly.* 18, 316-333.

Dekerle, J., Nesi, X., Lefevre, T., Depretz, S., Sidney, M., Huot-Marchand, F. & Pelayo, P. (2005). Stroking parameters in front crawl swimming and maximal lactate steady state speed. *International Journal of Sport Medicine.* 26, 53-58.

Deschodt, V.J. (1996). Paramètres cinématiques et niveau de performance en crawl. [Kinematical parameters and performance level in front crawl], Unpublished PhD thesis, University of Lyon, France.

Deschodt, V.J., Arsac, L.M., & Rouard, A.H. (1999). Relative contribution of arms and legs in humans to propulsion in 25 m sprint front crawl swimming. *European Journal of Applied Physiology.* 80, 192-199.

Diedrich, F.J. & Warren, W.H. (1995). Why change gaits? Dynamics of the walk-run transition. *Journal of Experimental Psychology: Human Perception and Performance.* 21, 183-202.

di Prampero, P.E., Dekerle, J., Capelli, C. & Zamparo, P. (2008). The critical velocity in swimming. *European Journal of Applied Physiology.* 102, 2, 165-71.

Fernandes, R.J., Cardoso, C.S., Soares, S.M., Ascensão, A., Colaço, P.J. & Vilas-Boas J.P. (2003). Time limit and VO_2 slow component at intensities corresponding to VO_{2max} in swimmers. *International Journal Sports Medicine.* 24, 576-81.

Fernandes, R.J., Marinho, D.A., Barbosa, T.M. & Vilas-Boas, J.P. (2006). Is time limit at the minimum swimming velocity of VO_{2max} influenced by stroking parameters? *Perceptual and Motor Skills.* 103, 67-75.

Fujishima, M. & Miyashita, M. (1999). Velocity degradation caused by its fluctuation in swimming and guidelines for improvement of average velocity. In K.L. Keskinen, P.V. Komi & A.P. Hollander (Eds.), *Biomechanics and Medicine in Swimming.* VIII (pp. 41-45), Jyvaskyla, University of Jyvaskyla.

Fulton, S., Pyne, D., Hopkins, W., & Burkett, B. (2009). Variability and progression in competitive performance of Paralympic swimmers. *Journal of Sport Sciences.* (in press)

Haljand, R. (2002). Race analysis of European Short Course Championships Riesa 2002. www.swim.ee/competition/2002_riesa/index.html

Hay, J.G. (2002). Cycle rate, length, and speed of progression in human locomotion. *Journal of Applied Biomechanics.* 18, 257-270.

Hellard, P., Dekerle, J., Avalos, M., Caudal, N., Knopp, K. & Hausswirth, C. (2008). Kinematic measures and stroke rate variability in elite female 200-m swimmers in the four swimming technique: Athens 2004 Olympic semi-finalists and French National 2004 Championship semi-finalists. *Journal of Sports Sciences.* 26, 1, 35-46.

Holt, K.G., Hamill, J. & Andres, R.O. (1991) Predicting the minimal energy costs of human walking. *Medicine and Science in Sports and Exercise.* 23, 4, 491-498.

Holt, K.G., Jeng, S.F., Ratcliffe, R. & Hamill, J. (1995) Energetic cost and stability during human walking at the preferred stride frequency. *Journal of Motor Behavior.* 27, 2, 164-178.

Hue, O., Benavente, H., & Chollet, D. (2003). The effect of wet suit use by triathletes: an analysis of the different phases of arm movement. *Journal of Sports Sciences.* 21, 1025-1030.

Kelso, J.A.S. (1995). Dynamic patterns, the self-organization of brain and behavior. MIT Press, Cambridge.

Keskinen, K.L. & Komi, P.V. (1988). Interaction between aerobic/anaerobic loading and biomechanical performance in freestyle swimming. In B.E. Ungerechts & K. Reischle (Eds.) *Swimming Science.* V (pp. 285-293), Champaign, Human Kinetics.

Keskinen, K.L., & Komi, PV. (1992). Effect of leg action on stroke performance in swimming. In D. MacLaren, T. Reilly, & A. Less (Eds.) *Swimming Science.* VI (pp. 251-255), London, E & FN SPON.

Kjendlie, P.L., Haljand, R., Fjortoft, O. & Stallman R.K. (2006). Stroke frequency strategies of international and national swimmers in 100 m races. *Portuguese Journal of Sports Sciences.* 6 (Supplement 2), 52-54.

Kolmogorov, S.V., Rumyantseva, O.A., Gordon, B.J. & Cappaert J. (1997). Hydrodynamic characteristics of competitve swimmers of different genders and performance levels. *Journal of Applied Biomechanics.* 13, 88-97.

Lavoie, J.P. & Montpetit, R.R. (1986). Applied physiology of swimming. *Sports Medicine.* 3, 3, 165-189.

Letzelter, H. & Freitag, W. (1983). Stroke length and stroke frequency variations in men's and women's 100 m freestyle swimming. In A.P. Hollander, P.A. Huijing & G. de Groot (Eds.), *Swimming Science.* IV (pp. 315-322), Champaign, Illinois: Human Kinetics Publishers.

Lighthill, M.J. (1975). Mathematical biofluid dynamics. Philadelphia: Society for Industrial and Applied Mathematics.

Maglischo, C.W., Maglischo, E.W., Sharp, RL., Zier, DJ. & Katz, A. (1984). Tethered and non tethered crawl swimming. In J. Terauds, E. Barthels, E. Kreighbaum, R. Mann & J. Crakes (Eds.) *Sports Biomechanics.* (pp. 163-167)

Maglischo, E.W. (2003). Swimming fastest, Champaign, Illinois, Human Kinetics.

Malenfant, E. (2007). Etude de la coordination motrice en crawl chez des nageurs spécialistes en natation longue distance lors d'un test exhaustif à vitesse incrémentée [Analysis of the motor coordination in long distance front crawl swimmers during an intermittent incremental protocol until exhaustion] Unpublished Master thesis, University of Rouen, France.

Malone, L. A., Sanders, R. H., Schiltz, J. H. & Steadward, R. D. (2001). Effects of visual impairment on stroke parameters in Paralympic swimmers. *Medicine and Science in Sports and Exercise.* 33, 12, 2098-2103.

Miller, D. (1975). Biomechanics of swimming. *Exercise Sport Science Review.* 3, 219-248.

Millet, G., Chollet, D., Chalies, S. & Chatard, J.C. (2002). Comparison of coordination in front crawl between elite swimmers and triathletes. *International Journal of Sports Medicine.* 23, 99-104.

Morais, P., Vilas-Boas, J.P., Seifert, L., Chollet, D., Keskinen, K.L. & Fernandes, R. (2008). Relationship between energy cost and the index of coordination in front crawl – a pilot study, *Journal of Sports Sciences.* 26, (Supplement 1), 11.

Nigg, B. (1983). Selected methodology in biomechanics with respect to swimming. In A.P. Hollander, P. Huijing & G. de Groot (Eds.), *Biomechanics and Medicine in Swimming.* (pp. 72-80), Illinois, Human Kinetics Books.

Ogita, F. (2006). Energetics in competitive swimming and its application for training. *Portuguese Journal of Sport Sciences.* 6 (Supplement 2), 117-121.

Osborough, C., Payton, C. & Daly, D. (2009a). Inter-arm coordination of competitive unilateral arm amputee front crawl swimmers. 7th Annual British Paralympic Association Sports Science, Medicine and Coaching Conference. Loughborough University, UK. 4-5 March 2009.

Osborough, C., Payton, C. & Daly, D. (2009b). Relationships between the front crawl stroke parameters of competitive unilateral arm-amputee swimmers, with selected anthropometric characteristics. *Journal of Applied Biomechanics.* (in press).

Pai, Y.C., Hay, J.G., & Wilson, B.D. (1984). Stroking techniques of elite swimmers. *Journal of Sports Sciences.* 2, 225-239.

Pelayo, P., Alberty, M., Sidney, M., Potdevin, F. & Dekerle, J. (2007). Aerobic potential, stroke parameters, and coordination in swimming front crawl performance. *International Journal of Sports Physiology and Performance.* 2, 347-359.

Pelayo, P., Sidney, M., Kherif, T., Chollet, D., & Tourny, C. (1996). Stroking characteristics in freestyle swimming and relationships with anthropometric characteristics. *Journal of Applied Biomechanics.* 12, 197-206.

Pendergast, D.R., Capelli C., Craig, A.B., di Prampero, P.E., Minetti, A.E., Mollendorf, J., Termin, A. & Zamparo, P. (2006). Biophysics in swimming. *Portuguese Journal of Sport Sciences.* 6 (Supplement 2), 185-189.

Pendergast, D.R., Mollendorf, J., Zamparo, P., Termin, A., Bushnell, D. & Paschke, D. (2005). The influence of drag on human locomotion in water. *Undersea and Hyperbaric Medicine.* 32, 45-58.

Potdevin, F., Bril, B., Sidney, M. & Pelayo, P. (2006). Stroke frequency and arm coordination in front crawl swimming. *International Journal of Sport Medicine.* 27, 193-198.

Potdevin, F., Delignières, D., Dekerle, J., Alberty, J., Sidney, M. & Pelayo, P. (2003). Does stroke frequency determine swimming velocity values and coordination? In J.C. Chatard (Ed.), *Biomechanics and Medicine in Swimming.* IX (pp. 163-167), Saint Etienne, France, University of Saint Etienne.

Pyne, D.B., Trewin, C.B. & Hopkins, W.G. (2004). Progression and variability of competitive performance of Olympic Swimmers. *Journal of Sports Sciences.* 22, 613-620.

Rouard, A.H. & Billat, R.P. (1990) Influences of sex and level of performance on freestyle stroke: an electromyography and kinematic study. *International Journal of Sports and Medicine.* 11, 2, 150-155.

Satkunskiene, D., Schega, L., Kunze, K., Birzinyte, K. & Daly, D. (2005). Coordination in arm movements during crawl stroke in elite swimmers with a locomotor disability. *Human Movement Science.* 24, 54-65.

Schleihauf, R.E. (1979). A hydrodynamic analysis of swimming propulsion. In J. Terauds & E.W. Bedingfield (Eds.), *Swimming Science.* III (pp. 71-109), Baltimore, University Park Press.

Schleihauf, R.E., Higgins, J.R., Hinricks, R., Luedtke, D., Maglischo, C., Maglischo, E.W., & Thayer, A. (1988). Propulsive techniques: front crawl stroke, butterfly, backstroke and breaststroke. In B.E. Ungerechts, K. Wilke, & K. Reischle (Eds.), *Swimming Science.* V (pp. 53-59), Champaign, Illinois, Human Kinetics Publishers.

Schnitzler, C., Seifert, L., Ernwein, V. & Chollet, D. (2008). Intra-cyclic velocity variations as a tool to assess arm coordination adaptations in elite swimmers. *International Journal of Sports Medicine.* 29, 6, 480-486.

Seifert, L., Boulesteix, L., Carter, M. & Chollet, D. (2005). The spatial-temporal and coordinative structure in elite men 100-m front crawl swimmers, *International Journal of Sports Medicine.* 26, 286-293.

Seifert, L., Boulesteix, L. & Chollet D. (2004a). Effect of gender on the adaptation of arm coordination in front crawl. *International Journal of Sport Medicine.* 25, 217-223.

Seifert, L. & Chollet, D. (2008). Inter-limb coordination and constraints in swimming: a review. In N.P. Beaulieu (Ed.) *Physical activity and children: new research.* (pp. 65-93), Nova Science Publishers, Hauppauge, New York.

Seifert, L. & Chollet, D. (2009). Modelling spatial-temporal and coordinative parameters in swimming. *Journal of Science and Medicine in Sport.* 12, 495-499.

Seifert, L., Chollet, D. & Bardy, B. (2004b). Effect of swimming velocity on arm coordination in front crawl: a dynamical analysis. *Journal of Sports Sciences.* 22, 651-660.

Seifert, L., Chollet, D. & Chatard, J.C. (2007a). Changes in coordination and kinematics during a 100-m front crawl. *Medicine and Science in Sports and Exercise.* 39, 1784-1793.

Seifert, L., Chollet, D. & Rouard, A. (2007b). Swimming constraints and arm coordination. *Human Movement Science.* 26, 68-86.

Seifert, L., Toussaint, H., Schnitzler, C., Alberty, M., Chavallard, F., Lemaitre, F., Vantorre, J. & Chollet D. (2008). Effect of velocity increase on arm coordination, active drag and intra-cyclic velocity variations in front crawl. In T. Nomura & B. Ungerechts (Eds.), *1st International Scientific Conference of Aquatic Space Activities.* (pp. 254-259), University of Tsukuba, Tsukuba, Japan.

Sidney, M., Delhaye, B., Baillon, M. & Pelayo, P. (1999). Stroke frequency evolution during 100 m and 200 m events front crawl swimming. In K.L. Keskinen, P.V. Komi & A.P. Hollander (Eds.), *Swimming Science.* VIII (pp. 71-75), Jyvaskyla, Finland.

Sparrow, W.A. & Newell, K.M. (1998). Metabolic energy expenditure and the regulation of movement economy. *Psychonomic Bulletin & Review.* 5, 173-196.

Swaine, I. & Reilly, T. (1983). The freely chosen swimming stroke rate in a maximal swim and on a biokinetic swim bench. *Medicine and Science in Sports and Exercise.* 15, 370-375.

Toussaint, H.M., Carol, A., Kranenborg, H. & Truijens, M. (2006). Effect of fatigue on stroking characteristics in an arms-only 100-m front-crawl race. *Medicine and Science in Sports and Exercise.* 38, 1635-1642.

Toussaint, H.M., & Truijens, M. (2005). Biomechanical aspects of peak performance in human swimming. *Animal Biology.* 55, 17-40.

Toussaint, H.M., & Hollander, A.P. (1994). Energetics of competitive swimming. Implications for training programmes. *Sports Medicine.* 18, 6, 384-405.

Toussaint, H.M., Hollander, A.P., van den Berg, C & Vorontsov, A. (2000). Biomechanics in swimming. In W.E. Garrett & D.T. Kirkendall (Eds.) *Exercise and Sport Science.* (pp. 639-660). Philadelphia: Lippincott, Williams & Wilkins.

Vaday, M. & Nemessuri, M. (1971). Motor pattern of freestyle swimming. In L. Lewillie & J.P. Clarys (Eds.), *Swimming Science.* I (pp. 167-173), Brussels, University of Brussels.

Wilke, K. (1992) Analysis of sprint swimming: the 50m freestyle. In D. MacLaren, T. Reilly, & A. Less (Eds.) *Swimming Science.* VI (pp. 33-46), London, E & FN SPON.

Zamparo, P., Pendergast, D.R., Mollendorf, J., Termin, A. & Minetti, A.E. (2005). An energy balance of front crawl. *European Journal of Applied Physiology.* 94, 134-44.

In: Handbook of Motor Skills
Editor: Lucian T. Pelligrino

ISBN: 978-1-60741-811-5
© 2009 Nova Science Publishers, Inc.

Chapter 4

EVALUATION OF MOTOR AND PROCESS SKILLS

Esra Aki[*]

Hacettepe University, Faculty of Health Sciences,
Physiotherapy and Rehabilitation Department, Ankara, Turkey

ABSTRACT

Skill is a task-specific ability that is influenced by task demands to achieve a task proficiently. Motor skills consist of both movement and interactions as an observable, goal-directed action and have a sequence that constitutes a routine. While skills are performed in a routine sequence, they are linked together by individualized habits.

The assessment of skills has significant importance because, as with skills, task demands and physical and social environment can affect habits.

Motor skills may be evaluated with non-standardized and standardized methods. Nonstandardized methods are informal evaluation based on observation of the performing of any task. After the observation is completed, the relevant motor skill is investigated carefully and systematically. Standardized methods are objective and well documented.

This chapter aims to explain this wide variety of evaluation methods.

INTRODUCTION

Motor skills comprise body position, obtaining and holding objects, moving the self and objects, and sustaining performance. Process skills are structured to maintain motor skills and comprise sustaining performance, applying knowledge, temporal organization, organizing space objects and adapting performance parameters. These two skill domain complement each other and bring about gross and fine motor skills [30].

Gross motor skills comprise the abilities attained by the large muscles of the body, such as controlling head movement, rolling, sitting, balancing, crawling, walking, maintaining equilibrium, jumping, lying, lifting and throwing.

---

[*] Tel: 00 90 312 305 15 77 / 157; E-mail: esraaki@hotmail.com or esraaki@hacettepe.edu.tr

Gross Motor	Fine Motor	Gross & Fine Motor	Handwriting	Screening
• Arm Motor Ability Test • Gross Motor Function Measure • Test of Gross Motor Development • Wolf Motor Function Test	• Beery-Buctenica Developmental Test of Visual-Motor Integration • Bennet Hand Tool Dexterity Test • Benton Constructional Praxis Test • Box and Block Test • Crawford Small Parts Dexterity Test • Fine Dexterity Test • Fine Motor Task Assessment • Grooved Pegboard Test • Jebsen Test of Hand Function • Minnesota Manual Dexterity Test • Nine Hole Peg Test • Purdue Pegboard • Stromberg Dexterity Test • Skills Assessment Module	• Assessment of Motor and Process Skills • Bruininks-Oseretsky Motor Proficiency Test • Lincoln-Oseretsky Motor Development Scale • McCarthy Scale of Children's Abilities • Miller Assessment for Preschoolers • Movement Assessment Battery for Children • Peabody Developmental Motor Scales-2 • Quality of Upper Extremity Skills Test	• Children's Handwriting Evaluation Scale • Children's Handwriting Evaluation Scale for Manuscript Writing • Denver Handwriting Analysis • Evaluation Tool of Children's Handwriting • Minnesota Handwriting Assessment • Test of Handwriting Skills	• Clinical Observations of Motor and Postural Skills • Denver Developmental Screening Test • FirstSTEP Developmental Screening Test

Figure 1. Standardized Skills Evaluation Tools.

Fine motor skills are fine motor movements used to complete tasks that require precision. Manipulating small objects, transferring objects from hand to hand, hand-eye coordination, writing, stringing beads, using a computer, turning pages, cutting with scissors and using a knife and fork are among the tasks that require high-level control and precision. Fine motor skills are not limited only to manual dexterity but also include attentiveness and stabilized posture.

EVALUATION OF THE SKILLS

Detailed assessment of motor skills, on which the functioning of people of all ages is based, is very crucial to identify the source of a dysfunction. An accurately and precisely identified dysfunction leads to a precise treatment procedure. Skills can be assessed by both non-standardized and standardized analysis methods.

Non-standardized analysis methods are based on observations. An individual is observed and analyzed in detail while performing an activity. Can the subject initiate the activity? Can the subject proceed and complete the activity? Does the subject need verbal or physical help in initiating, proceeding, or completing the activity? Is the subject willing or not? Does the subject need an auxiliary tool? Is the subject successful in reaching, grasping, lifting or manipulating objects? How is the subject's posture while performing the activity? Can the subject find alternative ways in case of unforeseen circumstances? This list could be expanded and detailed depending on the nature of the job, age, gender, roles and domains. A subjective judgment could be made regarding the subject's performance of the observed activity by answering such questions. The role of non-standardized analyses in realistic interpretation of standardized analyses is very important.

Standardized tests provide objective results. They enable us to estimate the level of impairment and to evaluate the treatment efficiency and to perform screening. There are tests for only gross motor skills or for only fine motor skills as well as for both skills. Furthermore, hand manipulation, visual-motor control, upper limb speed, dexterity and steadiness are the characteristics defining the quality of handwriting, and the quality of handwriting may be assessed by special standardized methods [28]. In addition, there are objective assessment methods enabling the developmental screening (figure 1).

In this part of the chapter, standardized assessment methods are analyzed.

GROSS MOTOR ASSESSMENT

Gross Motor Function Measure (GMFM)

The GMFM is a clinical measure that includes normal developmental samples. It is sensitive to changes of gross motor functions (lying, rolling, sitting, crawling, kneeling, standing, walking, running, jumping) in children five months to 16 years old with cerebral palsy and is also validated for children with Down syndrome [64, 87]. There are two versions of the GMFM: the original 88-item measure (GMFM-88) and the more recent 66-item GMFM (GMFM-66). There is a four-point scoring system for each item. The scoring of both

GMFM-88 and GMFM-66 is the same. The GMFM-88 item scores are calculated for raw and percent scores for each of the subtests of GMFM. The GMFM-66 requires a computer program called Gross Motor Ability Estimator (GMAE).

GMFM has good psychometric properties. The reliability of the test is 0.99 [57]. The test has been preferred frequently in investigating the effectiveness of several treatment modalities such as strength, walking training and ankle-foot orthotics in children with cerebral palsy [11, 21].

Test of Gross Motor Development

The Test of Gross Motor Development, which measures gross motor skills of children aged 3–11 years, was developed by Ulrich. It includes two subtests. The locomotor skills subtest assesses running, galloping, hopping, leaping, horizontal jumping, skipping and sliding skills. The other subtest is object control skills and measures two-hand striking, stationary bouncing and catching activities. It takes about 15 min to complete the task [101]. The reliability of the test is 0.88 [84].

Wolf Motor Function Test (WMFT)

The WMFT has three sections, namely, timed activities, functional ability and strength. As part of the timed activities, the subject's time of completion of a task is focused, whereas the movement quality of the subject during performing the task is focused in the functional ability section. The strength section deals with the subject's lifting ability against gravity. WMFT, which is generally used to assess moderately impaired hemiparetic stroke patients' upper extremity motor skill performance, has a reliability of 0.97–0.99 [75, 83, 109, 110]. Scoring of the test is between 0 and 4: "0" indicates that the impaired arm has no effect in the action and "4" indicates that the movement is performed normally [107].

The *Arm Motor Ability Test (AMAT),* which was developed as a supplement to WMFT, assesses the development in the activities of daily living [61]. The test focuses on the quality of the performance rather than the speed. AMAT includes 17 activities of daily living, namely, cutting meat, preparing a sandwich, eating with spoon, drinking from mug, combing hair, opening jar, tying shoelaces, using a telephone, wiping up spilled water, putting on a cardigan, putting on a t-shirt, propping on an extended arm, lighting switch/door, removing sweater from drawer, carrying sweater, putting on a mitten and washing hands. AMAT has the reliability of 0.95 to 0.99 [108].

FINE MOTOR ASSESSMENT

Beery-Buctenica Developmental Test of Visual-Motor Integration (BEERY™ VMI)

BEERY™ VMI assesses the integration of visual and motor skills in children and adults (2.9 to 19.8 years in the 4th Edition and 2.9 to 100 years in the 5th Edition). It is a reliable (r = 0.86) and valid measure. The test requires copying of geometric forms. It is scored using the test manual [68].

BEERY™ VMI is used frequently in optometric studies to investigate the visual analysis, motor coordination, and visual motor integration. The test reveals differences between various kinds of deficits [97].

Bennet Hand Tool Dexterity Test (H-TDT)

H-TDT was developed by George K Bennet in 1965. It provides quick determination of proficiency with manipulation of hand tools and safety skills that are independent of intellectual factors in adults. It takes approximately 10 min. The reliability coefficient of the H-TDT is .91. The test requires completing the task by removing the nuts and bolts from the left upright and mounting them on the right upright. The score is the amount of time spent for completing the task [9].

Benton Constructional Praxis Test (BCPT)

BCPT is a three-dimensional evaluation test. It was developed by Benton as a clinical praxis test in 1962 [10]. However, the use of BCTP is quiet limited today probably because there was no evidence-based knowledge when the test was developed and also opportunities to popularize the test were less than today.

Box and Block Test (BBT)

BBT is a quantitative, quick, sensitive, and easy-to-administer test that is standardized (r = 0.93 and 0.97 for left and right hand, respectively) and is used to evaluate gross manual skills. It can be used for children 7 years of age to adults. One hundred and fifty cubes (2.5 cm x 2.5 cm x 2.5 cm) are used in the test. The number of cubes the subject transfers from one side of the box to the other in one minute is determined. Each hand is tested separately. The test could also be used to test endurance by determining the number of cubes before signs of fatigue. The literature highlights that, because of its practicality, BBT has applicability in a wide range of fields. For instance, activities that are part of some treatments used with hemiplegic patients in the functional recovery after stroke—such as electric stimulation, mechanical arm training, exercise program, upper extremity intensive repetitive training, fully implanted cortical stimulation, music-supported training, and combination of botulinum toxin and exercise therapy—are assessed using the BBT [3, 45, 50, 59, 62, 90, 109]. Moreover, it is noted in the literature that the test is also preferred as a motor skill test determining the deterioration of motor skills occurring in intellectual disabilities, multiple sclerosis and in cerebral palsy [4, 18, 77]. Moreover, the Box and Block test could be used to support the computerized assessment of upper extremity skills [90]. Farrel and Weir stated that they used this instrument to be able to quantitatively observe the optimal daily usage potential of upper extremity prosthesis with sufficient speed and endurance [27]. The practitioners may choose BBT in clinics cause of wide range of application and easy to administer.

Crawford Small Parts Dexterity Test

The Crawford Small Parts Dexterity Test measures eye-hand coordination, dexterity, and fine motor skills in adults with small hand tools. It is a standardized reliable test that measures dexterity and is used in occupational assessment [76]. Test materials comprise pins, collars, screws, and a board with metal plates. There is a pair of screw-and-pin-compatible plates—one with 42 threaded holes and the other with 42 unthreaded holes. Pins and collars are placed into the holes using tweezers. The screws are inserted to a certain depth using a screwdriver. The time spent on the task is recorded. Split half reliabilities of the test are: pins $r = 0.86$ and screws $r = 0.92$. The literature shows that, in addition to occupational rehabilitation applications, this instrument could have been used in various fields. For instance, whether premenstrual period has any effect on women's manual dexterity was investigated and it was found to have the value of objective evaluation [81]. Various studies involving trainees and master surgeons investigated the eye-hand coordination and manual dexterity, which is very important for surgeons, using the Crawford Small Parts Dexterity Test [37, 89]. Similarly, it was emphasized that it could be used as a differential test in the evaluation of dental students' school performance [12].

Fine Dexterity Test (FDT)

FDT is a test material appropriate for 16 years to adults that measures fine finger and small tool dexterity. It is a quick assessment that mimics fine finger skills and provides precise information about job requirements. It is a sensitive tool especially in the electronics industry. The test comprises a board and 60 pins (plus nine pins for practice), collars, washers and a pair of forceps. The test is performed with the preferred hand and the number of collars and washes assembled is recorded.

Fine Motor Task Assessment (FMTA)

The Fine Motor Task Assessment provides a detailed picture of fine motor requirements in school-age children. Integrated fine motor tasks and academic and nonacademic activities may be assessed by FMTA. When it defines fine motor problems, it may also give information about handwriting problems [70].

Grooved Peg Board Test

The Grooved Pegboard is a manipulative dexterity test, which consists of 25 holes with different positioned slots. It was developed by Trites in 1989. There is a wide range of usage of the test and it can be applied to individuals from five years old to adults. It can be used in student labs, screening procedures in industry, and in evaluating the lateralized brain damage. This test requires more complex visual-motor coordination than most pegboard tests because pegs are rotated to match the hole, and also because differently positioned slots require cognitive functioning skills involving spatial perception. To that end, Kodl and co-workers used the Grooved Peg Board Test in their study to investigate the cognitive changes related to the central white matter dysfunction in patients with Type I diabetes mellitus. The authors state that this test reflects the white matter function very well [60].

Jebsen Test of Hand Function (JTHF)

JTHF is a standardized and reliable (r = 0.60–0.99) seven-item test that measures the functional capability. The purpose of the test is to evaluate hand functions with daily activities. The test involves several hand activities, such as writing a sentence, turning over cards, picking up small objects and putting them in a container, stacking checkers, simulated eating, moving empty cans, and moving heavy cans. These tasks, except writing a sentence, are performed by the non-dominant hand first and then the dominant hand. The test normally could be completed in about 15 min, but it could take as long as 45 min with slow performing subjects. It is scored by marking down the completion time for each task [53, 80].

JTHF is a simple and quick test that could be used with a wide age range for diagnosis, such as to assess the aging-related changes on hand functions and the effect of treatment methods on dexterity, functional performance after hand burns, and to measure performance in several conditions, such as low vision, neuropathy, stroke, multiple sclerosis, rheumatoid arthritis, wrist arthrodesis, and Duchenne muscular dystrophy [1, 3, 16, 34, 42, 46, 48, 58, 102, 103, 106]. Mathiowetz also acknowledges these advantages; however, he also argues that most of the daily living activities (e.g., tying shoelaces, fastening a button, etc.) are bilateral and JTHF is not sufficient in bilateral performance assessment [69]. On the other hand, easy access to the objects used in the test is one of the most important advantages of it.

Minnesota Manual Dexterity Test

The Minnesota Manual Dexterity Test is a standardized and reliable (r = 0.84 to 0.91) test that is used in prevocational assessment. The test includes a long board with 60 holes lined along four lines and 60 disks. The test comprises of two tasks: turning and placing. One of the important properties of this test is that it is adapted and standardized for the visually impaired people [8, 52]. Furthermore, Gloss and Wardle state that the test has the property of providing information regarding the disability rating of the hand [40]. This test can be used various problems related to upper extremity.

Nine-Hole Peg Test

The nine-hole peg test is a simple and quick test assessing finger dexterity. As part of the test, the subject is asked to place and then remove nine pegs (3.2 cm) into nine holes on a wooden board (12.7 cm X 12.7 cm), and the time of task completion is recorded. The test is performed for each hand individually. Test-retest reliability of the test is intermediate (left hand; r = 0.43, right hand; r = 0.69) and it may also reflect the subject's instruction taking and learning skills. The correlation between other clinical assessments (functional MRI, voxel-based morphometry, etc.) and the nine-hole peg test was investigated in respect to the degree of the effect of the changes caused by the cerebral structure on hand functions related with neurological diseases affecting the cerebral structure (atrophy, plates, etc.) [44]. The nine-hole peg test has been the choice of measurement instrument used as a performance benchmark in central and peripheral neurological complications such as in determining the effect of home-based rehabilitation applications on hand dexterity in stroke, traumatic brain injury, multiple sclerosis and Parkinson's patients; in determining the functioning and disability of finger dexterity in multiple sclerosis; and in determining the dexterity in patients with carpal tunnel syndrome [47, 51, 56, 111]. Lynch and co-workers stated that the nine-hole peg test is, along with other performance measures—namely, timed 25-foot walk and low-contrast letter acuity—one of the best ways of monitoring the progress of Friedreich ataxia [66]. Similarly, Felder and co-workers maintained that the nine-hole peg test is a suitable test to predict elderly people's oral care ability and tooth brushing ability. In the same study, the Box and Block test was also found as a suitable instrument to predict oral care ability [29]. The nine-hole peg test is also preferred in the evaluation of dexterity in orthopedic cases [7]. On the other hand, although the nine-hole peg test was developed for adults, because it is simple, comprehensible, and quick, it is widely used with children, too [15, 98]. Furthermore, Smith and co-workers argue that it is an effective tool in screening the fine motor dexterity amongst the school-age children [95]. It is observed very frequently in the literature that the nine-hole peg test is preferred by practitioners for describing the fine motor ability briefly in a short time.

Purdue Pegboard

The Purdue Pegboard is a finger dexterity test originally designed for selecting adult individuals for manual dexterity requiring professions. The test is composed of a board with two columns with 25 small holes each and three slots across the top containing pins, collars and gaskets. There are two subtests: placing the pins into the holes and placing a gasket, a collar, and a second gasket on the pin. It is scored by counting the parts placed in the holes correctly in a given time period. Reddon and co-workers maintain that the test is sensitive to changes in hand functions (r = 0.63–0.83) [82]. Furthermore, it is a reliable instrument for testing manual fine motor skills of people aged 60 and over [24].

The test, which is used in professional assessment in adults, could also be used to investigate the effects of professional exposure on hand functions and the treatment efficacy [92, 99]. Although this test was designed for adults, the literature indicates that it has been also used in the assessment of the manual ability of minors with cerebral palsy [4]. As a fine dexterity assessment tool, which has been widely used and studied scientifically, the Purdue Peg Test's use area has expanded in time.

Stromberg Dexterity Test (SDT)

It was developed by Eleroy Stromberg in 1985. SDT requires a special pattern of arm and hand movements. Hand and arm coordination is evaluated by having the subject insert 54 disks into appropriate slots on a form board as quickly as possible. The time is recorded as seconds. The test takes approximately 5 to 10 min [41]. It is a preferable test for vocational evaluation.

Skills Assessment Module (SAM)

SAM can be used for vocational evaluation and is related to motor, cognitive and affective demands of adults. This standardized test includes simulated jobs and asked from person to perform the tasks. These tasks can support information about learning styles, basic skills, vocational interests, aptitudes and work performances of the subject. Twelve hands-on activities measure clerical/numerical, motor coordination, finger dexterity, manual dexterity, form perception, color perception, clerical/verbal, following written instructions, following oral directions, measuring skills, spatial perception and following diagrammed instructions. Furthermore, the test also features career development plan, learning styles inventory, non-reading interest survey and basic functional skills assessment [86].

GROSS AND FINE MOTOR ASSESSMENT

Assessment of Motor and Process Skills (AMPS)

AMPS is a valid, reliable, and sensitive method for individuals 5 years of age and up. It is based on activities of daily living task performances with 85 standardized tasks. Each task consists of 16 motor and 20 process skill items that arranges from simple to complex items. The subject selects two activities of daily living to be observed by the person administering the test and these activities are evaluated against 16 motor skill items and 20 process skill items, separately. The motor and process skill measurement of the client is analyzed statistically on computer-scoring program of AMPS. AMPS is scored using a four-point scale: "4" competent performance, "3" questionable performance, "2" ineffective performance and "1" markedly deficient performance.

Liu and co-workers argue that AMPS is useful in determining the independency of dementia patients' activities of daily living [65]. Similarly, Linden and co-workers argue that, compared to neuropsychological tests, AMPS is more efficient in determining independent living skills of brain-injured patients [63].

The school version of the AMPS is used to observe the functional classroom dexterity of children. Fingerhut and co-workers maintain that AMPS is a useful instrument in the observation of school motor skills and school process skills of healthy children in naturalistic settings [33]. Munkhol and Fisher, and especially Fisher, who developed the test, state that the test is less effective than expected with students with mild disabilities [74].

The facts that AMPS is applicable to a wide age range and that activities to be tested are selected by the subject add an important dimension to the test, because the role of an individual has an important place in community involvement. An individual's self-selection of the most important activity/activities, or activity/activities that s/he wants to be able to do most would define the problem more definitely and provide more realistic solutions to the problem.

Bruininks-Oseretsky Motor Proficiency Test (BOMPT)

BOMPT is standardized, reliable (0.86 to 0.89), and valid test for children 4½ to 14½ years of age. The complete battery of the test includes eight subtests with 46 separate items. Eight subtests of the complete battery are the following: (1) Running speed and agility (one item): It measures running speed during a shuttle run. (2) Balance (eight items): Three items assess static balance while standing on one leg. Five items assess performance balance while various walking movements. (3) Bilateral coordination (eight items): Seven items assess sequential and simultaneous coordination of the upper limbs with the lower limbs. One item assesses coordination of upper limbs only. (4) Strength (three items): It assesses arm and shoulder strength, abdominal strength, and leg strength. (5) Upper limb coordination (nine items): Six items assess coordination of visual tracking with movements of the arms and hands. Three items assess precise movements of arms, hands, or fingers. (6) Response speed (one item): It measures the ability to respond quickly to a moving visual stimulus. (7) Visual motor control (eight items): It measures the ability to coordinate precise hand and visual movements. (8) Upper limb speed and dexterity (eight items): It measures hand and finger dexterity, hand speed, and arm speed. The Short Form uses 14 items from the complete battery and provides a brief survey of general motor proficiency. It also is reliable (.84 to .87) and valid. There are eight subtests. Four of the subtests assess gross motor skills, three assess fine motor skills and one assesses both gross and fine motor skills [2, 6 ,13].

BOMPT is used for measuring the motor performance of children with various clinical diagnosis such as bronchopulmonary dysplasia, low birth weight, HIV, Down syndrome, neuromuscular deficits, attention deficit hyperactivity disorder, low vision and developmental coordination disorder [20, 72, 78, 88, 91, 100]. It also has been used with healthy children in longitudinal and comparative studies [20, 26, 32, 67, 85].

Lincoln-Oseretsky Motor Development Scale

The Lincoln–Oseretsky Motor Development Scale was developed by Sloan for measuring unilateral and bilateral fine and motor development [93]. It is appropriate for six- to 14-year-old children. The test, which is a neuromotor assessment, consists of 36 specific tasks, arranged from easy to difficult, and requires speed and dexterity. Parts of the test are walking backwards, standing on one foot, touching one's nose, jumping over a rope, throwing and catching a ball, putting coins in a box, jumping and clapping, balancing on tiptoe while opening and closing one's hands, and balancing a rod vertically [105].

McCarthy Scale of Children's Abilities (MSCA)

MSCA assesses cognitive development and motor skills of children aged 2½–8½. The testing session is 45–60 min. MSCA includes five scales: Verbal Scale (five subtests) assesses comprehension and use of language, Quantitative Scale (three subtests) measures mathematical ability, Perceptual-Performance Scale (seven subtests) evaluates conceptualization, Memory Scale (four subtests) tests short-term memory and Motor Scale (five subtests) assesses both gross and fine motor coordination [19].

Miller Assessment for Preschoolers (MAP))

MAP identifies mild to moderate developmental delays. Five index of MAP examines foundation (basic motor tasks and awareness of sensation), coordination (complex gross, fine, and oral motor abilities), verbal (memory, sequencing, comprehension, association, and expression), nonverbal (mental manipulations, memory, sequencing, and visualization with not requiring spoken language) and complex tasks (sensory motor and cognitive abilities). MAP can be used in children aged two years nine months to five years eight months. It takes about 25–35 min to complete this 27-item test. Coefficient varies between 0.26 and 0.54.

Daniels argued in his study investigating the construct validity of MAP that it could be used to differentiate between groups composed of children with moderate to severe developmental delays caused by various diagnoses [22]. Parush and co-workers maintained that, if children also have sensory integration problems, MAP could be preferred as a testing instrument [79]. The fact that this instrument also includes a verbal component makes it superior to several other screening instruments.

Movement Assessment Battery for Children (Movement ABC)

Movement ABC identifies motor coordination problems of four- to 12-year-old children. The battery evaluates manual dexterity (shifting peg by rows, threading nuts on bolts, flower trial), ball skills (catching and throwing bean bag with both hands), static balance and dynamic balance (hopping in squares, ball balance), and problem-solving abilities. The total score of the test indicates if the child is impaired or under risk in terms of motor skills [43]. The reliability of the Movement ABC is 0.95 to 1.00 [96].

This test especially assesses the interaction of postural stability and coordination with motor skills in children with attention-deficit-hyperactivity disorder and developmental coordination disorder [31, 54, 55]. Furthermore, Movement ABC has recently been used in very different clinical conditions, such as Down syndrome or congenital strabismus [17, 104]. The fact that the test evaluates motor skills as well as problem solving and cognitive skills results in such flexible use areas for the test.

Peabody Developmental Motor Scales-2 (PDMS-2)

This is an individually administered test, which assesses gross and fine motor skills of children from birth to five years of age. It provides both qualitative and quantitative results and takes 45–60 min. PDMS-2 assesses the gross motor composite with four sub-tests that are composed of 151 items. These subtests are reflexes, stationary, locomotion, and object manipulation. On the other hand, the fine motor composite is assessed with two subtests including 98 items: grasping and visual-motor integration. This is a three-point score test: (2) child performs the item according to the specified item criterion, (1) the behavior is emerging but that criterion for successful performance is not fully met, or (0) the child can not attempt to perform the item. The reliability coefficients of the test are between 0.82 and 0.93 [35, 49].

Quality of Upper Extremity Skills Test (QUEST)

QUEST assesses upper extremity functions in four domains: dissociated movement (shoulder, elbow, wrist, independent movements, and arm position during grasping/releasing), grasping (body posture during grasp, grasping of a one-inch cube, grasping of cereal, and grasping of pencil/crayon), protecting extension (forward, side, and backward), and weight bearing (in prone, prone with reaching, sitting with hands forward, sitting with hands by side, and sitting with hands behind) in children with 18 months to eight years of age. The reliability of QUEST total score is 0.95. Every effort of subtests is scored as "yes", "no" or "not tested". It is a proper material for describing the upper extremity quality of movement and in planning intervention programs [23].

HANDWRITING ASSESSMENT

Children's Handwriting Evaluation Scale (CHES)

CHES provides reliable information about handwriting rate and quality of children in grades three to eight. Letter size consistency, letter formation, letters on the line, and spacing between letters and words are evaluated while copying a short story. The percentiles are the following: very good (90%–100%), good (76%–90%), satisfactory (25%–75%), poor (9%–24%) and very poor (8% or lower) [94].

Children's Handwriting Evaluation Scale for Manuscript Writing (CHES-M)

CHES-M is similar to CHES. CHES-M provides information about copying, taking notes, and presenting ideas by writing in children in grades one and two. The test gives a quality score at the end of copying a short story. Quality of functional levels are good (80–100), satisfactory (50–70) and poor (10–40).

Denver Handwriting Analysis (DHA)

DHA is an informal, criterion-referenced cursive handwriting scale designed for use with students in grades three to eight. Near-point copying, writing capitals, writing lower case, far-point copying, manuscript-cursive transition, and dictation skills can be evaluated by DHA. Parts I–III are the total, part IV is the manuscript cursive transition, and part V is dictation [5].

Evaluation Tool of Children's Handwriting (ETCH)

ETCH is a standardized tool that was developed by Amundson and evaluates writing speed and legibility of children in grades one to three. It includes six subtests: (a) alphabet production in uppercase and lowercase from memory, (b) numeral writing (1 through 12) from memory, (c) near-point copying, (d) far-point copying, (e) dictation and (f) sentence composition. Reliability coefficient is 0.77 for total letter legibility and 0.63 for total numeral legibility. The scoring of the child's performance is made by a checklist consisting of the following categories: above average, average, needs improvement or very poor [25].

Minnesota Handwriting Assessment

The test analyzes legibility, form, alignment, size, and spacing of handwriting of students in grades one and two. During the test, the subject is asked to copy the sentence printed on a writing pad with differently spaced lines to the line just below the sentence. In each category of the test, the score range is between 0 and 34. It takes less than 10 min with scoring [14].

Test of Handwriting Skills

This is a standardized handwriting assessment tool developed by Gardner [73]. The test assesses various areas of handwriting, such as cursive, writing from memory, writing from dictation, copying upper and lower case, copying words and sentences, speed of writing and spacing.

SCREENING TOOLS

Clinical Observations of Motor and Postural Skills (COMPS)

COMPS is a screening tool for identification of motor problems in children five to nine years old. It evaluates slow motion, rapid forearm rotation, finger-nose touching, prone extension, asymmetric tonic neck reflex and supine flexion. The reliability of the test is 0.87 [108].

Foulder and Cooke evaluated preterm children's motor skills using COMPS in their study investigating motor, cognitive, and behavioral disorders, and they stated that COMPS is a very effective instrument in the evaluation of motor disorders in preterm children [36]. As the clinical use of the test increases, there would be more available data regarding the test.

Denver Developmental Screening Test (DDST)

DDST was first standardized and published in 1967 [39]. The test, which evaluates child development multilaterally, could be used with children aged between one month and six years. A revised version, Denver-II, was developed in 1990 [38]. Denver II investigates development in four categories: personal-social, fine motor adaptive, language and gross motor. As a result of the evaluation, children are classified as developmentally delayed, caution, and within normal range. The test has a high reliability (r = 0.91) [112]. DDST is a suitable screening tool for comparing the effects of various cultural changes.

FirstSTEP Developmental Screening Test

The FirstSTEP Developmental Screening Test was developed by Miller to define the development deficiency in preschoolers between two years nine months and six years two months of age. FirstSTEP comprises 72 items in five domains, namely, cognition, communication, motor, social emotional and adaptive functioning. Each domain is scored separately [71].

REFERENCES

[1] Aki, E., Atasavun, S., & Kayihan, H. (2008). Relationship between upper extremity kinesthetic sense and writing performance by students with low vision. *Perceptual and Motor Skills. 106(3),* 963-966.

[2] Aki, E., Atasavun, S., Turan, A., & Kayihan, H. (2007). Training motor skills of children with low vision. *Perceptual and Motor Skills. 104,* 1328-1336.

[3] Alamri, A., Eid, M., Iglesias, R., Shirmohamadi, S., & El Saddik, A. (2008). Haptic virtual rehabilitation exercises for poststroke diagnosis. *IEEE Transactions on Instrumentation and Measurement. 57(9),* 1876-1884.

[4] Arnould, C., Penta, M., & Thonnard, J. L. (2007). Hand impairments and their relationship with manual ability in children with cerebral palsy. *Journal of Rehabilitation Medicine. 39(9),* 708-714

[5] Anderson, P. L. (1983). *Denver Handwriting Analysis.* Novato, CA: Academic Therapy Publication.

[6] Ayhan, A. B., Aki, E., Aral, N., & Kayihan, H. (2007). Correlations of conceptual development with motor skills for a Turkish sample of kindergarten children. *Perceptual and Motor Skills. 105,* 261-264.

[7]   Bamberger, H. B., Stern, P. J., Kiefhaber, T. R., Mcdonough, J. J., & Cantor, R. M. (1992). Trapeziometacarpal joint arthrodesis - a functional-evaluation. *Journal of Hand Surgery-American. 17A(4),* 605-611.

[8]   Bauman, M. K. (1958). A manual of norms for tests used in counseling blind persons. NY: *American Federation of the Blind Research Series.*

[9]   Bennet, G. K. (1965). Mechanical ability test. Canada: *The Psychological Corporation.*

[10] Benton, A. L., & Fogel, M. L. (1962). Three-dimentional constructional praxis. A clinical test. *Archieves Neurology. 7(4),* 347-354.

[11] Bjornson, K. F., Schmale, G. A., Adamczyk, A. F., & McLaughlin, J. (2006). The effect of dynamic ankle foot orthoses on function in children with cerebral palsy. *Journal of Pediatric Orthopaedics. 26(6),* 773-776.

[12] Boyle, A. M., & Santelli, J. C. (1986). Assessing psychomotor skills: the role of the Crawford Small Parts Dexterity Test as a screening instrument. *Journal of Dental Education. 50(3),* 176-179.

[13] Bruininks, R. H. (1978). *Bruininks-Oseretsky Test of Motor Proficiency, examiner's manual.* Circle Pines, MN: American Guidance Service.

[14] Bumin, G., & Kavak, S. T. (2008). An investigation of the factors affecting handwriting performance in children with hemiplegic cerebral palsy. *Disability and Rehabilitation. 30(18),* 1374-1385.

[15] Bumin, G., & Kayihan, H. (2001). Effectiveness of two different sensory integration programmes for children with soastic diplegic cerebral palsy. *Disability and Rehabilitation. 15(23),* 394-399.

[16] Bumin, G., Uyanik, M., Aki, E., Duger, T. & Kayihan, H. (2001). Kavrama kuvveti ve el fonksiyonlarında yaşlanma ile oluşan değişiklikler. *Fizyoterapi Rehabilitasyon. 12(1),* 21-25.

[17] Caputo, R., Tinelli, F., Bancale, A., Campa, L., Frosini, R., Guzzetta, A., Mercuri, E., &, Cioni, G. (2007). Motor coordination in children with congenital strabismus: Effects of late surgery. *European Journal of Paediatric Neurology. 11(5),* 285-291.

[18] Carmeli, E., Bar, Y. T., Ariav, C., Levy, R., & Liebermann, D. G. (2008). Perceptual-motor coordination in persons with mild intellectual disability. *Disability and Rehabilitation. 30(5),* 323-329.

[19] Cohen, L. G., & Spenciner, L. J. (1994). *Assessment of Young Children.* New York: Longman.

[20] Connolly, B. H., & Michael, B. T. (1986). Performance of retarded children, with and without Down syndrome, on the Bruininks Oseretsky Test of Motor Proficiency. *Physical Therapy. 66(3),* 344-348.

[21] Damiano, D. L., & Abel, M. F. (1998). Functional outcomes of strength traininig in spastic cerebral palsy. *Archieves Physical Medicine and Rehabilitation. 79,* 119-125.

[22] Daniels, L. E. (1998). The Miller Assessment for preschoolers: Construct validity and clinical use with children with developmental disabilities. *The American Journal of Occupational Therapy. 52,* 857-865.

[23] DeMatteo, C., Law, M., Russel, D., Poolock, N., Rosenbaum, P., & Walter, S. (1992). *QUEST Quality of Upper Extremity Skills Test, User's Manual.* Canada: CanChild Centre for Childhood Disability Research.

[24] Desrosiers, S. J., Hebert, R., Bravo, G., & Dutil, E. (1995). The Purdue Pegboard Test: Normative data for people aged 60 and over. *Disablity and Rehabilitation. 17(5),* 217-224.

[25] Diekema, S.M., Deitz, J., & Amundson, S.J. (1998). Test-retest reliability of the Evaluation Tool of Children's Handwriting – Manuscript. *American Journal of Occupational Therapy. 52,* 248-255.

[26] Duger, T., Bumin, G., Uyanik, M., Aki, E., & Kayihan, H. The assessment of Bruininks Oseretsky test of motor proficiency in children. *Pediatric Rehabilitation. 3(3),* 125-131, 1999.

[27] Farrel, T. R., & Weir, R. F. (2007). The optimal controller delay for myoelectric prostheses. *IEEE Transactions on Instrumentation and Measurement. 15(1),* 111-118.

[28] Feder, K. P., Majnemer, A., Bourbonnais, D., Blayney, M., & Morin, I. (2007). Handwriting performance on the ETCH-M of students in a grade one regular education program. *Physical and Occupational Therapy in Pediatrics. 27(2),* 43-62.

[29] Felder, R., James, K., Brown, C., Lemon, S., & Reveal, M. (1994). Dexterity testing as a predictor of oral care ability. *Journal of the American Geriatrics Society. 42(10),* 1081-1086.

[30] Fisher, A. (2006). Overview of performance skills and client factors. In H. M., Pendleton & W. S. Krohn (Eds.), *Pedretti's Occupational Therapy Practice Skills for Physical Dysfunction.* (6th Edition, pp. 372-403). St. Louis, Missouri: Mosby.

[31] Flapper, B. C. T., Houwen, S., & Schoemaker, M. M. (2006). Fine motor skills and effects of methylphenidate in children with attention-deficit-hyperactivity disorder and developmental coordination disorder. *Developmental Medicine And Child Neurology. 48(3),* 165-169.

[32] Flegel, J. & Kolbe, T. H. (2002).Predictive validity of the test of infant motor performance as measured by the Bruininks-Oseretsky test of motor proficiency at school age. *Physical Therapy. 82(8),* 762-771.

[33] Fingerhut, P., Madill, H., Darrah, J., Hodge, M., & Warren, S. (2002). Classroom-based assessment: Validation for the school AMPS. *American Journal of Occupational Therapy. 56(2),* 210-213.

[34] Floel, A., Vomhof, P., Lorenzen, A., Roesser, N., Breitenstein, C., & Knecht, S. (2008). Levadopa improves skilled hand functions in the elderly. *European Journal of Neuroscience. 27,* 1301-1307.

[35] Folio, M. K., & Fewel, R. (1983). *Peabody Developmental Motor Scales and Activity Cards.* Chicago, Ill : Riverside Publishing Corporation.

[36] Foulder-Hughes, L. A., Cooke, R. W. I. (2003). Motor, cognitive, and behavioural disorders in children born very preterm. *Developmental Medicine and Child Neurology. 45(2),* 97-103.

[37] Francis, N. K., Hanna, G. B., Cresswell, A. B., Carter, F.J., & Cuschieri, A. (2001). The performance of master surgeons on standard aptitude testing. *American Journal of Surgery. 182(1),* 30-33.

[38] Frankenburg, W. K., Dodds, J. B., Archer, P., Shapiro, H., & Bresnick B. (1992). The Denver-II: a major revision and restandardization of the Denver Developmental Screening Test. *Pediatrics. 89,* 91-97.

[39] Frankenburg, W. K., & Dodds, J. B. (1967). The Denver Developmental Screening Test. *The Journal of Pediatrics. 71,* 181-191.

[40] Gloss, D. S., Wardle, M, G. (1982). Use of the Minnasota Rate of Manipulation Test for disability evaluation. *Perceptual and Motor Skills. 55(2),* 527-532.

[41] Goldberg, A. E., Neifeld, J. P., Luke, G., Wolfe, M. S., & Goldberg, S.R. (2008). Correlation of manual dexterity with USMLE Scores and medical student class rank. *Journal of Surgical Research, 147(2),* 212-215.

[42] Hardin, M. (2002). Assessment of hand function and fine motor coordination in the geriatric population. *Topics in Geriatric Rehabilitation, 18(2),* 18-27.

[43] Henderson, S. E., & Sugden, D. A. (1992). *Movement assessment battery for children.* London: Psychological Corporation.

[44] Henry, R. G., Shieh, M., Okuda, D. T, Evangelista, A., Gorno-Tempini, M. L., & Pelletier, D. (2008). Regional grey matter atrophy in clinically isolated syndromes at presentation. *Journal of Neurology Neurosurgery and Psychiatry. 79(11),* 1236-1244.

[45] Hesse, S., Werner, C., Pohl, M., Mehrholz, J., Puzich, U., & Krebs, H.I. (2008). Mechanical arm trainer for the treatment of the severely affected arm after a stroke- A single-blinded randomized trial in two centers. *American Journal of Physical Medicine and Rehabilitation. 87(10),* 779-788.

[46] Hiller, L. B., & Wade, C. K. (1992). Upper extremity funciional assessment scales in children with Duchenne muscular-dystrophy - a comparison. *Archives of Physical Medicine and Rehabilitation. 73(6),* 527-534.

[47] Hoffmann, T., Russell, T., Thompson, L., Vincent, A., & Nelson, M. (2008). Using the Internet to assess activities of daily living and hand function in people with Parkinson's disease. *Neurorehabilitation. 23(3),* 253-261.

[48] Holavanahalli, R. K., Helm, P. A., Gorman, A. R., & Kowalske, K. J. (2007). Outcomes after deep full-thickness hand burns. *Archieves Physical Medicine and Rehabilitation. 88(12 Suppl),* 30-35.

[49] Hsiang, H. W., Hua, F. L., & Ching, L. H. (2006). Reliability, sensitivity to change, and responsiveness of the Peabody Developmental Motor Scale-Second Edition for children with cerebral palsy. *Physical Therapy. 86(10),* 1351-1359.

[50] Huang, M., Harvey, R. L., Stoykov, M. E., Ruland, S., Weinand, M., Lowry, D., & Levy, R. (2008). Cortical stimulation for upper limb recovery following ischemic stroke: A small phase II pilot study of a fully implanted stimulator. *Topics in Stroke Rehabilitation. 15(2),* 160-172.

[51] Huijgen, B. C. H., Volienbroek-Hutten, M. M. R., Zampolini, M., Opisso, E., Bernabeu, M., Van Nieuwenhoven, J., Ilsbrouk, S., Magni, R., Giacomozzi, C., Marcellari, V., Marchese, S. S., & Hermens, H. J. (2008). Feasibility of a home-based telerehabilitation system compared to usual care: arm/hand function in patients with stroke, traumatic brain injury and multiple sclerosis. *Journal of Telemedicine and Telecare. 14(5),* 249-256.

[52] Ittyerah, M. (2000). Hand skill and hand preference in blind and sighted children. *Laterality. 5(3),* 221-235.

[53] Jebsen, R. H., Taylor, N., Trieschmann, R. B., Trotter, M. J., & Howard, L. H. (1969). An objective and standardized test of hand function. *Archieves Physical Medicine and Rehabilitation. 50,* 311-319.

[54] Johnson, D. A., & Williams, H. G. (1988). Postural support and fine motor control in children with normal and slow motor development. In J. E. Clark & J. H. Humphrey (Eds.), *Advances in Motor Development Research.* New York: AMS Press.

[55] Johnston, L. M., Burns, Y. R., Brauer, S. G., & Richardson, C. A. (2002). Differences in postural control and movement performance during goal directed reaching in children with developmental coordination disorder. *Human Movement Science. 21*, 583–60.

[56] Keskin, D., Ucan, H., Babaoglu, S., Akbulut, L., Eser, F., Bodur, H., & Kose K. (2008). Evaluation of clinical, electromyographic parameters and quality of life in patients with carpal tunnel syndrome. *Türkiye Klinikleri Tıp Bilimleri Dergisi. 28(4),* 456-461.

[57] Ketelaar, M., Vermeer, A., & Helders, P. J. M. (1998). Functional motor abilities of children with cerebral palsy: a systematic literature review of assessment measures. *Clinical Rehabilitation. 12(5),* 369-380.

[58] Kitis, A., Altug, F., Cavlak, U., & Akdag, B. (2008). Comparison of the physical and non-physical functioning between the patients with multiple sclerosis and healthy subjects. *Neurosciences. 13(1),* 29-36.

[59] Knutson, J. S., Hisel, T. Z., Harley, M. Y., & Chae, J. (2009). A novel functional electrical stimulation treatment for recovery of hand function in hemiplegia: 12 week pilot study. *Neurorehabilitation and Neural Repair. 23(1),* 17-25.

[60] Kodl, C. T., Franc, D. T., Rao, J. P., Anderson, F. S., Thomas, W., Mueller, B. A., Lim, K. O., & Seaquist, E. R. (2008). Diffusion tensor imaging identifies deficits in white matter microstructure in subjects with type 1 diabetes that correlate with reduced neurocognitive function. *Diabetes. 57(11),* 3083-3089.

[61] Kopp, B., Kunkel, A., Flor, H., Platz, T., Rose, U., Mauritz, K. H., Gresser, K., McCulloch, K. L., Taub, E. (1997). The Arm Motor Ability Test: Reliability, validity, and sensitivity to change of an instrument for assessing disabilities in activities of daily living. *Archieves Physical Medicine and Rehabilitation. 78*, 615-620.

[62] Levy, C. E., Giuffrida, C., Richards, L., Wu, S., Davis, S., & Nadeau, S.E. (2007). Botulinium toxin A, evidence-based exercise therapy and constraint-induced movement therapy for upper-limb hemiparesis attributable to stroke: A preliminary study. *American Journal of Physical Medicine and Rehabilitation,* 86(9), 696-706.

[63] Linden, A., Boschian, K., Eker, C., Schalen, W., & Nordstrom, C.H. (2005). Assessment of motor and process skills reflects brain-injured patients' ability to resume independent living better than neuropsychological tests. *Acta Neurologica Scandinavica. 111,* 48-53.

[64] Linder-Lucht, M., Othmer, V., Walther, M., Vry, J., Michaelis, U., Stein, S., Weissenmayer, H., Korinthenberg, R. & Mall, V. (2007). Validation of the gross motor function measure for use in children and adolescents with traumatic brain injuries *Pediatrics. 120(4),* 880-886.

[65] Liu, K. P. Y., Chan, C. C. H., Chu, M. M. L., Ng, T. Y. L., Chu, L. W., Hui, F. S. L., Yuen, H. K., & Fisher, A. G. (2007). Activities of daily living performance in dementia. *Acta Neurologica Scandinavica. 116,* 91-95.

[66] Lynch, D. R., Farmer, J. M., Wilson, R. L., & Balcer, L. J. (2005). Performance measures in Friedreich ataxia: Potential utility as clinical outcome tools. *Movement Disorders. 20(7),* 777-782.

[67] MacCobb, S., Greene, S., Nugent, K., & O'Mahony P. (2005). Measurement and prediction of motor proficiency in children using bayley infant scales and the Bruininks-Oseretsky test. *Occupational Therapy in Pediatrics. 25(1-2),* 59-79.

[68]   Malloy, P., Belanger, H., Hall, S., Aloia, M., & Salloway, S. (2003). Assessing visioconstructional performance in AD, MCI and normal elderly using the Beery Visual Motor Integration Test. *The Clinical Neuropsychologist. 17(4),* 544-550.

[69]   Mathiowetz, V. (1993). Role of physical performance component evaluations in occupational therapy functional assessment. *American Journal of Occupational Therapy. 47,* 225-230.

[70]   McHale, K., & Cermak, S. A. (1992). Fine motor activities in elementary school, preliminary findings and provisional implications for children with fine motor problems. *American Journal of Occupational Therapy. 46,* 898-903.

[71]   Miller, L. J. (1993). *FirstSTEP Screening Test for Evaluating Preschoolers.* The Psychological Corporation. USA: Harcourt Brace Jovanovich Incorporation.

[72]   Miller, L. T., Polatajko, H. J., Missiuna, C., Mandich, A. D., & Macnab, J. J. (2001). A pilot trial of a cognitive treatment for children with developmental coordination disorder. *Human Movement Science. 20(1-2),* 183-210.

[73]   Morrison, F. G. (1998). *Test of Handwriting Skills Manual.* Hydesville, CA: Psychological and Educational Publications Corporation.

[74]   Munkholm, M., & Fisher, A. G. (2008). Differences in schoolwork performance between typically developing students and students with mild disabilities. *OTJR-Occupation Participation and Health. 28(3),* 121-132.

[75]   Ng, A. K. Y., Leung, D. P. K., & Fong, K. N. K. (2008). Clinical utility of the action research arm test, the Wolf Motor Function Test and the Motor Activity Log for hemiparetic upper extremity functions after stroke: A pilot study. *Hong Kong Journal of Occupational Therapy. 18(1),* 20-27.

[76]   Osborne, R. T. & Sanders, W. B. (1956). The Crawford Small Parts Dexterity Test as a time-limited test. *Personnel Psychology. 9(2),* 177-180.

[77]   Paltamaa, J., Sarasoia, T., Leskinen, E., Wikstrom, J., & Malkia, E. (2008). Measuring deterioration in international classification of functioning domains of people with multiple sclerosis who are ambulatory. *Physical Therapy. 88(2),* 176-190.

[78]   Parks, R. A., & Danoff, J. V. (1999). Motor performance changes in children testing positive for HIV over 2 years. *The American Journal of Occupational Therapy. 53(5),* 524-528.

[79]   Parush, S., Yochman, A., Jessel, A. S., Shapiro, M., & Karsenty, T. M. (2002). Construct validity of the Miller Assessment for Preschoolers and the Pediatric Examination of Educational Readiness for Children. *Physical and Occupational Therapy in Pediatrics. 22(2),* 7-27.

[80]   Poole, J. L. (2008). Measures of adult hand function. *Arthritis and Rheumatism (Arthritis Care and Research). 49(15),* 59-66.

[81]   Posthuma, B. W., Bass, M. J., Bull, S. B., & Nisker, J. A. (1987). Detecting changes in functional ability in women with premenstrual syndrome. *American Journal of Obstetrics and Gynecology. 156(2),* 275-278.

[82]   Reddon, J. R., Gill, D. M., Gauk, S. E., & Maers, M. D. (1988). Purdue Pegboard: test-retest estimates. *Peceptual and Motor Skills.* 66(2), 503-506.

[83]   Richards, L., Senesac, C., McGuirk, T., Woodbury, M., Howland, D., Davis, S., & Patterson, T. (2008). Response to intensive upper extremity therapy by individuals with ataxia from stroke. *Topics in Stroke Rehabilitation. 15(3),* 262-271.

[84] Rintala, P., Pienimaki, K., Ahonen, T., Cantell, M. & Kooistra, L. (1998). The effects of psychomotor training programme on motor skill development in children with developmental language disorders. *Human Movement Science. 17(4-5)*, 721-737.

[85] Rosenblum, S., & Josman, N. (2003). The relationship between postural control and fine manual dexterity. *Physical and Occupational Therapy in Pediatrics. 23(4)*, 47-60.

[86] Rosinek, M. (1985). Skills Assessment Module (S.A.M): A Unique & Practical Approach to the Assessment Process [http://www.pineymountain.com/sam.htm]

[87] Russell, D., Palisano, R., Walter, S., Rosenbaum, P., Gemus, M., Gowland, C., Galuppi, B., & Lane M. (1998). Evaluating motor function in children with Down syndrome: validity of the GMFM. *Developmental Medicine and Child Neurology. 40(10)*, 693-701.

[88] Salbenblatt, J. A., Meyers, D. C., Bender, B. G., Linden, M. G., & Robinson, A. (1989). Gross and fine motor development in 45, X and 47, XXX girls. *Pediatrics. 84 (4)*, 678-682.

[89] Schijven, M. P., Jakimowicz, J. J., & Carter, F. J. (2004). How to select aspirant laparoscopic surgical trainees: Establishing concurrent validity comparing Xitact L S500 index performance scores with standardized psychomotor aptitude test battery scores. *Journal of Surgical Research. 121(1)*, 112-119.

[90] Schneider, S., Schonle, P. W., Altenmuller, E., & Munte, T. F. (2007). Using musical instruments to improve motor skill recovery following a stroke. *Journal of Neurology. 254(10)*, 1339-1346.

[91] Short, E. J., Klein, N. K., Lewis, B. A., Fulton, S., Eisengart, S., Kerscmar, C., Bayley, J., & Singer, L. T. (2003). Cognitive and academic consequences of bronchopulmonary dysplasia and very low birth weight: 8 years old outcomes. *Pediatrics. 112(5)*, e359.

[92] Skinner, D. K., & Curwin, S. L. (2007). Assessment of fine motor control in patients with occupation-related lateral epicondylitis. *Manual Therapy. 12(3)*, 249-255.

[93] Sloan, W. (1955). The Lincoln-Oseretsky Motor Development Scale. *General Psychology Monographs. 51*, 183-252.

[94] Smith, J. C. (2001). *Occupational Therapy for Children.* St. Louis: Mosby.

[95] Smith, Y.A., Hong, E. S., & Presson, C. (2000). Normative and validation studies of the Nine-hole Peg Test with children. *Perceptual and Motor Skills. 90(3)*, 823-843.

[96] Smits-Engelsman, B. C. M., Fiers, M. J., Henderson, S. E., & Henderson, L. (2008). Interrater reliability of the movement assessment battery for children. *Physical Therapy. 88(2)*, 286-294.

[97] Sortor, J. M., & Kulp, M. T. (2003). Are the results of the Beery-Buctenica Developmental Test of Visual-Motor Integration and its subtests related to achievement test scores? *Optometry and Vision Science. 11*, 758-763.

[98] Speth, L., Leffers, P., Janssen-Potten, Y. J. M., & Vles, J. S. H. (2005). Botulinum toxin A and upper limb functional skills in hemiparetic cerebral palsy: a randomized trial in children receiving intensive therapy. *Developmental Medicine and Child Neurology. 47(7)*, 468-473.

[99] Thonnard, J. L., Masset, D., Penta, M., Piette, A., & Malchaire, J. (1997). Short-term effect of hand-arm vibration exposure on tactile sensitivity and manual skill. *Scandinavian Journal of Work Environment & Health. 23(3)*, 193-198.

[100] Tseng, M. H., Henderson, A., Chaw, S. M., & Yao, G. (2004). Relationship between motor proficiency, attention, impulse, and activity in children with ADHD. *Developmental Medicine and Child Neurology. 46(6),* 381-388.

[101] Ulrich, D. A. (2000). Test of Gross Motor Development, 2nd edition. Examiner's manual. TX: PRO-ED Incorpotation.

[102] Videler, A. J., Beelen, A., & Nollet, F. (2008). Manual dexterity and related functional limitations in hereditary motor and sensory neuropathy. An explorative study. *Disability and Rehabilitation. 30(8),* 634-638.

[103] Vlieland, T., VanderWijk, T. P., Jolie, I., Zwinderman, A. H., & Hazes, J. (1996). Determinants of hand function in patients with rheumatoid arthritis. *Journal of Rheumatology. 23(5),* 835-840.

[104] Volman, M. J. M., Visser, J. J. W., & Lensvelt-Mulders, G. J. L. M. (2007). Functional status in 5 to 7-year-old children with Down syndrome in relation to motor ability and performance mental ability. *Disability and Rehabilitation. 29(1),* 25-31.

[105] Walsh, W. B. & Betz, N. E. (1990). *Tests and Assessment.* Englewood Cliffs, NJ: Prentice Hall.

[106] Weiss, A., Wiedeman, G., Quenzer, D., Hanington, K.R., Hastings, H., & Strickland, J. W. (1995). Upper extremity function after wrist arthrodesis. *Journal of Hand Surgery-American Volume. 20A(5),* 813-817.

[107] Whitall, J., Savin, D. N., Harris-Love, M., & Waller, S. M. (2006). Psychometric properties of a modified Wolf Motor Function Test for people with mild and moderate upper-extremity hemiparesis. *Archieves Physical Medicine and Rehabilitation. 87,* 656-660.

[108] Wilson, B., Pollock, N., Kaplan, B. J., Law, M., & Faris, P. (1992). Reliability and construct-validity of the clinical observations of motor and postural skills. *American Journal of Occupational Therapy. 46(9),* 775-783.

[109] Wing, K., Lynskey, J. V., & Bosch, P. R. (2008). Whole-body intensive rehabilitation is feasible and effective in chronic stroke survivors: A retrospective data analysis. *Topics in Stroke Rehabilitation. 15(3),* 247-255.

[110] Wolf, S. L., Thompson, P. A., Morris, D. A., Rose, D. K., Winstein, C. J., Taub, E., Giuliani, C., & Pearson, S. L. (2005). The EXCITE trial: Attributes of the Wolf Motor Function Test in patients with subacute stroke. *Neurorehabilitation and Neural Repair. 19(3),* 194-205.

[111] Ytterberg, C., Johansson, S., Andersson, M., Holmqvist, L. W., & Von Koch, L. (2008). Variations in functioning and disability in multiple sclerosis - A two-year prospective study. *Journal of Neurology. 255(7),* 967-973.

[112] Xie, Z. H., Bo, S. Y., Zhang, X. T., Liu, M., Zhang, Z. X., Yang, X. L., Jl, S. R., Yan, H., Sui, X. L., Na, X., Guo, S. H., & Wu, Z. L. (2008). Sampling survey on intellectual disability in 0-6 year old children in China. *Journal of Intellectual Disability Research. 52(12),* 1029-1038.

In: Handbook of Motor Skills
Editor: Lucian T. Pelligrino

ISBN: 978-1-60741-811-5
© 2009 Nova Science Publishers, Inc.

Chapter 5

MOBILITY FUNCTION FOLLOWING STROKE: THE IMPACT OF MULTIPLE IMPAIRMENTS

A. C. Novak and B. Brouwer

Motor Performance Laboratory, School of Rehabilitation Therapy,
Queen's University; Kingston, Ontario, Canada

ABSTRACT

Stroke is a leading cause of adult disability and the number affected is increasing as the population ages and survival rates post-event improve. It is estimated that as many as 60% of stroke survivors live with significant physical deficits including muscle weakness, instability, poor motor coordination and cardiovascular compromise resulting in a loss of independence in performing activities required for daily living. This percentage has remained relatively constant over the past decades, which suggests that interventions to minimize or reverse the effects of stroke are not yet widely available. We propose that while most rehabilitation programs focus on reducing impairment they yield limited effect on mobility function because of inadequacies on two fronts. First, they often deal with impairments as isolated deficiencies and as such fail to consider stroke as a multisystem disorder that demands an integrated treatment approach for optimal restoration of function. Second, the minimum performance requirements of specific aspects of physical function including strength, balance, and aerobic capacity associated with every day activities are unknown. Consequently, clinicians are challenged to identify targets that if attained will translate into enhanced mobility. This chapter reviews the relevant literature and presents research findings to provide insight on these important issues.

The approach is to first discuss stroke related physical impairments and their association with mobility deficits. From our own research work and the growing body of literature examining the combined influence of muscle weakness, balance instability, and physiological cost on mobility we explore those factors that are important determinants of mobility function. Going a step further, the impact of reducing impairments on effecting positive change in mobility is discussed.

Stroke is a multisystem disorder and mobility is a complex construct dependent upon the integrity of individual physical systems as well as their capacity to work in concert. The research discussed in this chapter provides insight into the unique characteristics of these systems in stroke and their interactions which are fundamental to mobility.

OVERVIEW

Stroke, also referred to as a cerebrovascular accident (CVA), is the sudden loss of brain function caused by an interruption of blood flow to the brain (ischemic stroke) or rupture of the blood vessels in the brain (hemorrhagic stroke). Over 75% of strokes occur in people over 65 years of age and the incidence and prevalence are increasing as our population ages and more people survive the acute phase[1,2]. Depending on the severity and location of the stroke, survivors present with varying degrees of neurologic and functional deficits, including motor, sensory, cognitive, perceptual and language impairments making stroke the leading cause of adult disability[3,4]. With more than 85% of those who experience moderate to severe strokes and almost all who survive mild strokes living in the community[5], the risk of social isolation and dependency secondary to disability is high[6-9]. Indeed the majority of community-dwelling stroke survivors report restrictions in physical capacity and mobility that impact their reintegration into the community[9].

Mobility is fundamental to maintaining independence and regaining the ability to walk is the most frequently stated objective of stroke survivors. While most (approximately 60-70%)[10-12] recover the ability to walk by the time they are discharged from hospital, it is estimated that only about 7-22% regain the capacity to walk independently outside of their homes according to an audit of mobility outcomes post-stroke[13] and a one week follow-up of patients discharged home[10]. The reasons are many-fold, but of primary importance are the residual impairments in strength, coordination, balance and deconditioning that manifest in functional limitations. Deficits in one or more of these physical performance measures reflective of neuromuscular, postural and cardiorespiratory system capabilities can impact mobility and if reserve capacity to generate greater 'output' from any of these systems is limited, then compensatory strategies will be correspondingly constrained as will be the ability to perform more demanding tasks. Understanding the relationships among system impairments and functional ability is critical for the development and implementation of rehabilitation strategies that are optimally restorative. This chapter examines the physical deficits associated with stroke, their association with mobility and their collective contributions to mobility status.

STROKE RELATED PHYSICAL IMPAIRMENTS AND THEIR ASSOCIATION WITH MOBILITY

Muscle weakness, elevated muscle tone, poor motor coordination and postural instability characterize a large proportion of individuals with hemispheric stroke. In addition, up to 75% of stroke survivors have cardiovascular disease[14]. In combination these deficits contribute to the high energy cost of mobility estimated to be at least twice that of age-matched healthy individuals[15,16]. This being the case, there is logic to the traditional approach of early rehabilitation to reduce impairments as they are viewed as the primary factors limiting the recovery of mobility function. The abnormal walking patterns of individuals with stroke associated with weakness[17-20], hypertonia[19-22], incoordination[21,23,24], and instability[20,25] provide the scientific rationale to support the approach.

Mobility involves navigating over changing terrain, obstacle avoidance, stair negotiation and frequent modulation of speed and direction. Each task imposes different neuromuscular, postural and metabolic demands and the capacity to meet them is necessarily related to the integrity of the systems involved and their interactions. To facilitate understanding of how stroke related deficits in specific systems influence mobility function, the major contributors will be discussed in turn.

Muscle Function

Muscle weakness is among the most commonly reported and studied deficit following stroke. The force producing capacity of a muscle is dependent upon the characteristics of the muscle itself including the number and size of the motor units and muscle fibres, and the neural input to the muscle. The latter is affected as a direct consequence of the stroke associated brain lesion which disrupts the descending motor pathways thus limiting the capacity to bring spinal motor neurons to threshold and activate muscles (recruitment). Furthermore, damaged inhibitory circuits or neuromodulatory controls can adversely affect the ability to keep muscles silent or relax those previously activated (derecruitment). Co-activation between agonist and antagonist muscle groups is common in stroke resulting in increased joint stiffness, reduced net torque production and incoordination[23,26] . Unlike many other deficits, the abnormal temporal control of muscle activation patterns seems to persist despite observed improvements in function including gait and balance[27,28]. The characteristics of the muscle itself, however, can change considerably over time following stroke in response to the altered neural drive superimposed on naturally occurring age-related loss in muscle quality (structural integrity and contractility) and disuse atrophy secondary to activity restriction. These negative consequences can be attenuated and possibly reversed with appropriate regimens of physical activity and exercise[29-31].

It is well established that muscles contralateral to the stroke are significantly weaker than ipsilateral muscles though the extent of the paresis can vary widely. Isokinetic testing of concentric peak torque production following mild to moderate stroke has revealed that the paretic limb generates between 20% and 88% of the torque produced on the less-affected side with the greatest asymmetry occurring in the more distal muscles (table 1). The adoption of the term "less-affected" is deliberate as there are frequently strength deficits on the side ipsilateral to the lesion[29,32] that may reflect damage to the uncrossed corticospinal pathways, though this remains uncertain[33]. Our own data comparing peak torques of healthy controls with the less-affected side of an age and gender matched stroke group support this view (table 1).

The impact of muscle weakness is determined by the demands of the activities that individuals need or wish to perform. Bohannon[29] illustrated this point in the form of sigmoidal curves reflecting the theoretical relationship between strength and functional performance. A certain amount of strength is required to perform a given activity and until that level is attained, the individual will be unable to perform the task. Once the minimum strength requirement is met, further gains translate into better performance, though at some point performance plateaus regardless of continued improvements in strength. The absolute amount of strength required and the degree to which gains in strength are accompanied by improvements in performance differ in accordance with the task demands. In practical terms, these thresholds remain ill-defined but are compelling in the abstract and support muscle strengthening as a primary target for intervention. The focus on strengthening has certainly been fueled by the volume of research describing the relationships between strength and function. Some of this work is summarized below.

Table 1. Relative isokinetic strength of the affected side to the less-affected side. The shaded area reflects the relative strength of the less-affected side to age and gender matched healthy subjects

Muscle group	Kim and Eng	Hsu et al.	Pohl et al.	Our data	
Hip extensors	.88 (60°/s)			.74 (60°/s)[a]	
Hip flexors	.63 (60°/s)	.76 (30°/s)		.73 (60°/s)[a]	
Knee extensors	.47 (30-60°/s)		.63 (60°/s)	.64 (60°/s)[b]	.72 (60°/s)[b]
Knee flexors	.24 (30-60°/s)	.51 (90°/s)	.65(60°/s)	.62 (60°/s)[b]	.68 (60°/s)[b]
Plantarflexors	.20 (30-60°/s)	.51 (30°/s)	.44 (30°/s)	.55 (30°/s)[b]	.79 (30°/s)[b]
Dorsiflexors	.31 (30-60°/s)		.74 (30°/s)	.51 (30°/s)[b]	.72 (30°/s)[b]

[a] Barbic and Brouwer[34]
[b] Unpublished data from 22 stroke survivors and age- and gender-matched healthy controls.

Healthy adults are able to walk at a range of gait speeds and increase their walking cadence by generating progressively higher plantarflexor, hip flexor and hip extensor moments, which they are able to do because they have ample reserve strength[35]. In contrast, people with stroke tend to walk quite slowly and have limited capacity to increase their speed, perhaps due to insufficient residual strength. Nadeau and colleagues[36] evaluated the extent to which the plantarflexors were used during comfortable and fast walking by calculating the muscle utilization ratio (MUR). The MUR is an index of the amount of muscle force used during a task (biomechanical analysis) relative to the maximum force output (dynamometry), where 100% is total utilization. They found in their sample of 17 subjects with hemiparesis, that the plantarflexors worked at an average of 76.4% of their maximum at a walking speed of 0.8m/s and 85.9% at 1.09 m/s. This compares to 65.6% and 58.8% for healthy controls walking at their comfortable speed or at a comparable speed to those with stroke, respectively. The researchers concluded that weakness was a factor limiting gait speed, however this assumes that other muscle groups could not compensate for the limited plantarflexor output. Several studies have reported strong associations between hip flexor strength and gait speed in stroke[18,36-39] suggesting that the hip flexors could effectively pull the stance limb off the ground to compensate for limited plantarflexor push-off[20,39]. Considering that the strength of the hip flexors tends to be better preserved post stroke (see table 1) it is conceivable that they compensate for the weaker plantarflexors.

Significant associations have also been documented between gait speed and the affected knee extensor[40-42], knee flexor[41] and plantarflexor[17,18] torques (r values ranging from 0.57 to 0.85). Less attention has been paid to the relationships between gait speed and strength on the less affected side even though most mobility tasks like walking and stair climbing require the involvement of both sides and typically in near symmetrical fashion. From the limited data available, only the isokinetic strength of the less affected knee extensors and flexors, and ankle plantarflexors yielded significant correlations with walking and stair climbing (r values ranging from .48 to .61)[18,43] with the knee flexors and plantarflexors associated with the speed of stair ascent[18]. In combination these findings serve as a reminder that strength on both the affected and less-affected sides should be evaluated, but offer little insight to the clinician about their *relative* importance or how the muscle groups interact (including compensatory strategies) to maximize function. Furthermore, the relationship between lower limb strength and stair climbing ability is confounded when either reciprocal stepping is not possible or the upper limb provides support through hand rails as this alters the task demands.

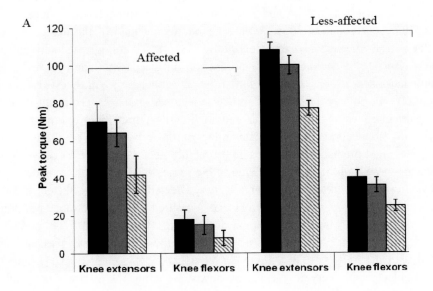

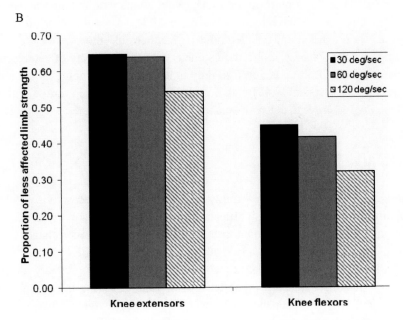

Figure 1. A. Mean peak concentric knee extensor and flexor torques generated isokinetically from each limb of 15 people with chronic stroke. B. The relative weakness of the affected to the less-affected limb. See Sharp and Brouwer[45] for study details.

Studies examining muscle output following stroke have almost exclusively assessed strength. Saunders and colleagues[44] contend that muscle power (product of torque and angular velocity) may in fact be more important than strength for the performance of mobility related tasks. The decline in force output as a function of the speed of contraction is a well documented characteristic of healthy muscle and would reasonably be expected to be exaggerated in stroke in association with deficits in motor unit recruitment, derecruitment and elevated tone. Indeed when measuring isokinetic torque production at the ankle in stroke, 18 of the 20 subjects tested in Kim and Eng's study[18] were unable to produce measurable torque at $60^\circ/s$, but could at $30^\circ/s$. Reviewing our own data[45], the degree of interlimb asymmetry in peak knee extensor and flexor torques increased at higher velocities attributable to an increased rate of decline in force production on the paretic side (figure 1). Velocity dependent increases in passive restraint from the antagonist muscles[21,46] and co-activation[24] can both reduce the net torque generated, and if severe could be extremely limiting, particularly when the task requires rapid directional transitions or large power bursts.

Revisiting Bohannon's theoretic description of the relationship between strength and function, one might predict that the capacity to rapidly generate muscle force would be most important for those mobility tasks demanding high rates of contraction. Saunders et al.[44] quantified lower-limb extensor power on the affected and less-affected sides in 66 independently ambulatory stroke survivors and measured their comfortable walking speed, timed up and go (TUG: rise from a chair, walk 3 metres, turn around, return and sit down), and time to rise from a chair. On the affected side, lower-limb power was most strongly associated with the TUG (r=0.68), followed by rising from a chair (r=0.63) then walking (r=0.54). Subjects with very low extensor power were unable to rise from a chair and therefore were also unable to perform the TUG. Older adults who require the use of mobility aids to walk or climb stairs have reportedly 42 - 54% less knee extensor power than those who perform these tasks independently[47]. Neither of these studies reported the corresponding torque measures so it remains unclear whether the rate of force production or weakness was the main limiting factor. Certainly in normal stair climbing power production is central to performance speed[47,48] and it may also be the case in stroke, although more research is required in order to determine its importance to mobility.

Balance Ability

Maintaining static and dynamic stability requires the integrated activity of sensory and motor systems and as such can be a significant challenge for stroke survivors. Balance control is essential in order to perform functional tasks and is strongly correlated with walking speed[45,49], endurance[50,51], and other mobility activities (sit-to-stand, stair climbing)[52,53]. Three key aspects are considered essential to recovery of function: i) maintenance of standing balance; ii) maintenance of balance during internal or self-initiated perturbation; and iii) maintenance of balance during external perturbation[54-56]. Rehabilitation efforts tend to target the first two in efforts to minimize sway, promote weight-bearing symmetry and stabilize posture in anticipation of voluntary movement[see 57 for review].

In stroke, quiet standing with eyes open is characterized by excessive body sway and asymmetrical weight support through the feet compared to healthy older[49,57-59]. It is axiomatic that standing balance is fundamental to mobility, yet the relationships between the excursion of the centre of pressure (COP) during quiet standing and measures of dynamic balance or gait speed in chronic stroke are poor (r = -0.38 and -0.21, respectively)[49]; the negative coefficient indicating that less sway is associated with better function. Suzuki et al.[40] however, reported moderately strong correlations between COP sway and maximum walking speeds (r = -0.683) after 4 weeks of gait training in people with subacute stroke (1.6 to 13 weeks post-stroke). The strength of the relationship declined after 8 weeks of training (r = -0.477) in conjunction with a 22% reduction in COP sway and nearly a doubling of gait speed. These findings are compatible with the view that there may be a ceiling effect in the performance of standing balance. Once a certain level of stability in quiet standing is achieved it is no longer likely to be a limiting factor of function and other "weak links", such as dynamic balance become critical.

Dynamic balance, the ability to maintain balance during voluntary activities (internal perturbations) or external perturbation is crucial to safe mobility under non-static conditions. At the most basic level, this requires the capacity to shift one's weight within the base of support to counteract a destabilizing force or to shift weight toward the limits of the base of support in preparation for the initiation of walking. While seemingly rudimentary, the task requires controlled translation of the centre of mass through appropriately timed and graded muscle activation. In stroke, efforts to shift weight toward the affected side or the limits of stability are often met with undesired muscle co-activation which increases joint stiffness[60]; the manifestation being slowed COP movement and limited excursion. Figure 2 illustrates the deficits in weight shifting capacity of a 63 year old woman who suffered an ischemic stroke 4.5 years prior to testing. Limitations in the ability to shift the COP while standing compromises mobility as reflected by the associations between gait speed and weight shifting (r values between 0.486 and 0.723)[49].

Stevenson and Garland[61] studied the muscle activation patterns associated with self-paced arm raises in a study involving 21 subjects with chronic hemiparesis. Subjects were asked to bring their non-paretic arm forward from their side and raise it above their head as fast as possible. An accelerometer measured the arm acceleration and activation of the hamstrings and triceps surae muscles was recorded bilaterally. They found that subjects who demonstrated anticipatory ipsilateral (less-affected) hamstring activation had the highest balance scores (Berg Balance Scale) which they attributed to the ability to modify postural stability as a countermeasure to upper limb mobility. They later reported that subjects adopt different strategies (bilateral or ipsilateral anticipatory hamstring activation) to achieve competency and highlighted the importance of feedforward control to minimize the effects of the perturbation[28]. Subjects who exhibited delayed (i.e. closer to movement onset) or no anticipatory activation compensated by limiting arm acceleration to reduce the impact of the perturbation on stability. Similar strategies may be employed to minimize instability associated with the performance of many functional activities including gait. Indeed, of the physical impairments due to stroke, impaired postural control has been described as having the greatest impact on activity and mobility[see 57 for review]. It must be recognized though that postural control is strongly associated to muscle function in healthy adults[61] and in stroke[62-64]. Kluding and Gajewski[65] suggest that strengthening lower extremity muscles can improve balance; however others have failed to demonstrate increases in balance ability with gains in strength[66,67]. Determining which impairment(s) limit function is an important step in selecting an appropriate rehabilitation strategy.

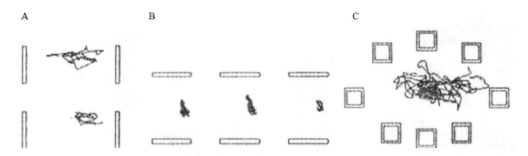

Figure 2. An individual with left hemiparesis follows instructions to shift their weight while standing; visual feedback of their centre of pressure position relative to the targets is provided. Side-to-side (A) and anterior-posterior (B) weight shifting requires subjects to track a cursor moving between targets at a 3 second pace. In C, a target is illuminated and the subject shifts their weight toward the target as quickly and accurately as possible (see Liston and Brouwer[49] and Walker et al[59] for study details).

Cardiorespiratory Function

Stroke rehabilitation focuses mainly on the neurologic impairments of muscle function (strength, coordination and tone) and balance; both discussed above. There is growing acknowledgment, however, that poor cardiovascular and cardiorespiratory health can limit recovery because of limited capacity to meet and respond to the demands of activity and mobility[see reviews:68,69]. It is well established that physical conditioning is markedly reduced in chronic stroke, in part due to restricted activity and a generally sedentary lifestyle. Recently though, research has indicated that the aerobic capacity early post-stroke (within 1-2 months) corresponds to 50%-60% of the normative values for age- and sex- matched sedentary healthy adults[70,71], thus indicating that deconditioning is not solely a consequence of long term stroke. Poor cardiorespiratory fitness and cardiovascular disease are risk factors for stroke and highly prevalent in the stroke population and deconditioning puts stroke survivors at risk of poor functional outcomes[68]; we have therefore included cardiorespiratory function as a stroke-related physical impairment.

Generalized fatigue affects about 70% of stroke survivors after accounting for symptoms of depression[72]. Macko and colleagues[73] have identified fatigue as a primary limitation of treadmill exercise; more important than paresis, although others have drawn different conclusions based on their own work[50,70]. Consistently though, research has shown that the energy cost associated with gait post-stroke is at least twice that of age matched, healthy individuals[70,74,75]. The abnormally low peak aerobic capacity in stroke estimated to be between 20-50% lower than healthy counterparts[50,70,71,76], paired with the elevated energy cost of walking on level ground can leave little reserve to handle higher demand activities or conditions such as curb and stair negotiation. The findings from a study comparing the metabolic demands of walking in 13 young stroke survivors (mean age $\pm$ SD: 40.7 $\pm$ 10.0 years) and age and gender matched healthy subjects highlights the extent of the stroke-related deficit[77]. Platts et al.[77] reported that the oxygen uptake is comparable between groups when they walk at their respective preferred speed, however taking gait speed into account (stroke: 0.39 $\pm$ 0.20 m/s, control: 1.22 $\pm$ 1.0 m/s) illustrated a marked discrepancy in oxygen uptake per unit distance (stroke: 0.63 $\pm$ 0.41 ml/kg/m, control: 0.16 $\pm$ 0.02 ml/kg/m). In community ambulation where both speed of walking and distance are important parameters[78], the low aerobic capacity in stroke can seriously compromise independence. It has been suggested that walking speeds of at least 0.66 m/s[78] and endurance of 300 to 500 m[79] are required for community ambulation; clearly the oxygen costs could be prohibitively high for many stroke survivors. The situation is further exacerbated when unlevel ground or stairs need to be negotiated due to the higher metabolic requirements.

Healthy older adults (average of 78 years) consume oxygen at a rate between 13.3 and 23.7 ml/kg/min while climbing stairs at a rate of 24 steps/min (44% of their VO_2max)[80] compared to 11.0 - 12.0 ml/kg/min during comfortable walking[77,81,82]. Young adults climb nearly 4 times faster, but at a higher O_2 cost of about 33.5 ml/kg/min or 83% of their VO_2max[83]. Stair descent requires about half the energy consumption[83] and our own data indicate that the reduced cost is paralleled by a reduction in muscle force requirements.

From the discussion above, deficits in cardiorespiratory function could pose a major limitation to stair negotiation in stroke. A recent systematic review of the effects of exercise training on walking competency following stroke reported evidence to support the utility of aerobic training in improving stair climbing ability[67]. Following 8 weeks of training using a leg cycle ergometer, the exercise group (n=46) demonstrated a significant increase in the ability to climb one flight of stairs compared to a control group (n=44)[84]. Logistic regression modeling confirmed the effect was due to the training, although it could be argued that corresponding training-related increases in strength (not measured) could have contributed to the outcome. Because weakness and poor cardiorespiratory function generally coexist in stroke it is important to determine the extent to which one or both factors contribute to mobility including stair negotiation and account for the fact that these two parameters are themselves related.

Reductions in muscle function and quality following stroke directly contribute to low cardiorespiratory fitness as a result of a loss in metabolically active tissue (fewer accessible motor units) and reductions in mitochondrial content[31,69]. Disuse atrophy secondary to limited activity exacerbates the problem, lowering the oxidative potential further. The interactions between neuromuscular and cardiorespiratory impairments compound their influence on mobility function making it challenging to determine their relative impact, yet it is important to do so to appropriately guide rehabilitation efforts.

Stroke is a multisystem disorder and mobility is a complex construct that is associated with muscle function, balance and cardiorespiratory function. While understanding the associations between specific impairments and mobility provides insight into which parameters are important it does not offer guidance on how to enhance mobility. The research by Roth et al.[85] clearly illustrates this point. They followed 400 stroke patients admitted for rehabilitation and monitored changes in impairment and function over time. Multivariate analysis indicated that changes in impairment levels explained only 2% to 36% of the gains in function but also noted that functional gains were detected in patients regardless of whether they exhibited reductions in impairment. The implication is that a more indepth understanding of the links between impairment and function is needed to determine if impairment influences function and if so, will reducing impairment translate into better function?

DETERMINANTS AND PREDICTORS OF MOBILITY IN STROKE

Physical capacity and mobility function are not static after stroke but are responsive to aging, recovery, activity level, as well as adaptive and compensatory strategies. It is likely that there is a natural order in which impairments must be reduced to achieve a certain level of mobility function that is dictated by the integrity of and interdependency among systems (e.g. strength and metabolic capacity) as well as the requirements of the mobility task itself (i.e. what is needed to succeed?). It follows that there could be a number of solutions to a mobility problem since individuals with stroke are unique in their physical capabilities and in their capacity to compensate. A global goal of rehabilitation is to maximize mobility, therefore it is essential that those factors that significantly influence specific mobility tasks (e.g. level ground walking, distance walking, stair-climbing, etc.) are identified.

Cross sectional correlation studies provide valuable contributions to our understanding of the associations between variables of interest; in our case impairment and mobility, but not their temporal or causal nature. In addition, the bivariate approach has two key limitations. First, depending on when the evaluation of impairment occurred in terms of the stage and extent of recovery, the assessment outcome could be more (or less) relevant to mobility, hence restricting generalizability of the findings and validity of the conclusions. Second, performance indicators of physiological systems are often related, therefore examining one aspect in isolation can misrepresent its significance to a complex behavior like mobility. Multivariate approaches allow the researcher to examine the relationship between a single dependent variable (mobility) and numerous independent variables (impairment related) while also assessing multicollinearity (shared variance) between independent variables. This is critical in stroke research given the importance of determining the unique contributions of individual variables to mobility function as well as their combined impact.

In this section, key findings derived from cross sectional and longitudinal studies that assessed multiple impairment-related outcomes to identify determinants and predictors of mobility function are discussed. A summary of selected studies is presented in table 2.

Mobility Early Post-Stroke

In the early stages of stroke recovery, walking status is extremely important to patients. Suzuki et al.[40] introduced a computer assisted gait training program targeting specific temporal-distance parameters of walking that needed improvement to a group of 34 men averaging 8.6 weeks post-stroke. After 4 weeks of training, significant gains were observed in maximum walking speed as well as secondary outcomes of knee extensor strength and balance (standing and weight-shifting); continued improvement was evident for all variables after 8 weeks of training. The determinants of walking speed changed over time with side-to-side weight-shifting capacity important at baseline and knee extensor strength at 4 and 8 weeks, yet it was initial walking speed, knee extensor strength and time post stroke (shorter is better) that predicted walking speed at 8 weeks. The early importance of standing weight-shifting ability to mobility and its lack of significance as predictor of walking speed is

Table 2. Summary of selected studies reporting regression models that considered multiple impairment-related outcomes

Mobility measure	Design	Sample	Outcome measures	Determinants / predictors of mobility	Study
Walking speed and maximum walking speed (m/s)	Cross sectional	n=16, 18-73 years, mean of 44 months post-stroke	Fugl-Meyer (motor function, sensation and balance), spasticity (composite of Modified Ashworth, tendon jerk, and clonus), peak isokinetic hip and ankle torques (30°/s)	Comfortable speed: hip flexor strength, $R^2 = .685$. Maximum speed: hip flexor strength ($R^2 = .770$) + plantarflexor strength ($R^2 = .040$) + sensation ($R^2 = .035$); total $R^2 = .845$	Nadeau et al.[89]
Walking speed (m/s)	Cross sectional	n=74, ≥ 40 years, > 6 months post-stroke	Berg Balance Scale, Modified Ashworth Scale (knee), 6 minute walk test, VO2max, average peak isokinetic knee extensor torque (30, 90 and 120°/s; eccentric, bilateral), body composition	VO2 max ($R^2 = .48$) + Balance ($R^2 = .09$) + affected knee extensor strength ($R^2 = .03$), total $R^2 = .60$. Slow walkers (≤ .48m/s): Balance, $R^2 = .42$; fast walkers (> .48m/s): VO2 max, $R^2 = .26$	Patterson et al.[92]
6 Minute walk test (m)	Cross sectional	n=63, ≥ 50 years, ≥ 1 year post-stroke	Berg Balance Scale, isometric knee extensor force (bilateral), Modified Ashwoth Scale (MAS; average of foot + leg), VO2max, % body fat.	Balance ($R^2 = .665$) + affected knee extensor strength ($R^2 = .036$) + MAS ($R^2 = .023$); total $R^2 = .725$	Pang et al.[50]
Change in Function Ambulation Category (FAC)	Longitudinal, part of a RCT to study effects of intensity of acute-care rehabilitation, baseline and 6 month data used.	n=101, 30-80 year olds ≤ 14 days post-stroke	Motricity index (MI, upper and lower extremity strength), timed balance test (TBT), Fugl-Meyer (FM, arm, leg, balance, motor performance)	In descending order of significance: change in: TBT, FM leg, MI leg strength and time post-stroke*: $R^2 = .18$	Kollen et al.[86]
Maximum walking speed (MWS) (m/min)	Longitudinal, pre– interim-post 8 week computer assisted gait training program (4-5 days/wk); identified determininants (point in time) and predictors (8 wk MWS)	n=34 males, 28-82 years, 1.5 to 13 weeks post-stroke, no cardiorespiratory dysfunction	Peak isokinetic knee extensor torque (30°/s, concentric, bilateral), standing balance (centre of pressure (COP) excursion, ability to shift COP side-to-side and forward-backward as a % of the base of support)	Determinants: Baseline MWS: side-to-side COP shift, $R^2 = .454$; 4 & 8 wk MWS: Affected knee extensor strength, $R^2 = .629$ (4wks), .545 (8wks). Predictors: initial MWS + affected knee extensor strength + time post stroke*, $R^2 = .734$	Suzuki et al.[40]
Change in 6 Minute walk test (m)	Secondary analysis of longitudinal data, pre-post 19 week leg or arm exercise program (1hr, 3x/wk),	n=60, ≥ 50 years, ≥ 1 year post-stroke	Change in: isometric knee extensor force (bilateral), Berg Balance Scale, Activities-specific Balance confidence, VO2max	Age*, gender, time post-stroke* and initial 6 minute walk distance ($R^2 = .048$) + change in knee extensor strength ($R^2 = .119$) + change in VO2max ($R^2 = .061$); total $R^2 = .229$	Pang and Eng[51]
Change in gait speed (m/s)	Secondary analysis of longitudinal data, pre-post 8-10 week physical conditioning program	n=28, > 20 years, ≥ 9 months post-stroke. All increased gait speed from baseline	Change in work produced by ankle, knee and hip flexors and extensors during natural speed walking (bilateral)	Model 1: change in affected hip extensor work ($R^2 = .660$) + change in affected plantarflexor work ($R^2 = .089$); total $R^2 = .749$. Model 2: change in affected hip extensor work ($R^2 = .660$) + change in less-affected hip extensor work ($R^2 = .083$); total $R^2 = .743$	Parvataneni et al.[39]

* Indicates a negative coefficient, i.e. inverse relationship between independent and dependent (mobility) variables.

shifting ability to mobility and its lack of significance as predictor of walking speed is interesting. Kollen and colleagues[86] found that improvements in standing balance, leg mobility and strength observed from ~2 weeks to 6 months post-stroke explained the change from dependent to independent ambulation. The variance in mobility status accounted for by each variable was not provided, though the authors did state that the change in balance was the most important factor. The combined findings of these two studies fuel our earlier speculation that there may be a ceiling of standing balance performance. In the first study, the minimum balance performance level compatible with walking may have been achieved at baseline; therefore any further gains were not instrumental in incrementing walking speed. At this stage other factors (strength) were critical to mobility function suggestive of a sequence in which impairments must be addressed to enable gains in walking ability.

Mobility in Chronic Stroke

Loss of independent ambulation is one of the most disabling aspects following stroke[87]. In the early stages of recovery survivors often experience improvements in physical function, but after discharge from hospital the gains erode and mobility function declines in the absence of appropriate activity[9,88]. Seventy-five percent of those discharged home consider getting out and walking in the community to be essential or very important[10] and the primary determinant of community ambulation is gait speed[78]. Using a cut-off of 0.66 m/s, van de Port and colleagues[78] accurately identified 93% of community ambulators and of those who walked more slowly, 57% were appropriately categorized as non-community walkers. The relationship between gait speed and community ambulation was however, significantly affected by activity-related balance ability, motor function (strength), walking endurance and the use of walking aids leading them to conclude that improving gait speed without addressing the other factors would not be sufficient to impact community mobility. To confirm whether this is the case requires a longitudinal design, although conventional wisdom dictates that the challenge of walking in the community would be influenced by factors other than solely gait speed, particularly when determined indoors, on level ground and over a short distance.

Cross sectional studies that have included measures related to impairments of several systems (muscular, balance, sensory and cardiorespiratory) as possible predictors of mobility have produced inconsistent results. Using walking speed as the dependent measure of mobility, Nadeau et al.[89] identified isokinetic hip flexor strength as the sole determinant of comfortable walking speed ($R^2 = .68$). Fast walking speed was primarily a function of hip flexor strength ($R^2 = .77$) but in addition, lower limb sensation and plantarflexor strength were major factors (total $R^2 = .84$). The importance of these two muscle groups is reasonable since the hip flexors advance the limb forward through swing and in stroke, larger flexor moments are strongly associated with faster walking particularly in the presence of limited plantarflexor contribution[36,90]. A companion paper by Nadeau et al.[36] documents that the fastest walkers yielded large hip flexor moments during gait and had high dynamometric torques. Parvatanini et al.[39] reported that increases in plantarflexor strength explained a significant portion of the gains observed in walking speed among stroke survivors, but that improvements in hip extensor strength (not flexor) was the major determinant of the observed gains in walking speed ($R^2 = .66$). The contrasting findings of these two studies highlights that the relationships between variables measured at a single point in time may not necessarily reflect their importance in effecting change.

Sensory function is seldom included in deterministic models of mobility as deficits rarely limit normal walking. The importance of sensation in fast walking was therefore notable[89] and may reflect that reduced sensory feedback is a deterrent to increasing speed if proprioceptive input is inadequate for controlling posture[56]. Other studies[40,86,91,92] have found balance to be an independent determinant of speed.

Patterson et al.[92] evaluated oxygen consumption, tone, strength and balance in 74 stroke survivors. Regression analysis identified balance as the second most important determinant of walking speed ($R^2 = .09$), but when they conducted separate analyses after splitting their sample into slow ($\leq .48$m/s) and fast ($> .48$m/s) walkers, balance was the major determinant of mobility only for those who walked slowly ($R^2 = .42$). People with stroke who have poor balance and abnormal postural control minimize destabilizing forces by limiting limb accelerations[28,57]; walking slowly would have the same effect. In contrast Pang et al.[50] reported that balance was the main contributor to mobility ($R^2 = .66$) in stroke survivors walking an average of $\sim .88$m/s. Their dependent measure, however, was the distance covered over a 6 minute period. Arguably the distance walked is a function of gait speed, but the demands on the contributing systems would be expected to differ with the added endurance component; the relative importance of balance being an example of this. Interestingly, in a longitudinal study this same group found that gains in balance performance did not contribute to improvements in distance walked[51]. This could indicate either that the magnitude of the balance improvement was insufficient to effect change in walking performance or that balance ability was adequate at the time of the first assessment such that any gains would not translate into enhanced walking capacity.

Muscle strength on the affected side is an important determinant of mobility[50,51,89,92] as shown above, although studies do not necessarily agree about their relative importance compared to other factors or which muscle groups are the main contributors. Peak knee extensor torque has been identified as the second or third ranking determinant of walking ability following balance or aerobic capacity and balance[50,92]. The knee extensors are not generally considered a major muscle group contributing to the work of gait, which might explain the low R^2 values (see table 2), but nonetheless the significance indicates their importance in stroke. Considering that strength measured at one joint correlates strongly with strength measured at other joints, the emergence of the knee extensors as a determinant of walking capacity might simply be by proxy, revealed because the strength of other muscle groups was not measured. Nadeau et al.[89] identified the hip flexors and ankle plantarflexor torques (at fast speed) as major contributors, which is compatible with their power generation profiles during gait, but they did not measure knee strength. Unpublished data from our own lab (table 3) derived from 72 chronic stroke survivors identified plantarflexor and knee flexor strength as determinants of gait speed (and stair climbing ability) after entering flexor and extensor strength for ankle, knee and hip joints into the model. We measured isometric strength rather than isokinetic, which may have impacted the results. In view of the differences in test protocols across studies and until more definitive results emerge, it may be reasonable to generalize that global lower limb strength is important in determining mobility status. Furthermore, gains in muscle work capacity[39] and strength[51] (see table 3) are significant independent factors associated with improvements in gait speed, distance walked and stair climbing emphasizing the value of improving muscle function to mobility.

Table 3. Determinants of walking speed and stair climbing
capacity in chronic stroke (n=72) and those impairment measures
that when improved translate into increased mobility

Dependent Variable	Independent Variable	Standardized β coefficient	R^2	Change in R^2	p-value
Walking speed	Affected plantarflexor strength	.376	.380		<.001
	Physiological cost index	-.354	.523	.143	<.001
	Affected knee flexor strength	.244	.557	.034	.026
Stairs climbed	Affected knee flexor strength	.234	.293		<.001
	Physiological cost index	-.333	.406	.113	.001
	Unaffected plantarflexor strength	.264	.455	.048	.017
	Ankle tone (modified Ashworth)	-.234	.499	.045	.017
Δ in walking speed	Δ affected knee flexor strength	.634	.402		<.001
Δ in number of stairs climbed	Δ affected dorsiflexor strength	.429	.184		.002

Aerobic capacity (VO_2max) was more important than balance or strength in determining gait speed in Patterson et al.'s study[92] (R^2 = .48) and was the sole variable retained in the model when subjects were categorized as fast walkers but not slow. Our data identified the physiological cost index (a proxy measure for oxygen cost[93]) after 2 minutes of walking as the second most important determinant of gait speed (R^2 = .143) in a stroke group walking at a speed of 0.78 $\pm$ 0.33 m/s. Paradoxically, neither oxygen cost or VO_2max were significant determinants of ambulatory activity (steps/day)[91] or walking distance (6 minute walk test)[50]; in both these studies balance was the main factor. It is possible that the speed of walking either throughout the day or over the six minute period was insufficient to challenge the aerobic system to the point that it influenced walking capacity. The average distance travelled in six minutes was about 57% of the age-related norm[94]. Indeed when the distance walked increased secondary to training (to about 70% of published norms), change in VO_2max explained a significant portion of the variance indicating its importance in improving mobility[51].

The combined contributions of muscle function, balance ability and cardiorespiratory function to mobility are significant although there are clearly other major factors to consider. The extent to which walking speed and distance are explained by measures reflective of these three systems ranges from 26% to 84% and the changes in mobility attributable to gains in system function range from 18% - 75% (table 2) leaving a large proportion unaccounted for. Ongoing research examining multiple physical parameters and other factors including cognitive and language function, emotional well-being and comorbidities will be instrumental to developing comprehensive approaches to the treatment of stroke-related disability.

SUMMARY

The research discussed in this chapter illustrates the association between and the relative importance of specific stroke related impairments to mobility function. The fact that specific impairments may be associated with mobility but not necessarily important determinants of walking capacity is an important distinction. Recognizing that the significance of a particular impairment (e.g. balance) varies with mobility status, with recovery status or time post-stroke and the demands of the mobility task (e.g. walking speed versus distance) is critical to ensure that appropriate interventions are introduced at appropriate times. Longitudinal studies that monitored changes in both residual impairments and mobility over time have shown that reducing the severity of impairments causally linked to mobility will not necessarily translate into walking faster or longer distances if they are not the limiting factor of enhancing mobility. Indeed other factors, not previously considered as important may prove instrumental in effecting changes to mobility function if they are a weak link in the progression toward recovery.

It is probable that there are minimum performance criteria for a given system for a specific mobility related task (level walking speed, distance, stair climbing). There are also likely maximum values beyond which further gains in ability will not translate into measurable mobility improvements although they could provide additional reserve capacity or compensatory potential. These "thresholds" remain to be determined, but recent research has contributed immensely to our understanding of the links between impairment and function in stroke and, perhaps more importantly, that the relationships are non static. Effective stroke rehabilitation must be multifaceted and responsive to the changes in the integrity of the neuromuscular, balance and cardiorespiratory systems. Furthermore, knowledge about the range of physical demands required across different mobility tasks is relevant to structuring interventions and to appropriately gauge the relative importance of specific impairments.

REFERENCES

[1] Langton-Hewer R. Rehabilitation after stroke. *Quarterly Journal of Medicine.* 1990; 76:659-674.

[2] Mayo NE. Hospitalization and case-fatality rates for stroke in Canada from 1982 through 1991. The Canadian collaborative study group of stroke hospitalizations. *Stroke.* 1996; 27:1215-1220.

[3] American Heart Association. Heart disease and stroke statistics: 2004 update. 2004. Dallas, AHA.

[4] Heart and Stroke Foundation of Canada. Just the Facts: 2002/2003 Edition. 2002.

[5] Stineman MG, Granger CV. Outcome, efficiency, and time-trend pattern analyses for stroke rehabilitation. *American Journal of Physical Medicine and Rehabilitation.* 1998; 77:193-201.

[6] Duncan PW, Goldstein LB, Horner RD, Landsman PB, Samsa GP, Matchar DB. Similar motor recovery of upper and lower extremities after stroke. *Stroke.* 1994; 25:1181-1188.

[7]   Hankey GJ, Jamrozik K, Broadhurst RJ, Forbes S, Anderson CS. Long-term disability after first ever stroke and related prognostic factors in the Perth community stroke study, 1989-1990. *Stroke.* 2002; 33:1034-1040.

[8]   Jorgensen HS, Nakayama H, Raaschou HO, Vive-Larsen J, Stoier M, Olsen TS. Outcome and time course recovery in stroke. Part I: Outcome. The Copenhagen Stroke Study. *Archives of Physical Medicine and Rehabilitation.* 1995; 76:399-405.

[9]   Mayo NE, Wood-Dauphinee S, Cote R, Durcan L, Carlton J. Activity, participation, and quality of life 6 months poststroke. *Archives of Physical Medicine and Rehabilitation.* 2002; 83:1035-1042.

[10] Lord SE, McPherson K, McNaughton HK, Rochester L, Weatherall M. Community ambulation after stroke: how important and obtainable is it and what measures appear predictive. *Archives of Physical Medicine and Rehabilitation.* 2004; 85:234-239.

[11] Thorngren M, Westling B, Norrving B. Outcome after stroke in patients discharged to independent living. *Stroke.* 1990; 21:236-240.

[12] Wade DT, Turnball GI. Walking after stroke. *Scandanavian Journal of Rehabilitation Medicine.* 1987; 19:25-30.

[13] Hill K, Ellis P, Bernhardt J, Maggs P, Hull S. Balance and mobility outcomes for stroke patients: a comprehensive audit. *Australian Journal of Physiotherapy.* 1997; 43:173-180.

[14] Roth E. Heart disease in patients with stroke. Part I: Classification and prevalence. *Archives of Physical Medicine and Rehabilitation.* 1993; 75:94-101.

[15] Corcoran PJ, Jebsen RH, Brengelmann GL, Simons BS. Effect of plastic and metal leg braces on speed and energy cost of hemiparetic ambulation. *Archives of Physical Medicine and Rehabilitation.* 1970; 51:69-77.

[16] Gerston J, Orr W. External work of walking in hemiparetic patients. *Scandanavian Journal of Rehabilitation Medicine.* 1971; 3:85-88.

[17] Bohannon RW. Strength of lower limb related to gait speed and cadence in stroke patients. *Physiotherapy Canada.* 1986; 38:204-206.

[18] Kim CM, Eng JJ. The relationship of lower-extremity muscle torque to locomotor performance in people with stroke. *Physical Therapy.* 2003; 83:49-57.

[19] Knutsson E, Richards C. Different types of disturbed motor control in gait of hemiparetic patients. *Brain.* 1979; 102:405-430.

[20] Olney SJ, Richards C. Hemiparetic gait following stroke. Part I: Characteristics. *Gait and Posture.* 1996; 4:136-148.

[21] Lamontagne A, Malouin F, Richards CL, Dumas F. Mechanisms of disturbed motor control in ankle weakness during gait after stroke. *Gait and Posture.* 2002; 15:244-255.

[22] Lin PY, Yang YR, Cheng SJ, Wang RY. The relation between ankle impairments and gait velocity and symmetry in people with stroke. *Archives of Physical Medicine and Rehabilitation.* 2006; 87:562-568.

[23] Den Otter AR, Geurts AC, Mulder T, Duysens J. Abnormalities in the temporal patterning of lower extremity muscle activity in hemiparetic gait. *Gait and Posture.* 2007; 25:342-352.

[24] Neckel N, Peliccio M, Nichols D, Hidler J. Quantification of functional weakness and abnormal synergy patterns in the lower limb of individuals with chronic stroke. *Journal of Neuroengineering and Rehabilitation.* 2006; 3:17-27.

[25] Chen G, Patten C, Kothari DH, Zajac FE. Gait differences between individuals with post-stroke hemiparesis and non-disabled controls at matched speeds. *Gait and Posture.* 2005; 22:51-56.

[26] Levin MF, Hui-Chan CW. Ankle spasticity is inversely correlated with antagonist voluntary contraction in hemiparetic subjects. *Electromyography and Clinical Neurophysiology.* 1994; 34:415-425.

[27] Den Otter AR, Geurts AC, de Haart M, Mulder T, Duysens J. Step characteristics during obstacle avoidance in hemiplegic stroke. *Experimental Brain Research.* 2005; 161:180-192.

[28] Garland SJ, WIllems DA, Ivanova TD, Miller KJ. Recovery of standing balance and functional mobility after stroke. *Archives of Physical Medicine and Rehabilitation.* 2003; 84:1753-1759.

[29] Bohannon RW. Muscle strength and muscle training after stroke. *Journal of Rehabilitation Medicine.* 2007; 39:14-20.

[30] Brouwer B. Strength training in long term stroke survivors. *BioMechanics.* 2000; 7:61-70.

[31] Brouwer B, Olney S. Aging skeletal muscle and the impact of resistance exercise. *Physiotherapy Canada.* 2004; 56:1-8.

[32] Andrews AW, Bohannon RW. Distribution of muscle strength impairments following stroke. *Clinical Rehabilitation.* 2000; 14:79-87.

[33] Kwon Y-H, Kim CS, Jang SH. Ipsi-lesional motor deficits in hemiparetic patients with stroke. *NeuroRehabilitation.* 2007; 22:279-286.

[34] Barbic S, Brouwer B. Hip strength in supine and standing in stroke. *Archives of Physical Medicine and Rehabilitation.* 2008; 89: 784-787.

[35] Requiao LF, Nadeau S, Milot MH, Gravel D, Bourbonnais D, Gagnon D. Quantification of level of effort at the plantarflexors and hip extensors and flexor muscles in healthy subjects walking at different cadences. *Journal of Electromyography and Kinesiology.* 2005; 15:393-405.

[36] Nadeau S, Gravel D, Arsenault B, Bourbonnais D. Plantarflexor weakness as a limiting factor of gait speed in stroke subjects and the compensating role of the hip flexors. *Clinical Biomechanics.* 1999; 14:125-135.

[37] Hsu AL, Tang PF, Jan MH. Test-retest reliability of isokinetic muscle strength of the lower extremities in patients with stroke. *Archives of Physical Medicine and Rehabilitation.* 2002; 83:1130-1137.

[38] Olney SJ, Griffin MP, McBride I. Work and power in gait of stroke patients. *Archives of Physical Medicine and Rehabilitation.* 1991; 72:309-314.

[39] Parvataneni K, Olney SJ, Brouwer B. Changes in muscle group work associated with changes in gait speed of persons with stroke. *Clinical Biomechanics.* 2007; 22:813-820.

[40] Suzuki K, Imada G, Iwaya T, Handa T, Kurogo H. Determinants and predictors of the maximum walking speed during computer-assisted gait training in hemiparetic stroke patients. *Archives of Physical Medicine and Rehabilitation.* 1999; 80:179-182.

[41] Flansbjer UB, Downham D, Lexell J. Knee muscle strength, gait performance, and perceived participation after stroke. *Archives of Physical Medicine and Rehabilitation.* 2006; 87:974-980.

[42] Nakamura R, Watanabe S, Handa T, Morohashi I. The relationship between walking speed and strength for knee extension in hemiparetic stroke patients: a follow-up study. *Journal of Experimental Medicine.* 1988; 145:335-340.

[43] Bohannon RW, Walsh S. Association of paretic lower extremity muscle strength and standing balance with stair climbing ability in patients with stroke. *Journal of Stroke and Cerebrovascular Diseases.* 1991; 1:129-133.

[44] Saunders DH, Greig CA, Young A, Mead GE. Association of activity limitations and lower limb explosive extensor power in ambulatory people with stroke. *Archives of Physical Medicine and Rehabilitation.* 2008; 89:677-683.

[45] Sharp SA, Brouwer B. Isokinetic strength training of the hemiparetic knee: effects on function and spasticity. *Archives of Physical Medicine and Rehabilitation.* 1997; 78:1231-1236.

[46] Rydahl SJ, Brouwer BJ. Ankle stiffness and tissue compliance in stroke survivors: a validation of myotonometer measurements. *Archives of Physical Medicine and Rehabilitation.* 2004; 85:1631-1637.

[47] Bassey EJ, Fiatarone MA, O'Neill EF, Kelly M, Evans WJ, Lipsitz LA. Leg extensor power and functional performance in very old men and women. *Clinical Science.* (London) 1992; 82:321-327.

[48] McFadyen BJ, Winter DA. An integrated biomechanical analysis of normal stair ascent and descent. *Journal of Biomechanics.* 1988; 21:733-744.

[49] Liston RAL, Brouwer B. Reliability and validity of measures obtained from stroke patients using the Balance Master. *Archives of Physical Medicine and Rehabilitation.* 1996; 77:425-430.

[50] Pang MYC, Eng JJ, Dawson AS. Relationship between ambulatory capacity and cardiorespiratory fitness in chronic stroke: influence of stroke-specific impairments. *Chest.* 2005; 127:495-501.

[51] Pang MYC, Eng JJ. Determinants of improvements in walking capacity among individuals with chronic stroke following a multi-dimensional exercise program. *Journal of Rehabilitation Medicine.* 2008; 40:284-290.

[52] Bohannon RW, Leary KM. Standing balance and function over the course of acute rehabilitation. *Archives of Physical Medicine and Rehabilitation.* 1995; 76:994-996.

[53] Cameron DM, Bohannon RW, Garrett GE, Owen SV. Physical impairments related to kinetic energy during sit-to-stand and curb climbing following stroke. *Clinical Biomechanics.* 2003; 18:332-340.

[54] Alexander NB. Postural control in older adults. *Journal of the American Geriatric Society.* 1994; 42:93-108.

[55] Berg K, Wood-Dauphine S, Williams JI, Gayton D. Measuring balance in the elderly: preliminary development of an instrument. *Physiotherapy.* Canada 1989; 41:311.

[56] Patla AE, Frank JS, Winter DA. Balance control in the elderly: implications for clinical assessment and rehabilitation. *Canadian Journal of Public Health.* 1992; 83:S29-S33.

[57] Geurts ACH, de Haart M, van Nes IJW, Duysens J. A review of standing balance recovery from stroke. *Gait & Posture.* 2005; 22:267-281.

[58] Laufer Y, Sivan D, Schwarzmann R, Sprecher E. Standing balance and functional recovery of patients with right and left hemiparesis in the early stages of rehabilitation. *Neurorehabilitation and Neural Repair.* 2003; 17:207-213.

[59] Walker C, Brouwer B, Culham E. Balance retraining following acute stroke: is visual feedback effective? *Physical Therapy.* 2000; 80:886-895.

[60] Duncan PW, Badke MB. Manual of Physical Therapy. New York: Churchill Livingstone; 1989.

[61] Stevenson TJ, Garland SJ. Standing balance during internally produced pertubations in subjects with hemiplegia: validation of the balance scale. *Archives of Physical Medicine and Rehabilitation.* 1996; 77:656-662.

[62] Binda SM, Culham EG, Brouwer B. Balance, muscle strength, and fear of falling in older adults. *Experimental Aging Research.* 2003; 29:205-219.

[63] Marigold DS, Eng JJ, Tokuno CD, Donnelly CA. Contribution of muscle strength and integration of afferent input to postural instability in persons with stroke. *Neurorehabilitation and Neural Repair.* 2004; 18:222-229.

[64] Tyson SF, Hanley M, Chillala J, Selley A, Tallis RC. Balance disability after stroke. *Physical Therapy.* 2006; 86:30-38.

[65] Kluding P, Gajewski B. Lower-extremity strength differences predict activity limitations in people with chronic stroke. *Physical Therapy.* 2009; 89:73-81.

[66] Chandler JM, Duncan PW, Kochersberger G, Studenski S. Is lower extremity strength gain associated with improvement in physical performance and disability in frail, community-dwelling elders? *Archives of Physical Medicine and Rehabilitation.* 1998; 79:24-30.

[67] van de Port IG, Wood-Dauphine S, Lindeman E, Kwakkel G. Effects of exercise training programs on walking competency after stroke: a systematic review. *American Journal of Physical Medicine and Rehabilitation.* 2007; 86:935-951.

[68] Ivey EM, Macko RF, Ryan AS, Hafer-Macko CE. Cardiovascular health and fitness after stroke. *Topics in Stroke Rehabilitation.* 2005; 12:1-16.

[69] Mackay-Lyons MJ, Howlett J. Exercise capacity and cardiovascular adaptations to aerobic training early after stroke. *Topics in Stroke Rehabilitation.* 2005; 12:31-44.

[70] Kelly JO, Kilbreath SL, Davis GM, Zeman B, Raymond J. Cardiorespiratory fitness and walking ability in subacute stroke patients. *Archives of Physical Medicine and Rehabilitation.* 2003; 84:1780-1785.

[71] Mackay-Lyons MJ, Makrides L. Exercise capacity early after stroke. *Archives of Physical Medicine and Rehabilitation.* 2002; 83:1697-1702.

[72] Ingles JL, Eskes GA, Phillips SJ. Fatigue after stroke. *Archives of Physical Medicine and Rehabilitation.* 1999; 80:173-178.

[73] Macko RF, DeSouza CA, Tretter LD, Silver KH, Smith GV, Anderson PA, Tomoyasu N, Gorman P, Dengel DR. Treadmill aerobic exercise training reduces the energy expenditure and cardiovascular demands of hemiparetic gait in chronic stroke patients: a preliminary report. *Stroke.* 1997; 28:326-330.

[74] Macko RF, Smith GV, Dobrovolny CL, Sorkin JD, Goldberg AP, Silver KH. Treadmill training improves fitness reserve in chronic stroke patients. *Archives of Physical Medicine and Rehabilitation.* 2001; 82:879-884.

[75] Potempa K, Lopez M, Braun LT, Szidon JP, Fogg L, Tincknell T. Physiological outcomes of aerobic exercise training in hemiparetic stroke patients. *Stroke.* 1995; 26:101-105.

[76] Mackay-Lyons MJ, Makrides L. Longitudinal changes in exercise capacity after stroke. *Archives of Physical Medicine and Rehabilitation.* 2004; 85:1608-1612.

[77] Platts MM, Rafferty D, Paul L. Metabolic cost of overground gait in younger stroke patients and healthy controls. *Medicine and Science in Sports and Exercise.* 2006; 38:1041-1046.

[78] van de Port IG, Kwakkel G, Lindeman E. Community ambulation in patients with chronic stroke: how is it related to gait speed? *Journal of Rehabilitation Medicine.* 2008; 40:23-27.

[79] Lerner-Frankiel MB, Vargas S, Brown MB, Krusell L, Schoneberger W. Functional community ambulation: what are your criteria? *Clinical Management in Physical Therapy.* 1986; 6:12-15.

[80] Reddy HK, McElroy PA, Janicki JS, Weber KT. Response in oxygen uptake and ventilation during stair climbing in patients with chronic heart failure. *American Journal of Cardiology.* 1989; 63:222-225.

[81] Parvataneni K, Ploeg L, Olney SJ, Brouwer B. Kinematic, kinetic and metabolic parameters of treadmill versus overground walking in healthy older adults. *Clinical Biomechanics.* 2009; 24:95-100.

[82] Waters RL, Hislop HJ, Perry J, Thomas L, Campbell J. Comparative cost of walking in young and old adults. *Journal of Orthopaedic Research.* 1983; 23:425-435.

[83] Teh KC, Aziz AR. Heart rate, oxygen uptake, and energy cost of ascending and descending the stairs. *Medicine and Science in Sports and Exercise.* 2001; 34:695-699.

[84] Katz-Leurer M, Shochina M, Carmeli E, Friedlander Y. The influence of early aerobic training on the functional capacity in patients with cerebrovascular accident at the subacute stage. *Archives of Physical Medicine and Rehabilitation.* 2003; 84:1609-1614.

[85] Roth EJ, Heinemann AW, Lovell LL, Harvey RL, McGuire JR, Diaz S. Impairment and disability: their relation during stroke rehabilitation. *Archives of Physical Medicine and Rehabilitation.* 1998; 79:329-335.

[86] Kollen B, van de Port I, Lindeman E, Twisk J, Kwakkel G. Predicting improvement in gait after stroke. A longitudinal prospective study. *Stroke.* 2005; 36:2676-2680.

[87] Pound P, Gompertz P, Ebrahim S. A patient-centred study of the consequences of stroke. *Clinical Rehabilitation.* 1998; 12:338-347.

[88] Mayo NE, Wood-Dauphinee S, Ahmed S, Gordron C, Higgins J, McEwen S, Salbach N. Disablement following stroke. *Disability and Rehabilitation.* 1999; 21:258-268.

[89] Nadeau S, Arsenault B, Bertrand A, Gravel D, Bourbonnais D. Analysis of the clinical factors determining natural and maximal gait speeds in adults with a stroke. *American Journal of Physical Medicine and Rehabilitation.* 1999; 78:123-130.

[90] Olney SJ, Griffin MP, McBride I. Temporal, kinematic and kinetic variables related to gait speed in subjects with hemiplegia: a regression approach. *Physical Therapy.* 1994; 74:872-885.

[91] Michael KM, Allen JK, Macko RF. Reduced ambulatory activity after stroke: the role of balance, gait, and cardiovascular fitness. *Archives of Physical Medicine and Rehabilitation.* 2005; 86:1552-1556.

[92] Patterson SL, Forrester LW, Rodgers MM, Ryan AS, Ivey FM, Sorkin JD, Macko RF. Determinants of walking function after stroke: differences by deficit severity. *Archives of Physical Medicine and Rehabilitation.* 2007; 88:115-119.

[93] Fredrickson E, Ruff RL, Daly JJ. Physiological cost index as a proxy measure for the oxygen cost of gait in stroke patients. *Neurorehabilitation and Neural Repair.* 2009.

[94] Steffen TM, Hacker TA, Mollinger L. Age- and gender-related test performance in community-dwelling elderly people: six-minute walk test, berg balance scale, timed up & go test, and gait speeds. *Physical Therapy.* 2002; 82:128-137.

In: Handbook of Motor Skills
Editor: Lucian T. Pelligrino

Chapter 6

IMPLICIT MOTOR LEARNING IN DISCRETE AND CONTINUOUS TASKS: TOWARD A POSSIBLE ACCOUNT OF DISCREPANT RESULTS

S. Chambaron[1], B. Berberian[1], L. Delbecque[2], D. Ginhac[3] and A. Cleeremans[1]

[1] Unité de Recherche Conscience, Cognition,
Computation (CO3) - Université Libre de Bruxelles, Belgique
[2] Service d'Analyse des Données (SAD) -
Université Libre de Bruxelles, Belgique
[3] Laboratoire d'Electronique, Informatique et Image (LE2I) –
Université de Bourgogne, France

ABSTRACT

Can one learn implicitly, that is, without conscious awareness of what it is that one learns? Daily life is replete with situations where our behavior is seemingly influenced by knowledge to which we have little access. Riding a bicycle, playing tennis or driving a car, all involve mastering complex sets of motor skills, yet we are at a loss when it comes to explaining exactly how we perform such physical feats. Thus, while it is commonly accepted and hence unsurprising that we have little access to the cognitive processes involved in mental operations, it also appears that knowledge itself can remain inaccessible to report yet influence behavior. Reber, who coined the expression "implicit learning" in 1967, defined it as "the process whereby people learn without intent and without being able to clearly articulate what they learn" (Cleeremans, Destrebecqz, & Boyer, 1998).

The research described in this chapter is positioned at the confluence of two different domains: Implicit Learning on the one hand, and Skill Acquisition on the other. The two domains have remained largely independent from each other, but their intersection nevertheless constitutes a field of primary import: the *implicit motor learning* field. The hallmark of implicit motor learning is the capacity to acquire skill through physical practice without conscious recollection of what elements of performance have improved. Unfortunately, studies dealing with implicit motor learning are not very abundant (Pew, 1974; Magill & Hall, 1989; Wulf & Schmidt, 1997; Shea, Wulf, Whitacre, & Park,

2001). These studies provide an apparently straightforward demonstration of the possibility of unconsciously learning the structure of a complex continuous task in a more efficient way than explicit learning allows. Nevertheless, other evidence seems to challenge this view. Indeed, recent studies (Chambaron, Ginhac, Ferrel-Chapus & Perruchet, 2006; Ooteghem, Allard, Buchanan, Oates & Horak, 2008) suggest that taking advantage from the repetition of continuous events may not be as easy as previous research leads us to believe. Indeed, these studies have suggested that sequence learning in continuous tracking tasks might be artefatctually driven by peculiarities of the experimental material rather than by implicit sequence learning per se.

Consequently, a central goal of this chapter will be to reconcile these discrepant results so as to better characterize the conditions in which implicit motor learning occurs. Moreover, understanding what facilitates or prevents learning of regularities in motor tasks will be useful both in sport and in motor rehabilitation fields.

INTRODUCTION

Can one implicitly learn a motor sequence, that is, without conscious awareness of what it is that one learns? Over the past few decades, a large number of studies has been conducted in the domains of implicit learning (for reviews see Cleeremans, 1993; Berry, 1997; Stadler & Frensch, 1998; Shanks, 2003) and motor learning (for reviews see Famose, 1995; Schmidt, 1988; 1993; 1999). However, few studies have addressed issues that involve the two fields, and the two domains have remained largely independent from each other, most likely because of historical contingencies. Their intersection nevertheless constitutes a field of primary import: the *implicit motor learning* field.

The goal of this chapter is to explore the question of implicit motor learning, and is thus positioned at the confluence of two different domains: Implicit learning on the one hand, and Skill acquisition and Motor learning on the other hand. We begin by reporting on research about implicit processes and particularly findings about implicit learning. In a second part, we will focus on skill acquisition and on the distinction between discrete and continuous abilities. The next two sections discuss the notion of implicit motor learning and suggest discrepancies between results obtained in discrete and continuous tasks. The closing section of this chapter describes an attempt to reconcile these discrepant results in order to better characterize the conditions in which implicit learning occurs in both discrete and continuous tasks. In this perspective, we will introduce some recent neuroimaging studies. To conclude, we briefly discuss the relevance of such findings for both sport psychology and rehabilitation.

IMPLICIT LEARNING

Daily life is replete with examples of situations where our behavior is seemingly influenced by knowledge to which we have little access. Riding a bicycle, playing tennis or driving a car, for instance, all involve mastering complex sets of motor skills, yet we are at a loss when it comes to explaining exactly how we perform such physical feats. Such "implicit motor control" has been demonstrated by an elegant experience led by Fourneret and Jeannerod (1998). By giving erroneous visual feedback about the trajectory of a hand movement, these authors observed that participants (who could not see their hands) were nevertheless able of reaching voluntarily the desired result when drawing a straight line on a computer screen. The movement of correction necessary for this achievement was produced unconsciously, the participants being (1) neither conscious to have produced a movement of correction, (2) nor conscious of having perceived some disturbance. In other words, the change is detected, this detection results in an adapted behavior but participants are neither conscious of the change itself nor of having adapted to it. Since then, many studies have confirmed that motor control can be achieved independently of conscious perception of movement, even for voluntary actions (for a discussion see Johnson and Haggard, 2005; see also Day & Brown, 2001; Goodale, Pélisson, & Prablanc, 1986; Desmurget, Epstein, Turner, Prablanc, Alexander, & Grafton, 1999; Varraine, Bonnard, & Pailhous, 2002).

Importantly, dissociations between our ability to report on cognitive processes and the behaviors that involve these processes are not limited to motor skills, but extend to higher-level cognition as well. Thus, most native speakers of a language are unable to articulate the grammatical rules that they nevertheless follow when uttering expressions of the language. Likewise, expertise in domains such as medical diagnosis or chess, as well as social or aesthetic judgments, involves intuitive knowledge that one seems to have little introspective access to. In particular, the last years have seen a great increase in research reporting on the implicit process involved in perception. For example, recent findings about implicit change detection (Fernandez-Duque, Grossi, Thornton, & Neville, 2003; Fernandez-Duque & Thornton, 2000, 2003; Laloyaux, Destrebecqz, & Cleeremans, 2006; Laloyaux, Devue, Doyen, David & Cleeremans, 2007; Thornton & Fernandez-Duque, 2000, 2002) have suggested the continued existence of visual information that is normally inaccessible to the mechanisms underlying conscious change detection. Thus, visuomotor systems can be controlled by stimuli that are not seen consciously (Bridgeman, Hendry, & Stark, 1975; Fourneret & Jeannerod, 1998), familiarity of unrecognized faces can influence skin conductance (Bauer, 1984), and forced-choice guessing of unseen stimuli can be better than chance (Fernandez-Duque & Thornton, 2000; Merikle & Daneman, 1998; Laloyaux, Destrebecqz, & Cleeremans, 2006).

Moreover, if it is commonly accepted and hence unsurprising that we have little access to the cognitive processes involved in mental operations, it also appears that learning itself can remain inaccessible to report yet influence behavior. Arthur Reber, who coined the expression "implicit learning" in 1967, defined it as "the process whereby people learn without intent and without being able to clearly articulate what they learn". Since then, implicit learning has become a major topic of interest for psychologists (for reviews, see Cleeremans, Destrebecqz, & Boyer, 1998; Shanks, 2005; Perruchet & Pacton, 2006). This growing interest for implicit learning stems from its crucial role in the acquisition of natural language and in the development of other cognitive, social and motor abilities. Another interesting feature of implicit learning is that it has proven to be relatively insensitive to age (e.g., Howard & Howard, 1989; 1997; 2001; Curran, 1997; Kotchoubey; Haisst; Daum; Schugens & Birbaumer, 2000) and is preserved in a number of neuropsychological disorders (e.g., McDowall & Martin, 1996; Smith, Siegert, McDowall, & Abernethy, 2001; Zilmer & Spiers, 2001; Stevens, Schwarz, Schwarz, Ruf, Kolter & Czekalla, 2002). As a consequence, the phenomenon is a focus of investigation not only for laboratory researchers, but also for those oriented towards educational or clinical objectives.

Most of the implicit learning literature has focused on three main experimental paradigms. The first is the serial reaction time (SRT) tasks designed on the basis of the Nissen and Bullemer (1987) paradigm. In a typical experiment, participants are presented with a sequence of visual stimuli displayed on a computer screen, and asked to respond by pressing a corresponding sequence of keys. Unknown to them, a specific sequence of stimulus locations recurs throughout the experiment. It was found that participants respond faster to such material than to random material. The reaction time speedup suggests that subjects have learned the patterns. The second paradigm, first investigated by Reber (e.g., 1967), involves artificial grammar learning. In a typical situation, participants are first exposed to a set of consonant letter strings generated based on a finite state grammar, without being asked to learn the rules or even without being informed of the structured nature of the material. A subsequent test is performed in order to reveal whether participants have learned about the grammar. Finally, tasks involving the control of complex and interactive systems find their origin in Broadbent's studies (e.g., Broadbent, 1977). Participants are placed in front of a computer simulating a complex system, such as a city transport system, and they are unaware that the parameters of the system are governed by a linear equation. The task consists of controlling the system, that is to say, participants have to manipulate a number of parameters in order to reach and maintain a predefined target state of the system. In each of these three situations, performance of participants trained with the repeated, or *rule-based* material has been found to be better than chance, or alternatively better than performance observed in participants trained on randomly generated materials, despite the fact that people are often unable to verbalize the learned regularities.

Although relevant research on these situations has led to important conclusions about implicit learning, it is worthwhile to examine whether those conclusions generalize over new experimental settings.

MOTOR LEARNING

Motor learning is defined as a set of processes associated with practice leading to a relatively permanent change in the capability for responding (Schmidt and Lee, 1999). In other words, motor learning is the process of improving the motor skills, the smoothness and accuracy of movements. It is obviously necessary for complicated movements such as speaking or playing the piano, but it is also important for calibrating simple movements like reflexes, as parameters of the body and environment change over time.

Whereas initial theoretical views of motor learning suggested that the motor commands and the sensory feedback were all that are needed to be stored in memory for learning to occur (Adam, 1987), more recent points of view highlight the important role of cognition in motor skills (Magill. 1993; Schmidt, 1988). Indeed, in order to accomplish a task, subjects must be able to anticipate, to plan, to regulate and to interpret the elements of their environment.

Moreover, different classifications of tasks suggest that the tasks are performed fundamentally differently, and that these tasks are learned with major different principles or methods. It is striking to note that almost no effort has been directed towards understanding the commonalities and differences between the learning processes involved in mastering the "continuous" skills requiring sensori-motor coordination and the "discrete" skills involved in more cognitive tasks such as Reber's Artificial Grammar Learning situation. Notice that movement behaviors have been classified in various ways. Here, we are interested in the distinction between discrete versus continuous skills. Discrete movements are those that feature a recognizable beginning and end (Schmidt, 1988). Kicking a ball, throwing, striking a match and shifting gears in a car are examples. Discrete skills can be very rapid, requiring only a fraction of second to complete (e.g., kicking, blinking an eye), but they can also require considerable time for completion. Discrete skills can also be quite cognitive in nature. Indeed, a common laboratory task is the well-known Serial Reaction Time paradigm (Nissen & Bullemer, 1987). In the standard SRT task, a target appears on successive trials in one of four possible locations on a computer screen, and participants are asked to react to the appearance of the target by pressing as fast as possible a key that spatially matches the location of the target. Unknownst to participants, the sequence of events typically consists in the repetition of the same sequence (e.g., a 12-trial sequence). A contrario, continuous movements are defined as movements that have no recognizable beginning and end (Schmidt, 1988), with behavior continuing until the movement is arbitrarily stopped. Example are swimming, running and steering a car. Continuous tasks tend to have longer movement times than do discrete tasks. A common class of continuous skills is the tracking tasks. The tracking task is characterized by a moving target that subject intends to follow with a device (joystick, computer mouse...). The subject attempts to keep tracking the moving target via certain limb movements. A very common laboratory task is the continuous tracking task. In this task, participants are asked to track a continuously moving target that follows a specific trajectory such sine-cosine wave patterns for example. Unknown to the participants, some segments of the target trajectory are predictable. To sum up, continuous tasks require continuous adjustment of the response based on a continually changing stimulus, whereas discrete tasks require discrete, punctuate responses.

Consequently, the differences between these two kinds of skills could have an impact on learning. Indeed, models of sequence learning, in general, assume that performance is facilitated in virtue of the fact that participants become progressively better able to anticipate the location where the next stimulus will appear, thus making it possible for them to achieve better motor preparation, and hence faster reaction times, for the next response. Such improved motor preparation is assumed to result from participants' progressive learning about the relationships between each sequence element and the temporal context in which it occurs. Different models make different assumptions about the nature of the representations that link each element with its temporal context. For instance, the Simple Recurrent Network (SRN, see Elman, 1990; Cleeremans & McClelland, 1991) assumes that such links are learned continuously over training as the network progressively learns to use self-developed increasingly richer representations of the contextual information to predict the location at which the next element will appear. In contrast, models such as Perruchet's PARSER (Perruchet & Vinter, 1998) assume that participants parse the sequence of successive locations that the stimulus visits into non-overlapping chunks that represent frequently observed fragments of the training material. These different assumptions have different consequences on the implicit vs. explicit nature of the acquired representations: Whereas models such as the SRN assume that preparation for the next event is largely implicit to the extent that it does not depend on declarative representations of the links between the temporal context and each sequence element, models such as PARSER assume in contrast that participants form episodic, declarative representations of such links. Consequently, it is interesting to find out if the SRN model, with its principle of anticipation, can be applied to continuous displacements. This model uses discrete components to predict the next location of a stimulus, so how can the SRN explain learning in continuous tasks? Actually, a series of experiments are in progress to bring new elements of response.

After presenting the characteristics of discrete and continuous skills, we will now focus on learning in discrete and continuous tasks. The next section will first present what implicit motor learning is. Secondly, it will describe relevant studies in the domain.

IMPLICIT MOTOR LEARNING

The hallmark of implicit motor learning is the capacity to acquire skill through physical practice without conscious recollection of what elements of performance have improved. According to Maxwell et al. (2000), implicit motor learning is characterized by "the acquisition of a motor skill without the concurrent acquisition of explicit knowledge about the performance of that skill". A classic example illustrating this process is learning to ride a bicycle. Unfortunately, studies dealing with implicit motor learning are not very abundant (Pew, 1974; Magill & Hall, 1989; Wulf & Schmidt, 1997; Shea, Wulf, Whitacre, & Park, 2001). These studies provide an apparently straightforward demonstration of the possibility of unconsciously learning the structure of a complex continuous task in a more efficient way than explicit learning allows. Such findings are in line with those obtained in implicit learning studies, using for instance the Serial Reaction Time paradigm (SRT). An impressive number of studies using the SRT task (Cleeremans & McClelland, 1991; Destrebecqz & Cleeremans, 2001; Howard & Howard, 1989; Reed & Johnson, 1994; Shanks, Wilkinson, & Channon, 2003; Willingham, Greeley, & Bardone, 1993) have shown that reaction times improve selectively for the repeated sequence.

Congruently, studies of implicit learning in continuous tasks provide an apparently straightforward demonstration of the possibility of unconsciously learning the structure of a complex continuous task in a more efficient way than explicit learning permits. In Pew (1974) and in Wulf and Schmidt (1997), participants were asked to track a moving target by acting on a hand-driven lever. The target moved along a horizontal axis, according to the y-value of a polynomial function. The experimental sessions consisted of a succession of trials, with each trial divided into three segments. Typically, the first and the third segment were generated by a function in which the coefficients were randomly drawn on each occasion, hence generating pseudo-random target displacements. The same function served to generate the second segment, but the coefficients were now fixed, and hence, the movement described by the target around the middle of each trial was the same across the whole training session. The tracking accuracy of participants improved only on the repeated segment. Shea, Wulf, Whitacre, and Park (2001) generalized these results to a situation in which participants had to track the target by moving the platform of a stabilometer on which they were standing.

The robustness of these results suggests that human participants are particularly prone to detect and exploit such sequential regularities. In sum, participants seem able to implicitly learn regularities embedded both in continuous tasks (*i.e*, a tracking task) and in discrete tasks (*i.e* SRT task).

Nevertheless, other evidence seems challenge this view. Indeed, recent studies (Chambaron, Ginhac, Ferrel-Chapus & Perruchet, 2006; Ooteghem, Allard, Buchanan, Oates

& Horak, 2008) suggest that benefiting from the repetition of continuous events may not be as easy as previous researches lead us to believe. In an attempted to replicate prior results in continuous tracking tasks, Chambaron et al. (2006) found that participants failed to learn the repeated segment in several experiments in which the design of the studies by Wulf and collaborators was followed, except that a different repeated segment was used for each subject in order to ensure a sound control over the idiosyncratic properties of this segment. A plausible explanation for the discrepancy between these different results could be relied on the properties of the repeated segment. In particular, Wulf and collaborators used the same repeated segment in most of their experiments. Unfortunately, the speed of displacement and the acceleration of the target in this segment were found to be lower than in the random segments used to assess the baseline. In other worlds, a possible alternative is that much of the evidence for implicit learning in a continuous tracking task could be due to the selection of a repeated segment that is especially easy to track. Such an alternative is supported by recent result of Ooteghem and collaborators (2008) which shows that sequence learning in continuous tracking tasks might be driven in part by peculiarities in the repeated segment and not implicit sequence learning per se Implicit learning in discrete and continuous motor tasks

IMPLICIT LEARNING IN DISCRETE MOTOR TASKS: CONSENSUAL RESULTS

Although several tasks have been used to investigate implicit learning (e.g.,artificial grammar learning task proposed by Reber, 1967, dynamic control task used by Berry and Broadbent, 1984) , the motor sequence learning tasks are increasingly popular. In the most typical paradigm, usually coined as the Serial Reaction Time (SRT) task developed by Nissen and Bullemer (1987), a target stimulus appears on successive trials at one of a limited number of positions. Participants are asked to react to the appearance of the target by pressing a key that spatially matches the location of the target on a keyboard. Unknown to participants, the sequence of events is not random. It usually consists of the continuous cycling of the same sequence. Learning is attested by the fact that reaction times (RTs) progressively decrease with practice of the repeated sequence and suddenly increase when a random sequence is unexpectedly inserted (Destrebecqz & Cleeremans, 2001; Reed & Johnson, 1994; Shanks & Johnstone, 1999). This indicates that participants have acquired knowledge about the structured nature of the repeated sequence. However, even if it has been shown that participants have demonstrated sequence learning, the debate about the nature of the acquired knowledge (implicit versus explicit) remains open, but we do not develop these considerations here.

Moreover, several reasons justify the current success of the SRT paradigm. There is no doubt that sequential behavior is involved in virtually any real-world abilities, from language processing to the organization of movements, thus ensuring good ecological validity to sequential tasks. The use of a visual-motor implementation makes a quantitative assessment of learning easy to obtain, and robust learning has proven to be possible within a short time in a large variety of populations, from children (Vinter & Perruchet, 2000) to elderly people (Howard & Howard, 1997). Another advantage of the SRT task over some other tasks of implicit learning is that participants are in truly incidental conditions of learning, because the effect of regularities can be assessed without participants having been informed about the presence of hidden regularities (Cleeremans, 1993; Destrebecqz & Cleeremans, 2001). Finally, it has been shown that the reliability of SRT tasks is pretty good when compared with other tasks of implicit learning (Salthouse, McGuthry & Hambrick, 1999). This latter property is essential when the aim of the researcher is to compare the learning abilities of different samples of participants, and moreover when the residual learning abilities of patients need to be assessed on an individual basis.

Since the initial study by Nissen and Bullemer (1987), SRT tasks have been the object of a huge number of investigations, which have led to both the emergence of a number of variants and the growing sophistication of methodological controls (e.g., Curran & Keele, 1993; Perruchet, Bigand & Benoit-Gonnin, 1997; Ziessler & Nattkemper, 2001; Bischoff-Grethe, Goedert, Willingham, & Grafton, 2004; Osman, Bird & Heyes, 2005; Chambaron, Ginhac, & Perruchet, 2008). Nevertheless, all the studies agree that implicit learning in discrete tasks is remarkably robust whatever the procedural or methodological modifications carried out in the SRT task. We can thus conclude that a consensus emerges concerning the robustness of implicit sequential learning.

Do the results obtained with discrete tasks generalize to continuous motor tasks? This is the object of the next section.

IMPLICIT LEARNING IN CONTINUOUS MOTOR TASKS: DISCREPANT RESULTS

The studies exploring implicit motor learning in continuous tracking tasks (Pew, 1974, Exp. 1; Shea, Wulf, Whitacre, and Park, 2001; Wulf and Schmidt, 1997) are of particular interest. In the studies by Pew (1974) and by Wulf and Schmidt (1997), participants were asked to track a moving target by acting on a hand-driven lever. The target moved along a horizontal axis, according the y-value of a polynomial function. The experimental sessions consisted of a succession of trials, with each trial divided into three segments. Typically, the first and the third segment were generated by a function in which the coefficients were randomly drawn on each occasion, hence generating pseudo-random target displacements. The same function served to generate the second segment, but the coefficients were now fixed, and hence, the movement performed by the target around the middle of each trial was the same across the entire training session (in another condition, the repeated segment was the third one). Participants' tracking accuracy improved over the experiment, but only for the repeated segment. Shea et al. (2001) generalized those results to a situation in which participants had to track the target by moving the platform of a stabilometer on which they were standing. In a first experiment, in each of four successive practice sessions, participants performed two blocks of seven 75-s trials. Unknown to the subjects, each trial was divided into three 25-s segments. The target moved pseudo-randomly during the first and the last segments of each trial, whereas the middle segment was the same throughout the four sessions. A fifth session included a retention test, in which it appeared that Segment 2 was completed with fewer errors than Segments 1 and 3. In a subsequent interview, none of the participants mentioned that a segment had been repeated, even when they were directly questioned about this possibility. Furthermore, participants responded randomly when they were informed about the repetition of a segment and asked to identify whether this was the first, second, or third segment. Finally, the participants were unable to select the repeated segment better than chance would predict when this segment was displayed again among randomly generated segments in a subsequent forced-choice recognition test. These results essentially replicated those obtained by Pew (1974) and Wulf and Schmidt (1997) in a simpler task involving manual pursuit tracking. These studies also showed that the participants selectively improved the accuracy of their tracking on the repeated segment, although they were found to be unaware of the repeated segment and its location within a trial in subsequent recall and recognition tests. Shea et al.'s (2001) Experiment 2 used the same task as that in Experiment 1, except that the random segment was now the middle segment, and the repeated identical segments were the initial and final ones. The authors manipulated the information given to the participants about the structure of the task. Half of the participants were informed that the first third of each trial was repeated, whereas the other half were informed that the repetition concerned the last third of each trial. In a subsequent interview, only one out of the 16 participants mentioned that another segment was repeated in addition to the one designated during the instructions. Thus this design made it possible to compare performance in instructed and non-instructed conditions, without any confound due to the position of the repeated segments within the sequence. It turned out that explicit instructions produced better performances in the early phase of practice, although not at a significant level. However, this pattern was reversed with practice. In the retention test in Session 5, there were significantly fewer errors on the repeated-unknown segment than on the repeated-known segment. Thus these results show that explicit information about the structure of the task has a detrimental effect on performance.

These studies provide an apparently straightforward demonstration of the possibility of unconsciously learning the structure of a complex task in a more efficient way than explicit learning allows.

Although the occurrence of learning in this situation is not surprising given the close parallel between continuous tracking tasks and other implicit learning situations, and especially SRT tasks (Rosenbaum, Carlson, & Gilmore, 2001), there is at least one intriguing point of departure between the results collected in the new and in the classical situations. With the latter, most studies report some degree of explicit knowledge about the regularities of the material when this knowledge was investigated in post-experimental tests (e.g., Dulany, Carlson, & Dewey, 1984; Perruchet, Bigand, & Benoit-Gonin, 1997; Shanks & St.John, 1994; Shanks & Perruchet, 2002). Studies on continuous tracking report a different outcome. In Shea et al. (2001) for instance, none of the participants mentioned that a segment had been repeated in a subsequent interview, even when they were directly questioned about this possibility. Furthermore, participants responded randomly when they were informed about the repetition of a segment and asked to identify whether this was the first, second or third segment. Finally, the participants were unable to select the repeated segment better than chance would predict when this segment was displayed again among randomly generated segments in a subsequent forced-choice recognition test. These results essentially replicate those previously obtained by Pew (1974) and Wulf and Schmidt (1997). These studies also suggested that the participants were unaware of the repeated segment and of its location within a trial in subsequent recall and recognition tests.

In an earlier comment, Perruchet, Chambaron, & Ferrel-Chapus, (2003) suggested that this discrepancy could be due to the fact that the knowledge explored in the post-experimental tests in pursuit tracking experiments did not match the knowledge that was actually responsible for the behavioural improvement. The features explored in the post-experimental tests were (1) the fact that the very same segment is repeated throughout the study phase and (2) the location of this segment within the overall sequence (first, second, or third segment). Perruchet et al. (2003) demonstrated that neither of those features is necessary for performance improvement and, furthermore, they pointed out that neither of these features was actually learned in conventional SRT tasks. Rather, participants in SRT tasks gain knowledge of small chunks composed of 2 or 3 trials (e.g., Buchner, Steffens, & Rothkegel, 1998; Perruchet & Amorim, 1992).

What about the possibility that the conclusions made based on SRT tasks are in fact tightly linked to a very specific experimental setting? A prior study of Chambaron and colleagues (2006) indeed suggests that benefiting from the repetition of events may not be as easy as SRT research leads us to believe. They found that participants failed to learn the repeated segment in several experiments in which the design of the studies by Wulf and collaborators was followed, except that a different repeated segment was used for each subject in order to ensure sound control over the idiosyncratic properties of this segment. A plausible explanation for the discrepancy between Chambaron's results and those of Wulf and collaborators is that most of the experiments by Wulf and collaborators used the same repeated segment, and that the speed of displacement and the acceleration of the target in this segment were found to be lower than in the random segments used to assess the baseline. In support of this hypothesis, Chambaron and colleagues obtained positive results when using this same repeated segment for all participants. Overall, these results suggest that much of the evidence for implicit learning in a continuous tracking task could be due to the selection of a repeated segment that is particularly easy to track. The consequences of this for our concern are straightforward: Learning from event repetitions may not be as easy as studies involving SRT tasks seem to suggest. Such a finding is supported by recent results from Ooteghem and collaborators (2008). These authors examined changes in the motor organization of postural control in response to continuous, variable amplitude oscillations evoked by a translating platform and explored whether these changes reflected implicit sequence learning. Results showed similar improvements for the random and repeated segments, indicating that participants did not exploit the sequence of perturbations to improve balance control. They concluded that implicit sequence learning does not occur for compensatory posture control under conditions where other regularities exist in the perturbation environment. Finally, they argued that sequence learning in continuous tracking tasks might be driven in part by peculiarities in the repeated segment and not by implicit sequence learning per se.

IMPLICIT MOTOR LEARNING: TOWARD A POSSIBLE ACCOUNT OF DISCREPANT RESULTS

A large body of neuroimaging studies has explored motor skill learning. Studies in animals and humans have shown that motor cortical regions, the cerebellum, and the basal ganglia are significantly involved in learning skilled movements (Graybiel, 1995; Thach, 1996; Doyon, 1997; Karni et al., 1998; Van Mier, 2000). Current models suggest that different networks of cortical and subcortical regions are preferentially involved in the early and late phases of skill acquisition (Karni et al., 1998; Hikosaka et al., 1999; Van Mier, 2000; Doyon and Ungerleider, 2002). Neuroimaging studies of motor sequence learning have shown decreasing cerebellar activation as a task is learned, accompanied by increased activation in the basal ganglia, primary motor cortex (M1), and in the supplementary motor area (SMA) (Grafton et al., 1994; Jenkins et al., 1994; Karni et al., 1995; Doyon et al., 1996, 1999; Van Mier et al., 1997; Toni et al., 1998).

Recently, Doyon, Penhune and Ungerleider (2003) showed that changes in the brain depend not only on the stage of learning (Doyon and Ungerleider, 2002) but also on whether subjects are required to learn a new sequence of movements (motor sequence learning) or to learn to adapt to environmental perturbations (motor adaptation). This model of Doyon and collaborators proposes that the cortico-striatal and cortico-cerebellar systems contribute differentially to motor sequence learning and motor adaptation. It is therefore interesting to ask whether different cerebral systems are also involved in learning in discrete vs. continuous tasks.

Concerning continuous tasks, a convincing study by Maquet and collaborators (Maquet, Schwartz, Passingham, & Frith, 2003) seems to contrast with earlier results obtained by Chambaron et al. (2003, 2006). In this study, subjects were trained on a pursuit task in which the target can move along the two dimensions, that is to say on the horizontal and vertical axes. This task was a particular version of the pursuit task (Frith, 1973) in which the target trajectory was predictable on the horizontal axis but not on the vertical axis. Moreover, in this study, the authors were also interested in the impact of sleep deprivation on the learning. Participants were tested during a functional magnetic resonance imaging (fMRI) scanning session. Functional magnetic resonance imaging revealed task-related increases in brain responses to the learned trajectory, as compared with a new trajectory. According to the findings obtained by Maquet and collaborators, positive learning results were obtained using a two-dimensional tracking task. Such results contrast with previous results obtained by Chambaron et al. (2003, 2006). Thus it seems that the introduction of a second dimension in the experimental material makes it possible for participants to learn about the regularities contained in the target's movements. Adding a second dimension seems permit a better identification because, we can suppose that, it is a more "ecological" situation. This is an argument leading to a possible explanation of discrepant in continuous tasks.

Consequently, it is interesting to ask if different cerebral systems are involved in learning of discrete and continuous tasks. To further investigate this issue, we (Chambaron, Ginhac, Cleeremans and Peigneux, in prep) have attempted to test subjects in comparable SRT and continuous tracking situations, using strictly identical material in which the 2D target trajectory (tracking) or stimulus moves (SRT) were predictable on one of the two dimensions: axes. In other words, a perfect matching exists between these two tasks concerning the design; only the nature of the task differs. For half of the participants, the target trajectory was predictable on the horizontal but not on the vertical axis, and vice versa for the other half. The subjects will perform both the tracking task and the SRT task in the scanner. A mirror box will allow them to view the display. Subjects will be simultaneously shown the positions of a moving target and of a joystick. By manipulating a custom made joystick with their non-dominant hand (left hand), the subjects can move the position of the joystick on the screen. The left hand is chosen to ensure that performance on the tasks does not rely on preexisting motor skills such as writing or drawing. Participants do not know that the trajectory followed by the target is manipulated in a similar way as in Maquet, Schwartz, Passingham, & Frith

(2003). The trajectory followed by the target was easily predictable along the horizontal axis but very difficult to predict along the vertical axis. With such a protocol, we will be able to explore the neural bases of learning in discrete and continuous conditions. Thus, we can hypothesize that two distinct cerebral systems are implied in these two kinds of tasks. If this indeed proves to be the case, we would be able to understand why discrepant results exist in the literature. Succeed in reconciling these discrepant results in order to better characterize the conditions in which implicit learning occurs in both discrete and continuous tasks would be an important result. Indeed, understand what facilitates or prevents learning of regularities in motor tasks will be useful both in sport and in motor rehabilitation fields.

CONCLUSION

The main goal of this chapter was to explore the field of implicit motor learning. As we mentioned, an abundant literature exists concerning both implicit learning and motor learning, but the literature concerning specifically implicit motor learning is more limited. We have reported on the main findings in these domains. Whereas consensual results emerge when discrete tasks are used, continuous tasks have led to divergent findings. Consequently, neuroimaging studies represent an interesting way of understanding (and maybe resolving) these discrepancies.

Theories and results stemming from the fields of implicit learning and of motor learning represent a valuable source of support for problems encountered in rehabilitation. Indeed, a large portion of the rehabilitation experience after stroke relies on implicit learning. Boyd and Winstein (2006) concluded that for healthy participants, explicit information appears helpful for learning. A contario, after stroke, some forms of explicit information are less beneficial for the patients. Consequently, it is important that therapists adapt their interventions to facilitate motor skill learning. It is likely that to optimize rehabilitation outcomes alternative methods of prescriptive information may be more useful to the learner than are explicit instructions. Clearly, success in exploring and circumscribing conditions enabling better implicit motor learning in healthy people and after stroke represent a challenge both for researchers and therapists. Obviously, much more research is needed in the behavioral and neuroimaging domains.

REFERENCES

Adams, J. A. (1987). Historical review and appraisal of research on the learning, retention, and transfer of human motor skills. *Psychological Bulletin. 101*, 41-74.
Bauer, R. (1984). Autonomic recognition of names and faces in prosopagnosia: A neuropsychological application of the guilty knowledge test. *Neuropsychologia. 22*, 457-469.
Berry, D. C. (1997). *How implicit is implicit learning.* Oxford: Oxford University Press.
Berry, D. C. & Broadbent, D. E. (1984). On the relationship between task performance and associated verbalizable knowledge. *Quarterly Journal of Experimental Psychology. 36A*, 209-231.

Bischoff-Grethe A., Goedert K.M., Willingham D.T., Grafton S.T. (2004). Neural substrates of response-based sequence learning using fMRI. *Journal of Cognitive Neurosciences. 16(1),*127-138.

Boyd, L.A. & Winstein, C.J. (2006). The interaction between explicit knowledge, task demand and focal brain damage on implicit motor sequence learning. *Journal of Neurologic Physical Therapy.* 30, 46-57.

Bridgeman, B., Hendry, D., & Stark, L. (1975). Failure to detect displacement of the visual world during saccadic eye movements. *Vision Res. 15*(6), 719-722.

Broadbent, D. E. (1977). Levels, hierarchies, and the locus of control. *Quarterly Journal of Experimental Psychology. 29,* 181-201.

Buchner, A., Steffens, M. C. & Rothkegel, R. (1998). On the role of fragmentary knowledge in a sequence learning task. *Quarterly Journal of Experimental Psychology. 51A,* 251-281.

Chambaron, S., Ginhac, D., Ferrel-Chapus, C. & Perruchet, P. (2006) Implicit learning of a Repeated Segment in Continuous Tracking: A Reappraisal. *The Quarterly Journal of Experimental Psychology.* 59A, 845-854.

Chambaron, S., Ginhac, D., Cleeremans, A., & Peigneux, P. (in prep). Learning discrete and continuous regularities in two-dimensional settings.

Chambaron, S., Ginhac, D., & Perruchet, P. (2008) gSRT-Soft: A generic software and some methodological guidelines to investigate implicit learning through visual-motor sequential tasks. *Behavior Research Methods. 40(2)*, 493-502.

Cleeremans, A. (1993). Mechanisms of implicit learning : Connectionist models of sequence processing. Cambridge: MIT Press.

Cleeremans, A., Destrebecqz, A., & Boyer, M. (1998). Implicit learning: news from the front. *Trends in Cognitive Sciences. 2,* 406–416.

Cleeremans, A. & McClelland, J. L. (1991). Learning the structure of event sequences. *Journal of Experimental Psychology-General, 120,* 235-253.

Curran, T. (1997). Effects of aging on implicit sequence learning: Accounting for sequence structure and explicit knowledge. *Psychological Research, 60,* 24–41.

Curran, T., and Keele, S.W. (1993)Attentional and non attentional forms of sequence learning. *Journal of Experimental Psychology: Learning, Memory, and Cognition. 19,* 189-202.

Day, B. L., & Brown, P. (2001). Evidence for subcortical involvement in the visual control of human reaching. *Brain. 124*(Pt 9), 1832-1840.

Desmurget, M., Epstein, C. M., Turner, R. S., Prablanc, C., Alexander, G. E., & Grafton, S. T. (1999). Role of the posterior parietal cortex in updating reaching movements to a visual target. *Nat. Neurosci. 2*(6), 563-567.

Destrebecqz, A. & Cleeremans, A. (2001). Can sequence learning be implicit? New evidence with the Process Dissociation Procedure. *Psychonomic Bulletin & Review.* 8 (2), 343-350.

Doyon J (1997) Skill learning. In: The cerebellum and cognition (Schmahmann J, ed), pp 273-294. San Diego: Academic

Doyon J, Owen A, Petrides M, Sziklas V, Evans A (1996) Functional anatomy of visuomotor skill learning in human subjects examined with positron emission tomography. *Eur. J. Neurosci.* 8:637-648.

Doyon, J., Penhune, V., and Ungerleider, L. (2003) Distinct contributions of the cortico-striatal and cortico-cerebellar systems to motor skill learning, *Neuropsychologia. 41*, 252–262.

Doyon J, Song A, Lalonde F, Karni A, Adams M, Ungerleider L (1999) Plastic changes within the cerebellum associated with motor sequence learning: an fMRI study. *NeuroImage. 9*:S506.

Doyon, J., & Ungerleider L. Functional anatomy of motor skill learning. (2002) In: L. Squire and D. Schacter, Editors, *Neuropsychology of Memory.* Guilford Press, New York , 225–238.

Dulany, D. E., Carlson, R. A. & Dewey, G. I. (1984). A case of syntactical learning and judgement : How conscious and how abstract? *Journal of Experimental Psychology-General. 113*, 541-555.

Elman, J. (1990) Finding structure in time. *Cognitive Science. 14,* 179-211.

Famose, J. P. (1995). L'apprentissage moteur. In R. Thomas (Ed.), *Sciences et techniques des activités physiques et sportives.* Paris: P.U.F.

Fernandez-Duque, D., Grossi, G., Thornton, I. M., & Neville, H. J. (2003). Representation of change: separate electrophysiological markers of attention, awareness, and implicit processing. *J.Cogn. Neurosci. 15*(4), 491-507.

Fernandez-Duque, D., & Thornton, I. M. (2000). Change detection without awareness: Do explicit reports underestimate the representation of change in the visual system? *Visual Cognition. 7*(1-3), 323-344.

Fernandez-Duque, D., & Thornton, I. M. (2003). Explicit mechanisms do not account for implicit localization and identification of change: An empirical reply to Mitroff et al. (2002). *Journal of Experimental Psychology: Human Perception and Performance. 29*(5), 846-858.

Fourneret, P., & Jeannerod, M. (1998). Limited conscious monitoring of motor performance in normal subjects. *Neuropsychologia. 36*(11), 1133-1140.

Frith, C. (1973) Learning rhythmic hand movements. *The Quarterly Journal of Experimental Psychology. 25,* 253–259.

Goodale, M. A., Pelisson, D., & Prablanc, C. (1986). Large adjustements in visually guided reaching do not depend on vision of the hand or perception of target dispalcement. *Nature. 320*, 748-750.

Grafton S, Woods R, Tyszka M (1994) Functional imaging of procedural motor learning: relating cerebral blood flow with individual subject performance. *Hum. Brain Map.* 1:221-234.

Graybiel, A.M. Building action repertoires: memory and learning functions of the basal ganglia, *Curr. Opin. Neurobiol. 5,* 733–741.

Hikosaka O, Nakahara H, Rand M, Sakai K, Lu X, Nakamura K, Miyachi S, Doya K (1999) Parallel neural networks for learning sequential procedures. *Trends Neurosci. 22*:464-471

Howard, D.V. & Howard, J.H. (1989). Age differences in learning serial patterns: Direct versus indirect measures. *Psychology and Aging. 4*, 357-364.

Howard, J.H., Jr., & Howard, D.V. (1997). Age differences in implicit learning of higher-order dependencies in serial patterns. *Psychology and Aging. 12*, 634-656.

Howard, D.V., & Howard, J.H., Jr. (2001). When it does hurt to try: Adult age differences in the effects of instructions on sequential pattern learning. *Psychonomic Bulletin and Review.* 8(4), 798-805.

Jenkins I, Brooks D, Nixon P, Frackowiak R, Passingham R (1994) Motor sequence learning: a study with positron emission tomography. *J. Neurosci. 14*:3775-3790

Johnson, H., & Haggard, P. (2005). Motor awareness without perceptual awareness. *Neuropsychologia. 43*(2), 227-237.

Karni A, Meyer G, Jezzard P, Adams M, Turner R, Ungerleider L (1995) Functional MRI evidence for adult motor cortex plasticity during motor skill learning. *Nature. 377*:155-158

Karni A., Meyer G., Rey-Hipolito C., Jezzard P., Adams M.M., Turner R., Ungerleider L.G. (1998). The acquisition of skilled motor performance: fast and slow experience-driven changes in primary motor cortex. *Proc. Natl. Acad. Sci. U.S.A. 95*:861– 868

Kotchoubey, B., Haisst, S., Daum, I., Schugens, M., & Birbaumer, N. (2000). Learning and self-regulation of slow cortical potentials in older adults. *Experimental Aging Research. 26*(1), 15-35.

Laloyaux, C., Destrebecqz, A., & Cleeremans, A. (2006). Implicit change identification: a replication of Fernandez-Duque and Thornton (2003). *J. Exp. Psychol. Hum. Percept. Perform, 32*(6), 1366-1379.

Laloyaux, C., Devue, C., Doyen, S., David, E., & Cleeremans, A. (2008). Undetected changes in visible stimuli influence subsequent decisions. *Conscious Cogn. 17*(3), 646-656.

Magill, R.A. (1993). Motor Learning. Concepts and applications. Madison, Wisconsin: Brown & Benchonrk.

Magill, R. A. & Hall, K. G. (1989). *Implicit learning in a complex tracking skill.* Paper presented at the 30th annual meeting of the psychonomic society, Atlanta.

Maquet, P., Schwartz, S., Passingham, R., & Frith, C. (2003). Sleep-Related Consolidation of a Visuomotor Skill: Brain Mechanisms as Assessed by Functional Magnetic Resonance Imaging. *J. Neurosci. 23,* 1432-1440.

Maxwell, J.P., Masters, R.S.W. & Eves, F.F. (2000) From novice to know-how: A longitudinal study of implicit motor learning. *Journal of Sports Sciences. 18,* 111–120

McDowall, J. and Martin, S. (1996) Implicit learning in closed head injured subjects: evidence from an event sequence learning task. *New Zealand Journal of Psycholoy. 25,* 1-6.

Merikle, P. M., & Daneman, M. (1998). Psychological investigations of unconscious processing. *Journal of Consciousness Studies. 5,* 5-18.

Nissen, M.J. & Bullemer, P. (1987). Attentional requirements of learning: Evidence from performance measures. *Cognitive Psychology. 19,* 1-32.

Osman, M., Bird, G., & Heyes, C.M. (2005) Action observation supports effector-dependent learning of finger movement sequences. *Experimental Brain Research. 165(1),* 19-27.

Ooteghem, K., Frank, J.S., Allard, F., Buchanan, J.J., Oates, A.R., & Horak, F.B. (2008). Compensatory postural adaptations during continuous, variable amplitude perturbations reveal generalized rather than sequence-specific learning. *Experimental Brain Research. 187(4),* 603-11.

Perruchet, P. & Amorim, M. A. (1992). Conscious knowledge and changes in performance in sequence learning : Evidence against dissociation. *Journal of Experimental Psychology-Learning Memory and Cognition. 18,* 785-800.

Perruchet, P., Bigand, E. & Benoit-Gonnin, F. (1997a). The emergence of explicit knowledge during the early phase of learning in sequential reaction time. *Psychological Research. 60,* 4-14.

Perruchet, P., Chambaron, S., & Ferrel-Chapus, C. (2003). Learning from implicit learning literature: Comment on Shea, Wulf, Whitacre, and Park (2001). *The Quarterly Journal of Experimental Psychology. 56A,* 769-778.

Perruchet, P. & Vinter, A. (1998). PARSER: A model for word segmentation. *Journal of Memory & Language. 39,* 246-263.

Perruchet, P., & Pacton, S. (2006). Implicit learning and statistical learning: Two approaches, one phenomenon. *Trends in Cognitive Sciences.* 10, 233-238

Pew, R.W. (1974). Levels of analysis in motor control. *Brain Research. 71,* 393-400.

Reber, A. S. (1967). Implicit learning of artificial grammars. *Journal of Verbal Learning and Verbal Behavior. 5,* 855-863.

Reed, J. & Johnson, P. (1994). Assessing implicit learning with indirect tests : Determining what is learned about sequence structure. *Journal of Experimental Psychology-Learning Memory and Cognition. 20,* 585-594.

Rosenbaum, D. A., Carlson, R. A. & Gilmore, R. O. (2001). Acquisition of intellectual and perceptual-motor skills. *Annual Review of Psychology. 52,* 453-470.

Salthouse, T. A., McGuthry, K. E., & Hambrick, D. Z. (1999). A framework for analyzing and interpreting differential age patterns: Application to three measures of implicit learning. *Aging, Neuropsychology, & Cognition. 6,* 1-18.

Schmidt, R. A. (1988). *Motor control and learning: a behavioral emphasis.* (2nd ed.). Champaign, IL.: Human Kinetics Publishers.

Schmidt, R. A. (1993). *Apprentissage moteur et performance.* Paris: Vigot.

Schmidt, R. A. & Lee, T. D. (1999). *Motor Control and Learning: A Behavioral Emphasis, 3ème édition.* Champaign, IL: Human Kinetics.

Shanks, D. R. (2003). Attention, awareness, and implicit learning. In L. Jimenez (Ed.), *Attention and implicit learning.* (Vol. 48, pp. 11-42). Amsterdam and Philadelphia: John Benjamins.

Shanks, D. R. (2005). Implicit learning. In K. Lamberts and R. Goldstone, *Handbook of Cognition.* (pp. 202-220) . London: Sage.

Shanks, D. R., Johnstone, T. (1999). Evaluating the relationship between explicit and implicit knowledge in a sequential reaction time task. *Journal of Experimental Psychology: Learning, Memory, & Cognition. 25,* 1435-1451.

Shanks, D. R. & Perruchet, P. (2002). Dissociating between priming and recognition in the expression of sequential knowledge. *Psychonomic Bulletin & Review. 9,* 362-367.

Shanks, D. R. & St. John, M. F. (1994). Characteristics of dissociable human learning systems. *Behavioral and Brain Sciences. 17,* 367-447.

Shanks, D. R., Wilkinson, L., & Channon, S. (2003). Relationship between priming and recognition in deterministic and probabilistic sequence learning. *Journal of Experimental Psychology: Learning, Memory, and Cognition. 29,* 248–261.

Shea, C.H., Wulf, G., Whitacre, C.A., & Park, J-H. (2001). Surfing the implicit wave. *The Quarterly Journal of Experimental Psychology. 54A,* 841-862.

Smith, J., Siegert, R., McDowall, J., & Abernethy, D. (2001). Preserved implicit learning on both the serial reaction time task and artificial grammar in patients with Parkinson's disease. *Brain and Cognition. 45,* 378-391.

Stadler, M. A. & Frensch, P. A. (1998). Handbook of Implicit Learning and Implicit Memory. In P. A. Frensch & M. A. Stadler (Eds.). Thousand Oaks: SAGE.

Stevens A, Schwarz J, Schwarz B, Ruf I, Kolter T, Czekalla, J. (2002) Implicit and explicit learning in schizophrenics treated with Olanzapine and with classic neuroleptics. *Psychopharmacology. 160*, 299-306.

Thach, W. On the specific role of the cerebellum in motor learning and cognition: clues from PET activation and lesion studies in man, *Behav. Brain Sci. 19* , 411–431.

Thornton, I. M., & Fernandez-Duque, D. (2000). An implicit measure of undected change. *Spatial Vision. 14*(1), 21-44.

Thornton, I. M., & Fernandez-Duque, D. (2002). Change blindness and transsacadic integration. In J. Hyönä, D. P. Munoz, W. Heide & R. Radach (Eds.), *Progress in Brain Research.* (Vol. 140). Amsterdam: Elsevier.

Toni I, Krams M, Turner R, Passingham R (1998) The time course of changes during motor sequence learning: a whole-brain fMRI study. *NeuroImage. 8*:50-61.

Van Mier H (2000) Human learning. In: *Human brain mapping: the Systems.* (Mazziota J, ed), pp 605-662. Academic.

Van Mier H, Ojemann J, Miezin F, Akbudak E, Conturo T, Raichle M, Peterson S (1997) Practice-related changes in motor learning measured by fMRI. *Soc. Neurosci. Abstr. 23*:1051.

Varraine, E., Bonnard, M., & Pailhous, J. (2002). The top down and bottom up mechanisms involved in the sudden awareness of low level sensorimotor behavior. *Brain Res. Cogn. Brain Res. 13*(3), 357-361.

Vinter, A., Perruchet, P. (2000). Unconscious learning in children is not related to age: Evidence from drawing behavior. *Child Development. 71*, 1223-1240.

Willingham, D. B., Greeley, T., & Bardone, A. (1993). A dissociation of awareness and performance using a more sensitive declarative measure: Reply to Perruchet and Amorim. *Journal of Experimental Psychology: Learning, Memory, and Cognition. 19*, 1424-1430.

Wulf, G., & Schmidt, R.A. (1997). Variability of practice and implicit motor learning, *Journal of Experimental Psychology: Learning, Memory and Cognition. 23*, 987-1006.

Ziessler, M. & Nattkemper, D. (2001): Learning of event sequences is based on response-effect learning: Further evidence from a serial reaction task. *Journal of Experimental Psychology: Learning, Memory and Cognition. 27*, 595-613

Zilmer, E. & Spiers, M. (2001). *Principles of Neuropsychology.* Belmont, CA: Wadsworth.

In: Handbook of Motor Skills
Editor: Lucian T. Pelligrino

ISBN: 978-1-60741-811-5
© 2009 Nova Science Publishers, Inc.

Chapter 7

ON THE INABILITY TO PREDICT THE PERFORMANCE OF PROFESSIONAL GOLFERS

Russell D. Clark III
University of North Texas, Denton TX, USA

ABTRACT

This chapter reviews a growing number of studies that indicate it is difficult to predict fluctuations in the performance of professional golfers from their immediate preceding performance. Results indicate that the scores of professional golfers do not cluster together where successful performance follows successful performance ("hot streaks") and/or poor performance follows poor performance ("cold Streaks"). Professional golfers show little consistency in either their round-to-round performance or their hole-to-hole performance. Contrary to popular belief, choking under pressure is not a common occurrence among professional golfers. Evidence is presented that that the unreliability of golf scores for professional golfers is due to restriction of range. Professional golfers who play on professional tours are so nearly equal in ability that it is mainly a matter of chance who will have either better scores or the best score on any given day.

Keywords: Hot-hand phenomenon, choking under pressure, reliability, restriction of range.

INTRODUCTION

Picture each of the following scenarios. First, a professional golfer has scored par or better in his/her last ten rounds. Is the player more or less likely to score par or better on the next round? Second, another professional golfer has just performed poorly on three consecutive holes. Will the player continue to perform poorly on the next hole or will the player's performance improve. Third, a professional golfer has played well and is leading the tournament going into the last round. Will the player continue to play well and maybe win the tournament or will the player's performance be significantly worse in the last round? The critical question being asked in each scenario is can we use a player's immediate, past performance to predict the player's future performance?

In this chapter, we review a growing body of evidence that demonstrates it is very difficult to predict the performance of professional golfers (and other highly skilled athletes as well) from their immediate prior performance. Evidence exists that performance of professional golfers on any hole or round in a tournament is not a reliable predictor of their performance in the preceding hole or round. The scores of professional golfers do not cluster together where successful performance follows successful performance and poor performance follows poor performance. We cannot predict the performance of professional golfers from their immediate preceding performance. Moreover, contrary to popular belief, choking is not a common occurrence among professional golfers. The evidence for each of these assertions is reviewed, and an explanation based on the restricted range of scores for professional golfers is offered for the unreliability of golf scores for professional golfers. It is my hope that this chapter will shed light on why it is so difficult to predict the future performance of professional golfers.

THE HOT HAND IN GOLF

Gilovich, Vallone, and Tversky (1985) referred to belief that an athlete's performance during a particular period is significantly better than could be expected on the basis of the player's overall record as the "hot hand" or "streak shooting." Forthofer (1991) further classified "streak shooting" into three categories: players with "hot hands" show a significant tendency to perform better during a particular period than could be expected on the basis of their overall record; players with "cold hands" perform worse during a particular period than would be expected; and players with "hot and cold streaks" exhibit greater than expected periods where success follows success ("hot streaks") and failure follows failure ("cold streaks"). Despite the widespread belief among athletes, coaches, announcers, and sports fans that "streak shooting" occurs (Gilovich et al., 1985), the evidence for "hot and cold streaks" for highly-skilled athletes in basketball, baseball, and golf is not convincing (Bar-Eli, Avugos, & Raab, 2006).

Gilovich et al. (1985) conducted three studies that questioned the validity of streak shooting or the hot hand phenomenon among highly skilled basketball players. Evidence for streak shooting would be a positive correlation between the outcomes of previous shots and a clustering of shots such that hits follow hits and misses follow misses. Whether the study involved the field goal records of the Philadelphia 76ers during the 1980-1981season, the free-throws records of the Boston Celtics, or the performance in a controlled shooting exercise with the men and women varsity teams from Cornell University, detailed analyses failed to find support for streak shooting. There was no evidence for a positive correlation between the outcomes of successive shots. Players were just as likely to hit a basket following a miss as make a basket following a hit. Similarly, there was no evidence of systemic streaks with misses following misses and hits following hits. These results strongly suggest that successive shots by highly skilled basketball players are independent, and the sequence of hits and misses that occur for any given player is random.

Similar studies have been conducted in baseball, and the results do not support the existence of streak hitters. Siwoff, Hirdt, and Hirdt (1987) found that the probability of hitting well or poorly in a game was independent of a batter's previous performance at bat. Albright (1993) analyzed streak hitting in batting by examining the sequences of plate appearances for 501 players during an entire season. The results indicated that none of the players were consistently streaky, and the sequences of successful at bats or unsuccessful at bats did not depart significantly from randomness.

Although the results from the baseball and basketball studies failed to find the existence of streaks for individuals players, there is some evidence that streaks do exists if players as a group are analyzed as a group rather than individually. Wardrop (1995) reanalyzed the Gilovich et al. (1985) free throw data for nine members of the Boston Celtics. Although none of the individual players were streaky, the players as a group were: they hit a free throw 79% of the time after a hit compared to 74% of the time after a miss. Similarly, when Stern (1995) reexamined Albright's (1993) baseball data, evidence was found for streak scoring when players were analyzed as a group rather than individually.

Vergin (2000) extended the investigation of "hot" and "cold" streaks to include the outcomes of team sport games. Vergin (2000) analyzed the winning and losing streaks of the 28 Major League Baseball (MLB) teams over the 1996 season and the 29 National Basketball Association Teams over the 1996-1997 and 1997-1998 seasons; each of the 28 MLB teams played 162 games, and there were 82 games per season for the 29 NBA teams. Vergin (2000) did not find evidence for streaks or momentum effects: wins and losses were shown to be independent of the outcomes of previous games, and winning and losing streaks did not significantly differ from chance. Thus, whether we consider the outcomes for individual players or the outcomes for team sports, there is no evidence that successful performance is followed by successful performance or poor performance is followed by poor performance.

Clark (2003a) suggested that golf may be a more suitable sport to investigate streakiness than either basketball or baseball. Since shooting a basketball or hitting a baseball is such a fast paced activity, involving quick reflexive movements, there is little time for players to analyze their body movements, consider the range of potential outcomes or reflect on their previous performance. In contrast, the golfer must consciously decide when the time is right to begin the execution of a shot, and there are many opportunities for negative and positive thoughts to enter the golfer's mind. Standing over the ball, the golfer can eye the middle of the fairway but ponder the water lining the left side of the fairway and the out of bounds area off to the right. The player can also think about whether the ball will be struck cleanly. Because golf is a game that consists of many miss-hits and well-executed shots, a player's memory will contain all the ugly and also all the beautiful possibilities. In short, players have more than enough time to recall and reflect on past performance and think about the current situation as they consider the unpredictable outcome of the shot at hand. This may very well set the stage for prior performance to affect future performance.

Numerous investigators have argued that self-conscious attention to the process of performance can disrupt the performance of skilled behaviors (Baumeister & Steinhilber, 1984; Lewis & Linder, 1997; Nideffer, 1993; Zaichkowsky & Baltzell, 2001). Conscious attempts to ensure or control the behaviors that are necessary for the execution of an athletic behavior by monitoring the process of performance (e.g., the exact body and muscle movements) are likely to lead to decrements in performance, because consciousness does not contain the knowledge of the skills (e.g., muscle memory) that is necessary to successfully carry out the skilled behaviors. Well-skilled behaviors are performed best when they are carried out in an automated fashion, with as little conscious attention as possible. Compared to basketball and baseball players, the golfer has much more time to dwell on the execution of shots---worry about performing up to one's potential, revive past failures, and mentally rehearse all the mechanical thoughts—which are likely to produce poor shots and poor rounds. On the other hand, reviving past successes, expecting to hit well-executed shots, and paying minimal attention to the process of performance should lead to better shot making and lower scores.

Clark (2003a, 2003b) found streakiness over a 2-year period from 1997 to 1998 for a random group of players on the PGA Tour, Senior PGA Tour, and the LPGA Tour. For every player a sequence of rounds was formed beginning with their first round of the year and ending with their last; this was done separately for rounds in 1997 and 1998. Rounds were either coded as par or better or above par. For each tour there was a significant tendency for players' par or better rounds to cluster together and for players' above par rounds to cluster together. However, the significance of players' par or better rounds to occur together and for their above par rounds to occur together was related to the difficulty of courses rather than to any inherent tendency or disposition of players to streak. When the difficulty of courses was taken into account, the results showed that the clustering of par or better rounds was more likely to occur on easy than on difficult courses, and the clustering of above par rounds was more likely to occur on difficult than on easy courses.

The data used in the Clark (2003a, 2003b) studies were 18-hole round scores. Round scores, however, may not be the best unit of measurement when investigating streakiness. Hole-to-hole scores within tournaments may be a more sensitive measure of streakiness. A clustering of par or better holes and above par holes might be more likely to occur within tournaments because a player's performance within a round of golf should be harder to ignore than a player's performance between rounds, particularly when there have been days or even weeks between rounds as sometimes occurs. A poor shot or bad hole should be particularly salient for a player and difficult at times to ignore. When either there is excessive concern with a shot or things start to go bad, it may be difficult either to avoid recalling past failures or making conscious attempts to control the outcomes of successive shots. As a result, the player's performance suffers. On the other hand, after several consecutive par or better holes, it may be easier for a player to recall past successes, expect good shot making, and pay minimal attention to the process of performance, all of which should lead to better shot making and lower scores. Thus, an analysis of hole-to-hole scores within tournaments should identify streakiness among professional golfers, if it, in fact, occurs.

Clark (2005a) investigated streak scoring among professional golfers by examining their hole-to-hole performance within golf tournaments. For a random sample of 1997 PGA Tour players, a sequence of hole-to-hole scores beginning with a player's first hole score of each tournament and ending with his last hole score was recorded as either par or better and above par. Evidence for streakiness would occur if players' par or better holes were more likely to follow their par or better holes than if their par or better holes were to follow above par holes. The results showed no evidence for streakiness. The professional golfers were just as likely to score a par or better following an above par hole as score par or better after a par or better hole.

In the Clark (2005a) study, each hole score was recorded as either par or better and above par. Since professional golfers are supposed to score par or better on any given hole, a player who has a series of par or better holes would not be considered to have a "hot hand" or "hot streaks," but a clustering of consecutive above par holes could be considered poor performance that could represent a "cold streak." Thus, when Clark (2005a) did not find evidence for streakiness, one could say that professional golfers are not prone to have "cold streaks," i.e., they are just as likely to have an above par hole follow a par or better hole as have an above par hole follow an above par hole. Thus, Clark (2005a) investigated the occurrence of "cold streaks" in golf.

For "hot streaks" or a "hot hand" to occur in golf, a golfer's successive performance during a period of time would have to be clearly better than would be expected from the player's overall record. In golf, birdie or better scores on holes are considered exceptional performance. Evidence for "hot streaks" or a "hot hand" in golf would occur if players' birdie or better holes were more likely to follow their birdie or better holes than if their birdie or better holes were to follow par or worse holes. In a follow-up study, Clark (2005b) recoded players' hole scores in the Clark (2005a) study as either birdie or better or par or worse. Analyses gave no evidence for "hot streaks" or the "hot hand." Players were just as likely to score a birdie or better following a par or worse hole as make a birdie or better following a birdie or better hole.

In summary, the results from studies on basketball, baseball, and golf do not support the belief that highly skilled athletes have "hot streaks," "cold streaks, " or both "hot" and "cold streaks." Rather, the evidence indicates that the sequence of hits and misses for collegiate and professional basketball players, hits and outs by professional baseball players and par or better holes and above par holes or birdie and better holes and par or above holes for professional golfers do not differ from chance. Thus, the literature on "hot" and "cold streaks" indicate that we are not able to use immediate, prior performance to predict future performance.

INDEPENDENCE OF GOLF SCORES

Research has yielded little consistency in round-to-round performance for professional golfers. Mosteller and Youtz (1993) found a mean correlation of .06 between the third and forth round scores of players from 33 tournaments on the 1990 PGA Tour. Clark (2004) computed correlations between all golfers' scores on consecutive rounds within tournaments on the 1999 PGA Tour, 1999 LPGA Tour, and 1999 Senior PGA Tour; the mean correlation between scores on consecutive rounds was -.08 for players on the PGA Tour, -.03 for players on the LPGA Tour, and .27 for players on the Senior PGA Tour.

Although the results from these studies indicate that it is very difficult for professional golfers to be consistent from round to round, the golfers were investigated as a group rather than individually. It is not known whether the same lack of consistency between consecutive rounds would be evident had performance of individual players been followed through the season. Even if players in general are not very consistent from day to day, it is still possible that some individual players are.

Clark (2005c) followed the performance of 35 randomly selected players on the three major American tours from 1997 through 2000 and investigated individual player's consistency in round-to-round performance. Although the number of players showing consistency for most years exceeded chance expectations, evidence for round-to-round consistency from one year to the next was small. On no tour did any of the players show round-to-round consistency in each of the four years. No player on the LPGA Tour and Senior PGA Tour and only 6% of the players from the PGA Tour showed round-to-round consistency in any three consecutive years. Moreover, only 11% of the PGA Tour sample, 20% of the LPGA Tour, and 3% of the senior PGA Tour displayed round-to-round consistency in any two consecutive years. Thus, whether players' round scores are analyzed as a group or individually, players' round scores on any given day will be a poor predictor of their performance on the next day.

Clark (2006) investigated whether the lack of player consistency that occurs in medal play also occurs in golf's traditional format of match play, where the winner is not the player with the fewest number of strokes but the player who wins the greater number of holes. Analyses of matches from the 1999 through 2006 World Golf Championships---Accenture Match Play Championship showed that higher seeded players won only 54% of the time, and the correlation between higher seeded players winning and the difference in World Ranking between players was .17. With such a slight advantage for higher seeded players, it appears that on any given day any one of the top professional golfers in the world can beat any other over 18 holes.

Clark (2008) investigated whether the slight advantage of higher seeded players to win in match play on the PGA Tour generalizes to the LPGA Tour. The results from the three-year history of the HSBC Women's World Match Play Championship from 2005-2007 showed no significant advantage for the higher seeded player in match play.

Since the evidence indicates that the outcomes of consecutive rounds within tournaments for professional tour players are unrelated, particularly for players on the PGA Tour and LPGA Tour, the best predictor of how a professional Tour player will perform on any given day is the player's average performance for the year. For example, if a player has an overall record of scoring par or better 80% of the time, the best predictor for the player scoring par or better on any given day is 80%, adjusted for any relevant factors such as weather, injury, difficulty of course, *et cetera*.

In summary, research has yielded little consistency in the round-to-round performance of professional golfers. Whether the round-to-round performance of professional golfers is analyzed individually or players are analyzed as a group, it is evidently extremely difficult for players to be consistent from round to round. Rather, the evidence strongly suggests that the performance of professional golfers on any round in a tournament is not a reliable predictor of their performance in a preceding round. Variability in round-to-round performance is more the rule than the exception for professional golfers who play on the American professional tours.

CHOKING UNDER PRESSURE

We have all heard the term "choking" before. We talk about "choking" when a collegiate or professional basketball player badly misses a free throw to win the game, when a field goal kicker misses the extra point to win the game, and when a professional golfer when leading a tournament plays poorly in the final round, plays poorly on the final hole or misses a short putt on the last hole to win the tournament. We even say a person "choked" if the person's performs more poorly than expected during an important job interview or when taking tests to enter college or graduate study.

"Choking under pressure" is a common phrase used to describe inferior performance despite situational demands for superior performance and high motivation to succeed. Baumeister (1984, p. 610) has defined pressure as "any factor or combination of factors that increases the importance of performing well on a particular occasion" and choking as "performance decrements under pressure circumstances." Thus, choking under pressure is suboptimal performance when under pressure to perform well (Lewis & Linder, 1997; Linder, Lutz, Crews, & Lochbaum, 1999).

Findings from the laboratory studies have consistently shown that choking under pressure occurs in situations in which the desire for high-level performance is maximal (Linder et al., 1999; Beilock & Carr, 2001), in situations where individuals become overly self-conscious, extremely preoccupied with the process of performance, and distracted from the task at hand (Baumeister, 1984; Baumeister, Hamilton, & Tice, 1985; Schlenker, Weigold, & Doherty, 1991; Lewis & Linder, 1997), and in situations when supportive audience expectations are high, but performers' private internal expectations are low (Baumeister, et al., 1985; Butler & Baumeister, 1998). For a recent, thorough review of the laboratory literature on "choking under pressure", see Beilock and Gray (2007).

Although research has shown consistent support for choking under pressure in the laboratory, the participants should be considered to be slightly to moderately skilled at best. The literature on choking for highly skilled athletes in actual competition is less supportive and more controversial. Support for choking under pressure among highly skilled athletes was first demonstrated by Baumeister & Steinhilber (1984). The authors hypothesized that, when a team plays in front of a supportive, home crowd, being close to a highly desired goal (e.g., playing for a national championship) may be harmful to team performance. To test this home-field disadvantage view, Baumeister and Steinhilber (1984) analyzed the outcomes of baseball World Series From 1924-1982. They found the home team won 60% of the time in the first two games of the series but only 41% of the time in the last game; when the series went seven games, the home team won 39% of the time. However, when Schlenker, Phillips, Boniecki, & Schlenker (1995) updated the Baumeister and Steinhilber (1984) data set by including World Series played in the decades following the Baumeister and Steinhilber analysis and included data from the league championships from 1985-1993, they found the decreased performance in front of home crowds no longer occurred. In the World Series data the home team won 60% of the time in the first two games of the series compared to 47% of the time in the last game; when the game went seven games, the home team won 48% of the time. For the league championships, the home team won 63% of the time in the first two games, 50% of the time in the last game, and 67% of the time when the seventh game was necessary.

Conflicting evidence for the home field disadvantage has also been found for hockey. Gayton, Matthews, and Nickless (1987) compared Games 1-4 with the last game in the semifinal and final Stanley Cup Championship series between 1960-1985. The results supported a home field advantage: the home team won 54% of Games 1-4, 53% of the time in the last game, and 58% of the time when the seventh game was necessary. However, Wright, Voyer, Wright, and Roney (1995) found that the home team tended to win Games 1 and 3 of the Stanley Cup playoffs but lose the last game. It is difficult to reconcile these findings with those of Gayton, *et al.* (1987), because Wright *et al.* (1995) did not report either the years studied for the Stanley Cup playoffs or the percentage of wins by the home and visiting teams.

Conflicting results for the home disadvantage have also been found for professional golfers. Following the lead of Baumeister and Steinhilber (1984), Wright, Jackson, Christie, McGuire, and Wright (1991) were interested in the performance of players who had a chance to win a major championship. These investigators compared the performance of British and foreign players who were nine strokes away from the leader in each of the British Opens from 1946 to 1980. The analysis indicated the performance of the British players deteriorated more from round 1 to round 4 than did the performance of the foreign players, supporting a home-course disadvantage.

Although the greater impaired performance of the British players in the Wright *et al.* (1991) study could have been the result of playing in front of very supportive and attractive crowds, the authors encountered methodological problems that precluded unambiguous support for a choking hypothesis. The foreign players could have been better player as evidenced by their overall lower scores; there could have been other differences among the players or characteristics of British Opens (links-style course) that were responsible for the results.

Clark (2002a) investigated the existence of choking among professional golfers on the PGA Tour, Senior PGA Tour, and LPGA Tour for the year 1999. Clark (2002a) hypothesized that, if choking was prevalent among professional golfers, the player who is one stroke away from the lead going into the final round of a tournament and to a lesser extent players who were leading should have higher final round scores than those players who are three to five strokes from the lead—there should be less pressure on the latter players because they have less chance of winning. The results did not support a choking hypothesis. In both top-tier and second-tier tournaments there were no differences in final round scores for players who either were leading going into the final round or who were within five strokes of the lead. Moreover, players who entered the final round leading won the majority of the time.

The lack of choking for professional golfers in the Clark (2002a) study may be due to the veteran status of many of the players who were leading going into the final round. They have many years of experience in pressured situations and have shown themselves to be resistant to the effects of pressure on their game. This view suggests that professional golfers with less experience may be more susceptible to choking. An ideal setting may be the annual PGA Tour Qualifying Tournament (Q-School), where exemplary performance earns players a tour card that allows players automatically to enter most tour events in the coming year. If we can take the opinions of players who have successfully completed the Q-School and have gone on to have successful careers on the PGA Tour at face value, the Q-School is a highly pressured event. A truism among veterans on the PGA Tour, including players who have won the most prestigious tournaments, is that the Q-School was the most pressure-packed tournament in which they have ever played (Sampson, 2000). Given that the majority of players who enter each year's Q-School have never played on the PGA Tour and getting on the getting on the Tour may induce more stress than trying to win on Tour, the Q-School may be an ideal setting to investigate choking among professional golfers.

Clark (2002b) compared the final round scores for 775 who entered the annual PGA Tour Q-School during 1989-1995 and 1997-2000 and who entered the final round either at the cutoff for receiving a Tour card or within five strokes lower or higher than the cutoff. Clark (2002b) hypothesized that the least amount of pressure with little decrement in performance should occur for players whose scores are either four of five strokes better or worse from players at the cutoff for receiving a tour card because in the former players are likely to win earn a tour card and in the latter players are unlikely to do so. The pressure should be increased with a decrement in performance for players whose scores are either at the cutoff or one or two strokes better, because any performance less than good will likely fail to earn a tour card. The most pressure with the largest decrement in performance should be for players whose scores are one or two strokes worse than the cutoff going into the final round. Pressure should be particularly great for these players because any performance less than superb will most likely end their chances of obtaining a tour card.

The results failed to find support for choking under pressure. Final round scores for professional golfers in the PGA Tour Qualifying Tournaments who were near or at the cutoff for earning a tour card did not significantly differ from the final round scores of players who were within five strokes better or worse than players at the cutoff.

One potential serious limitation to the choking under pressure studies for professional golfers is their nomothetic perspective. The analyses in these studies were based on groups of individuals and groups of scores. These analyses do not allow for the discovery of ideographic examples of performing poorly under pressure. Data on a group of individuals make it difficult or impossible to show some very important and memorable cases of individuals performing very poorly, dramatically so, under extreme pressure. For example, in 1999 the French golfer Jean Van de Velde played the final hole of the British Open in a manner that many believe can only be viewed as choking under pressure. He lost a three-shot lead on the final hole. For a player of his ability, a very difficult golf hole should have become fairly easy if he attempted to make a five (bogey) on that par-four hole. Instead, he shot a seven by attempting to make one difficult shot after another. Although the results from most golf studies suggest that choking under pressure occurs far less frequently than most people believe, following the performance of single professional golfers over time may identify some players who do choke under pressure.

In a recent study, Clark (2007) followed the performance of 35 players who played on the PGA Tour from 1997 to 2004 and investigated whether any players were prone to choke when they were either leading or one stroke from the lead going into the final round. Choking was defined as a player having significantly higher than expected final round scores and being less likely than other professional golfers to win when either leading or one stroke from the lead. The results provided no evidence for a choking under pressure hypothesis. None of the players when in contention to win were both more likely to have higher than expected final round scores and less likely to win than other professional golfers in the sample.

Although the Clark (2007) failed to find evidence for choking under pressure, cases of individuals performing very poorly, even dramatically so, under extreme do occur. As mentioned earlier Jean Van de Velde lost a three shot lead on the last hole of the 1999 British Open and more recently Phil Mickelson shot two over par on the last hole of the 2006 U. S. Open to lose the tournament. What can be said in these graphic and vivid cases? First, vivid and dramatic events are so compelling that it is easy to assume they are commonplace (Tversky & Kahneman, 1973). To identify choking under pressure, we need to know how often a player performs poorly when both in and out of contention. It is quite possible that the two players above are just as likely to score a double or triple-bogey when out of contention as when in contention. Second, based on the data presented on Mickelson in the Clark (2007) study, one should be cautious in attributing any tendency for Mickelson to "choke." During the eight year period from 1997 to 2004, Mickelson won 63% of the time when leading going into the final round. This is hardly a sign of "choking." In short, vivid and cases like van de Velde and Mickelson example may tell us more about the powerful effects of dramatic and vivid events on individuals' memories and beliefs than they tell us about any tendency for professional golfers to choke under pressure.

In summary, the results for choking under pressure for professional baseball and hockey players are mixed with an equal number of studies finding support and no support. The bulk of choking studies for professional golfers suggest that choking under pressure is not a common occurrence on the PGA Tour. Once again, we cannot reliably use immediate prior performance to predict future performance.

IS GOLF PERFORMANCE REALLY UNPREDICTABLE? : A CASE FOR RESTRICTION OF RANGE

The restricted range of scores may be responsible for the lack of consistency in the performance of professional golfers. Professional golfers are clustered together at the extreme end of the distribution of golf ability. Round scores in a typical PGA Tour tournament are normally distributed with a SD of approximately 2.50 (Mosteller & Youtz, 1993). Thus, in any round on a Par 72 course, about two-thirds of the players would be expected to score between 69 and 75. With such a restricted range of ability among professional golfers, it is therefore mainly a matter of chance who will have the best round score or win any match play event on any given day. In other words, golf scores for professional golfers are so nearly equal for any particular round that the reliability of scores from one occasion to the next is bound to be low or quite limited (Nunnally & Berstein, 1994).

One way to directly test the plausibility of a restriction of range explanation is to compare reliability estimates of athletic performance from groups of athletes who are more variable in athletic ability and performance. Clark, Woodward, and Wood (2008) examined reliability estimates of athletic performance on hole-to-hole scores for PGA Tour players, senior club professionals, and female and male amateurs who had won their course or club championships. Compared to PGA Tour players, the authors argued that senior club professionals are likely to be both less skilled and more varied in their skills because they spend most of their time either giving lessons and/running the pro shop. Whereas some of the amateurs who have won their course or club championship may be as equally skilled as senior club professionals, many of the amateurs will be less skilled. If restriction of range explains the lack of consistency in the performance for Tour professionals, we should see low estimates of reliability for hole-to-hole performance for players on the PGA Tour. However, due to the greater variability in skills and performance of the senior club professionals and amateurs, the reliability estimates for hole-to-hole performance should be substantially higher for these two groups.

Clark et al. (2008) computed reliability estimates (e.g. Cronbach coefficient alpha) for hole-to-hole scores from 150 rounds on the 1997 PGA Tour, from one round for the 32 senior club professionals who in 2006 played in a one-day Texas Senior Qualifier for the Texas Senior Open, from three tournament rounds for the 62 male amateurs and from two tournament rounds for the 49 female amateurs—both the female and male amateurs played in the 2006 North Texas Tournament of Champions. The results supported a restriction of range hypothesis. Reliability estimates for hole-to hole scores were very small and negative for the PGA tour but positive and substantially higher (.50's and high 60's) for senior club professional and amateurs. Thus, with the greater variability in skills and performance of the senior club professionals and amateurs, there was a greater reliability of performance.

CONCLUSION AND APPLICATION

We have reviewed studies that indicate that performance of professional golfers cannot be reliably predicted from their immediate preceding performance. The performance of professional golfers on any given hole is not reliable predictor of their performance on the preceding hole. For both holes and rounds, the scores of professional golfers do not cluster together where successful performance follows successful performance and poor performance follows poor performance. Moreover, the evidence indicates that "choking" is not a common occurrence for professional golfers. The failure to predict the performance of professional golfers from immediate preceding performance is most likely due to the statistical concept of restriction of range. Professional golfers who play on tour are so nearly equal in ability that it is mainly a matter of chance who will have the better performance on any hole or round on any given day.

Whether golf performance can be predicted will depend upon the variability in ability among golfers. The reliability of golf scores will be positively related to the variability of golf ability among golfers in a given population. In a population where there are sufficient differences in golf skills, such as usually occurs with amateurs, one would expect the more skilled players to consistently have lower scores or win more matches than lesser skilled players. However, when a population consists of golfers who are so nearly equal in ability, such as occurs on the PGA Tour, it is mainly a matter of chance who will either have the better scores or win a match on any given day. We suspect as parity of skills increases in any sport, chance will be the major factor in the determination of outcomes.

It should be noted that the observed independence between successive outcomes for individual tour players extends to amateurs. Scheid (1990) computed correlations between the outcomes of previous scores for individual amateurs in a study of 3000 amateurs and found no evidence for a positive correlation between the outcomes of previous scores. The mean correlation between successive rounds was .08, and the mean correlation between successive holes was .04. The observed independence between successive outcomes simply means that within any player's range of scores any single outcome will be independent of the player's preceding outcome. That is, the scores for any individual golfer will be so restricted in range that it is mainly a matter of chance what score within any player's range of scores will be shot on any given day. Thus, the best predictor of what any individual golfer will score on any hole or round will be the player's average performance, adjusted for any relevant factors such as weather, difficulty of hole or course, injury, *et cetera*.

With athletic performance being highly dependent upon athletic skills—the greater the athlete's skills, the more successful the athlete's performance---golfers would be wise improve their skills. Using proper clubs, getting instruction, and learning and using arousal controlling techniques and strategies are proven pathways to improving skills (Crews,

Lochbaum, & Karoly, 2001). With improved skills, lower scores will follow. Yet, when the restriction of range of golf scores is an issue, as occurs for players of similar ability or for any single golfer, the ability to predict performance from the immediate preceding performance will continue to elude us. However, there is a bright side here. The inability to predict any golfer's future performance from their immediate prior performance probably plays a huge role in making golf among the most challenging and frustrating activities in which humans engage.

REFERENCES

Albright, S. C. (1993). A statistical analysis of hitting streaks in baseball. *Journal of the American Statistical Association. 88*, 1175-1183.

Bar-Eli, M., Avugos, S., & Raab, M. (2006). Twenty years of 'hot hand' research: Review and critique. *Psychology of Sport and Exercise. 7*, 525-553.

Baumeister, R. F. (1984). Choking under pressure: Self-consciousness and paradoxical effects of incentives on skilled performance. *Journal of Personality and Social Psychology. 46*, 610-620.

Baumeister, R. F., Hamilton, J. C., & Tice, D. M. (1985). Public versus private expectancy of success: confidence booster or performance pressure? *Journal of Personality and Social Psychology. 48*, 1447-1457.

Baumeister, R. F., & Steinhilber, A. (1984). Paradoxical effects of supportive audiences on performance under pressure: The home field disadvantage in sports championships. *Journal of Personality and Social Psychology. 47*, 85-93.

Beilock, S. L., & Carr, T. H. (2001). On the fragility of skilled performance: What governs choking under pressure? *Journal of Experimental Psychology: General. 130*, 701-725.

Beilock, S. L., & Gray, R. (2007). Why do athletics choke under pressure? In G. Tenebaum & R. C. Eklund (Eds.), *Handbook of sport psychology. (3rd edition)*. Hoboken, New Jersey: John Wiley & Sons, Inc. Pp. 425-444.

Butler, J. L., & Baumeister, R. F. (1998). The trouble with friendly faces: Skilled performance with a supportive audience. *Journal of Personality and Social Psychology. 75*, 1213-1230.

Clark, R. D. III (2002a). Do professional golfers choke? *Perceptual and Motor Skills. 94*, 1124-1130.

Clark, R. D. III (2002b). Evaluating the phenomenon of choking in professional golfers. *Perceptual and Motor Skills. 95*, 1287-1294.

Clark, R. D. III (2003a). Streakiness among professional golfers: Fact or fiction? *International Journal of Sport Psychology. 34*, 63-79.

Clark, R. D. III (2003b). An analysis of streaky performance on the LPGA Tour. *Perceptual and Motor Skills. 97*, 365-370.

Clark, R. D. III (2004). On the independence of golf scores for professional golfers. *Perceptual and Motor Skills. 98*, 675-681.

Clark, R. D. III (2005a). An examination of hole-to-hole scores on the PGA Tour. *Perceptual and Motor Skills. 100*, 806-814.

Clark, R. D. III (2005b). An examination of the "hot hand" in professional golfers. *Perceptual and Motor Skills. 101*, 935-942.

Clark, R. D. III (2005c). An analysis of players' consistency among professional golfers: A longitudinal study. *Perceptual and Motor Skills. 101*, 365-372.

Clark, R. D. III (2006). The beauty of match play. *Perceptual and Motor Skills. 102*, 815-818.

Clark, R. D. III (2007). A longitudinal study of "choking" in professional golfers. *Perceptual and Motor Skills. 105*, 827-837.

Clark, R. D. III (2008). Parity of match play: An LPGA replication. *Perceptual and Motor Skills. 107*, 222-224.

Clark, R. D. III, Woodward, K. L., & Wood, J. M. (2008). On the unreliability of golf scores for professional golfers: A case for restriction of range. *Perceptual and Motor Skills. 107*, 683-690.

Crews, D. J., Lochbaum, M. R., & Karoly, P. (2001). Self-regulation: Concepts, methods, and strategies in sport and exercise. In R. N. Singer, H. A. Hausenblas, & C. M. Janelle (Eds.), *Handbook of sport psychology.* (2nd ed.). New York: Wiley. Pp. 566-581.

Forthofer, R. (1991). Streak shooter—The sequel. *Chance. 4*, 46-48.

Gilovich, T., Vallone, R., & Tversky, A. (1985). The hot hand in basketball: On the misperception of random sequences. *Cognitive Psychology. 17*, 295-314.

Gayton, W. F., Matthews, G. R., & Nichols, C. (1987). The home field disadvantage in sports championships: Does it exist in hockey? *Journal of Sports Psychology. 9*, 183-185.

Lewis, B. P., & Linder, D. E. (1997). Thinking about choking? Attentional processes and paradoxical performance. *Personality and Social Psychology Bulletin. 23*, 937-944.

Linder, D. E., Lutz, R., Crews, D., & Lochbaum, M. (1999). Who chokes and when? Situational and dispositional factors in failure under pressure. In M. R. Farrally & A. J. Cochran (Eds.*), Science and golf: III.* London: E & FN Spon. Pp. 207-212.

Mosteller, F., & Youtz, C.)1993). Where eagles fly. *Chance. 6*, 37-42.

Nideffer, R. M. (1993). Concentration and attention control training. In J. M. Williams (Ed.), *Applied sport psychology: Personal growth to peak performance.* London: Mayfield Publishing Company. Pp. 243-261.

Nunnally, J. C., & Bernstein, I. H. (1994). *Psychometric theory. (3rd ed.)* New York: McGraw-Hill.

Sampson, C. (2000). Under pressure. *Golf Magazine.* January. 137-140.

Schlenker, B. R., Phillips, S. T., Boniecki, K. A., & Schlenker, D. R. (1995). Championship pressures: Choking or triumphing in one's own territory? *Journal of Personality and Social Psychology. 68*, 632-643.

Schlenker, B. R., Weigold, M. F., & Doherty, K. (1991). Coping with accountability: self-identification and evaluative reckonings. In C. R. Snyder & D. R. Forsyth (Eds.), *The handbook of social and clinical psychology.* New York: Pergamon. Pp. 96-115.

Scheid, F. (1990). On the normality and independence of score scores, with applications. In A. J. Cochran (Ed.), *Science and golf: Proceedings of the first world scientific congress of golf.* London: F & FN Spon. Pp. 147-152.

Siwoff, S., Hirdt, S., & Hirdt, P. (1987). *The 1987 Elias baseball analyst.* New York: Collier Books.

Stern, H. S. (1995). Who's hot and who's not: Runs of success and failure in sports. *In 1995 Proceedings of the Section on Statistics in Sports. American Statistical Association.* 26-35.

Tversky, A., & Kahneman, D. (1973). Availability: A heuristic for judging frequency and probability. *Cognitive Psychology.* 5, 207-302.

Vergin, R. C. (2000). Winning streaks in sports and the misperception of momentum. *Journal of Sport Behavior.* 23, 181-197.

Wardrop, R. L. (1995). Simpson's paradox and the hot hand in basketball. *The American Statistician. 49,* 24-28.

Wright, E. F., Jackson, W., Christle, S. D., McGuire, G. R., & Wright, R. D. (1991). The home-course disadvantage in golf championships: Further evidence for the undermining effect of supportive audiences on performance under pressure. *Journal of Sport Behavior. 14*, 51-60.

Wright, E. F., Voyer, D., Wright, R. D., & Roney, C. (1995). Supporting audiences and performance under pressure: The home-ice disadvantage in hockey championships. *Journal of Sport Behavior. 18*, 21-28.

Zaichkowsky, L. D., & Baltzell, A. (2001). Arousal and performance. In R. N. Singer, H. A. Hausenblas, & C. M. Janelle (Eds.), Handbook *of sport psychology. (2nd ed.)* New York: John Wiley and Sons, Inc. Pp. 319-339.

In: Handbook of Motor Skills
Editor: Lucian T. Pelligrino

ISBN: 978-1-60741-811-5
© 2009 Nova Science Publishers, Inc.

Chapter 8

MOVEMENT RELATED BRAIN MACROPOTENTIALS AND SKILLED MOTOR ACTIONS

Giuliano Fontani*, Silvia Migliorini,
Leda Lodi and Fausto Corradeschi
Department of Physiology, University of Siena, Siena, Italy

ABSTRACT

Background: Movement Related Brain Macropotentials (MRBMs) are electrical brain potentials occurring before, during and after skilled movements. Specific components of these potentials have been described and it has been reported that they can be recorded also during mental motor imagery and can be influenced by practice. To understand the exact relationship between MRBMs and skilled actions and to verify the hypothesis that motor training could modify MRBMs profile and influence specific components an experiment has been performed in which MRBMs were recorded during the execution of different skilled performance tasks and before and after a period of training.

Methods: The experiment has been carried out with 31 healthy male subjects, divided into three groups. Eleven performed the Alert test (A), a simple reaction time test, in which the subject had to press in a precise sequence three keys of a keyboard when a figure appeared on the computer monitor. Ten subjects performed the Choice test (CH), a complex reaction time test, in which they had to press the three keys in a different order when one of two different figures appeared randomly on the screen. Ten subjects performed the Choice test with the addition of a Go/No-Go paradigm (CHNG) in which participants had also to repress an unsuitable response. All subjects were tested before and after 10 days of training. During the trials EEG, EMG and other physiological parameters were recorded. The time of the recorded test was divided into three periods: prestimulus, motor (premotor, motor action, motor completion) and postmotor. Data were collected, averaged and compared by appropriate statistical methods.

---

* Corresponding author: Prof. Giuliano Fontani, Dipartimento di Fisiologia, Università di Siena, Via A. Moro 3, I-53100 Siena, Italy; Tel.: +39 0577 234036; Fax: 0577234037; e-mail: fontanig@unisi.it

Results: The time of EMG activation and Reaction Time (RT) were lower in A then in CH and CHNG. Training did not influenced A, but was followed by a significant reduction of RT in CH and CHNG. The profile of MRBMs was different in the motor period in the three tests. The duration of Premotor Potential (PMP), a positive wave recorded in the premotor component of the motor period, increased passing from A to CHNG, but after training, it was reduced only in the CHNG test. During motor action the duration of the negative wave Motor Cortex Potential (MCP) increased from A to CHNG and was reduced after training in all tests. In CHNG training reduced the latency of N1 and N2, the negative peaks recognizable in the MCP profile, and the latency of the Skilled Performance Positivity (SPP), a wave occurring in the postmotor period. Moreover, after training the period preceding the stimulus showed an increase of negativity in the last 200 msec.

Conclusions: MRBMs can change their profile in relation to the characteristics of the test and the skilled motor action. The increase of duration and latency of the motor period waves, passing from A to CHNG, can be considered as picture of increased information processing and response selection brain activity. Moreover, training can affect the profile of the waves, reducing their duration and latency, particularly when the performance requires high mental effort.

Keywords: MRBMs, Motor action, Brain activity, Reaction Time, Training.

INTRODUCTION

Motor behavior can be divided into two groups: simple action movements and complex motor tasks. These are goal-directed and require strategies of learning and training which often influence performance results. For this reason, many strategies have been developed to improve skilled movements, not only by means of detailed study and practice of motor execution (Yan & Dick, 2006), but also by trying to develop precise mental representations of the motor ability (Solodkin, Hlustik, Chen, & Small, 2004). Skilled movements development is associated with variations of brain activity (Fontani, et al., 2007). In particular, the profiles of some cortical potentials can change concomitantly with acquisition and learning of motor behavior. For example, it is possible to associate specific indices of brain activity, e.g., event-related potentials (ERP), with a sequence of motor acts, such as motor preparation and execution. Some electrical brain potentials seem to be closely related to movement (Kornhuber & Deecke, 1965; Shibasaki, Barret, Halliday, & Halliday, 1980) and in particular to skilled motor activities (Papakostopoulos, 1978; Fattapposta, Amabile, Cordischi, Di Venezio, Foti, Pierelli, D'Alessio, Pigozzi, Parisi, & Morrocutti, 1996).

In some studies, many using an interactive task or skilled performance task, the time of the recorded test was divided into three periods: premotor, motor and postmotor. Moreover, the motor period was divided into a motor sensory period and a subsequent motor completion period. In these periods, a sequence of brain potentials, Movement Related Brain Macropotentials (MRBMs), occurs in relation to execution of the skilled movement (figure 1) (Chiarenza, 1991; Fattapposta, et al., 1996). MRBMs have been recognized during skilled performance tasks in normal, developmental and pathological conditions (Chiarenza, Papakostopolous, Giordana, & Guareschi Cazzullo, 1983; Chiarenza, 1986) and have been studied in trained and untrained subjects, where differences have been described as a consequence of long-term practice (Fattapposta, et al., 1996; Di Russo, Pitzalis, Aprile, &

Spinelli, 2005). Scalp and cortical recordings have shown that many of these potentials are easily recognizable when recorded in the precentral and central regions of the brain, in particular, via electrodes placed at Cz and Fz (Papakostopoulos & Crow, 1984; Fattapposta, et al., 1996).

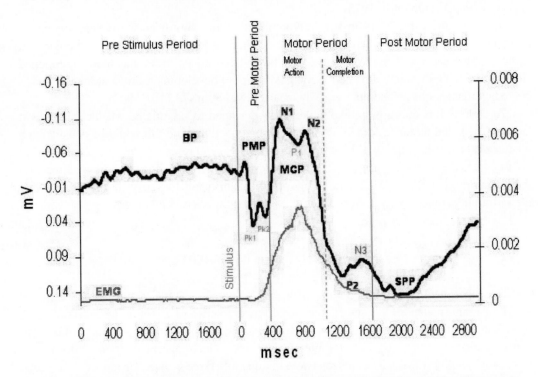

Figure 1. Movement Related Brain Macropotentials (MRBMs) recorded during the following periods: Pre Stimulus, Pre motor, Motor (Motor action, Motor completion) and Post motor. BP: Bereitschaftspotential (Readiness Potential); PMP: Pre motor Potential; MCP: Motor cortex Potential; SPP: Skilled Performance Positivity. Bottom: EMG of the forefinger flexor muscle.

Specific components occurring during premotor, motor and postmotor periods have been described. In particular, a negative phase potential called Bereitschaftspotential (Readiness Potential) has been recorded in the premotor period (Kornhuber & Deecke, 1965). This potential, that reflects different motor and non motor neural processes linked to motor preparation (Brunia, 1988; van Boxtel & Brunia, 1994), has been widely studied but the results have been controversial. In some cases, a reduction of BP amplitude was described in association with continuous repetition of motor activities (Kristeva, 1977) or with increased performance (Fattapposta, et al., 1996). In other studies, BP increased after acquisition of a skilled motor task (Taylor, 1978) or with attention (Grunewald & Grunewald-Zuberbier, 1983) and a higher level of preparation for voluntary movements (Papakostopoulos, 1978; Kristeva, 1984). In the motor period, premotion positivity has been described (Deecke, Scheid, & Kornhuber, 1969), followed by a series of potentials related to the onset and execution of the movement (figure 1). In particular, Motor Cortex Potential (MCP), a negative potential occurring in the first part of the motor period, has been considered an index of response-generated reafferent activity from muscles (Papakostopoulos, Cooper, & Crow, 1975), although it seems to be related to cortical activity and is affected by practice

(Fattapposta, et al., 1996). Less is known about the other potentials recorded during the motor period. N1 has been described as an exogenous component and P2, recorded during the motor completion period, as a somatosensory component (Chiarenza, 1991), while SPP, a positive wave occurring in the postmotor period, seems to increase when the accuracy of performance is greater (Papakostopoulos, 1978).

Despite some differences in the interpretation of the significance of these potentials (Chiarenza, 1991), they can be considered interesting markers of movement, particularly of skilled motor actions. However, some questions have arisen from the above-mentioned studies. The main question is related to the possibility of developing training strategies which could be effective and measurable, e.g., by means of variations in MRBMs.

To address this question an experiment was designed to investigate whether short term training of skilled motor actions could influence brain activity and this could be considered a marker of the effect of training. Electromyogram (EMG) and reaction times were recorded to try to understand if there were effects of training and in which period of the motor reaction they occurred. MRBMs were recorded and analyzed in detail to verify the hypothesis that motor training could modify their profiles and influence specific components.

MATERIALS AND METHODS

The experiment was carried out on 31 healthy volunteers, 20 males and 11 females, aged 21 to 53 years (mean 36±8). The subjects performed a series of attention tests according to the Zimmermann & Fimm Attention Test procedure (Zimmermann & Fimm, 1992), with concomitant recording of physiological activities: electroencephalogram (EEG) and electromyography (EMG). The subjects were divided into three groups: Group 1 (11 subjects) performed the Alert test (A), Group 2 (10 subjects) performed the Choice test (CH) and Group 3 (10 subjects) performed the Choice + No-go test (CHNG). They were tested on day 1 (Test 1). Then each group performed its specific test training daily for 16 minutes. The training lasted 8 days (from day 2 to day 9) and A, CH and CHNG groups were tested a second time on day 10 (Test 2).

Before the beginning of the experiment, all subjects signed an informed-consent form and filled in a questionnaire concerning their habits, health, diet, sleep, smoking, use of drugs, alcohol and caffeine, sport activity and work. All subjects were familiar with a computer (they spent more than 1 hour per day with the computer, with no significant differences between the groups), but they were not skilled in video-games or other computer-ability performances which could affect their reaction times. Only subjects in good health, free of drugs and medications, and with negative psychiatric and endocrine histories were enrolled in the experiment. Other criteria for exclusion from the study were heavy smoking (more than 8 cigarettes per day), drinking (more than two glasses of spirits per day) and caffeine consumption (more than two cups of coffee per day). The experimental design complied with the current laws of Italy. The study protocol was approved by the Ethical Review Board of the University of Siena.

Experimental Procedure

On day 1, all subjects underwent a medical visit in the morning (8:00 am). Then, each subject met the dietician and received a personalized diet to avoid excesses. In the following days they filled in a diary card to record their psychological and mood state and other general information used by the investigators to assess if any protocol violation occurred during the study (e.g. deviations from diet, use of drugs).

Subjects were tested on day 1 and 10 in homogeneous environmental and physiological conditions. Each subject sat in a comfortable reclining chair, 1 metre in front of a computer screen and with the forefinger of the dominant hand on one key (starting position) of a modified computer keyboard (SuperLab Pro, Cedrus Corporation, USA) (Fontani, Maffei, Cameli & Polidori, 1999; Fontani, Lodi, Felici, Corradeschi & Lupo, 2004). There was an interval of 5 minutes between the tests.

The tests were performed in the following order:

1. Alert (A): this test involved the measurement of a simple reaction to a stimulus considered not to require significant central analysis. The test was presented in one period of 80 trials. Each trial lasted 8 seconds with an intertrial interval of 2 seconds. It started with a warning stimulus (sound) and after 4 seconds a red number appeared on the computer monitor (imperative stimulus). The subject had to press three keys as soon as possible in the following sequence: first, the key under the forefinger of the dominant hand (key 1: reaction time 1, RT1), then the key on the right (key 2: reaction time 2, RT2) and then the key on the left (key 3: reaction time 3, RT3). At the end of each trial, the subject positioned the finger on the first key. Reaction times were recorded and analysed.

2. Choice (CH): this test assessed the subject's ability to react to different stimuli. This ability requires substantial central analysis of the stimulus properties. The number of trials was 120. Each trial lasted 8 seconds with an intertrial interval of 2 seconds, started with a warning stimulus (sound) and after 4 seconds a number was presented on the monitor screen (imperative stimulus). There was a sequence of numbers, presented one by one, and the subject had to recognize if the number presented (1, 2 or 3) was equal to the previous one in either colour (red, green, yellow), shape (1, 2, 3) or size (large, medium, small). When there was a match in any of the criteria, the subject pressed three keys as soon as possible in the following sequence: first, the key under the forefinger of the dominant hand (key 1: reaction time 1, RT1), then the key on the right (key 2: reaction time 2, RT2) and then the key on the left (key 3: reaction time 3, RT3). When there was not a match in any of the criteria, the subject pressed three keys as soon as possible in the following sequence: first, the key under the forefinger of the dominant hand (key 1: reaction time 1, RT1), then the key on the left (key 2: reaction time 2, RT2) and then the key on the right (key 3: reaction time 3, RT3). At the end of each trial, the subject positioned the finger on the first key.

3. Choice + No-go (CHNG): this test analysed the subject's ability to react to stimuli activating a complex go/no-go paradigm, i.e. the specific ability of the subject to repress an unsuitable response and to react only to some stimuli and not to others. This ability requires significant central intervention. Each of the 120 trials lasted 8 seconds with an intertrial interval of 2 seconds. It started with a warning stimulus

(sound) and after 4 seconds a number was presented on the monitor screen (imperative stimulus). There was a sequence of numbers, presented one by one, and the subject had to recognize if the number presented (1, 2 or 3) was equal to the previous one in either colour (red, green, yellow), shape (1, 2, 3) or size (large, medium, small). When there was a match in the shape and colour criteria, the subject pressed three keys as soon as possible in the following sequence: first, the key under the forefinger of the dominant hand (key 1: reaction time 1, RT1), then the key on the right (key 2: reaction time 2, RT2) and then the key on the left (key 3: reaction time 3, RT3). When there was a match in the size criterion, the subject did not perform any movement. When there was not a match in any of the criteria, the subject pressed three keys as soon as possible in the following sequence: first, the key under the forefinger of the dominant hand (key 1: reaction time 1, RT1), then the key on the left (key 2: reaction time 2, RT2) and then the key on the right (key 3: reaction time 3, RT3). At the end of each trial, the subject positioned the finger on the first key. Go trials (with stimuli requiring a response) were 70% of the total number and no-go trials (with stimuli not requiring a response) were 30%. They were divided and analysed separately.

For each attention test, three reaction times (RT1, RT2 and RT3) were collected, averaged and compared (RT - time in milliseconds from the stimulus to the response: pressing of the key). The RT variability for each test was indicated by the Variability Index (VI=SD/(1000/mean RT)) (Fontani, Maffei, Cameli & Polidori, 1999). Errors were a criterion to exclude the trial from analysis.

Physiological Recordings

Electrophysiological data were recorded contemporaneously during each attention test and analysed with the BIOPAC integrated system (Biopac Systems Inc., Santa Barbara, CA, USA). The electroencephalogram (EEG) was recorded using thin moulded electrodes mounted in custom-made electrode cups with 20 standard EEG references (Meditec, Parma, Italy). Recordings were made from the Cz, Fz, C3 and C4 scalp sites, referred to linked mastoids (Fattapposta, et al., 1996; Ranganathan, Siemionow, Liu, Sahgal & Yue, 2004). Additional electrodes were positioned superior and lateral to both eyes to monitor eye-related potentials. The impedance of the electrodes was kept below 5 kΩ. The electromyography (EMG) of the forefinger flexor muscle was recorded with Ag/AgCl surface electrodes. EEG and EMG recordings were digitized. The EEG signal was amplified (20,000x) and the data were digitized at a sampling rate of 500 Hz and passed through a 0-100 Hz band pass filter (24 dB/octave roll-off). The recording period lasted for the duration of the entire test. Different digital markers in separate channels of the recording system signalled the warning ring, the imperative stimulus and the response for each trial. Waveforms were recorded, processed and averaged by the BIOPAC software.

To study the movement-related brain macropotentials (MRBMs), averaged waveforms were divided into two periods: the period preceding the stimulus, in which we looked for a negativity similar to the Bereitschaftspotential (BP) and the period following the stimulus, including the premotor, motor and postmotor period, in which a series of negative and positive peaks was recorded (figure 1) (Fattapposta, et al., 1996; Fontani, et al., 2007). The motor period was divided into motor action period and motor completion period.

The first wave in the pre-motor period was a positive wave, the pre-motor potential (PMP). This potential could show one or two positive peaks (Pk1, Pk2). It was followed by a large negative wave, the motor cortex potential (MCP), presenting one or two peaks (N1-N2). N1 occurred between 200 and 350 msec in the A test and after 400 msec in the CH and CHNG tests. A subsequent positive peak (P2) corresponded to the motor completion period. The negative peak following P2 (N3) divided the motor period from the post-motor period, which presented a large positive wave, the skilled performance positivity (SPP) (figure 1). The amplitude and latency of the peaks were calculated. BP was referred to a baseline of 500 msec following the warning stimulus. The amplitude and latency of the peaks following the stimulus were calculated and referred to a pre-imperative stimulus baseline of 500 msec. PMP duration was calculated measuring the time (msec) between the first negative peak occurring after the stimulus and the midpoint between the last PMP positive peak and N1. MCP duration was calculated measuring the time (msec) between the midpoint PMP last peak-N1 and P2.

The EMG activation period was considered the time in milliseconds lasting from the imperative stimulus to EMG onset.

Statistical Analysis

Data were collected, averaged and compared by non-parametric statistical methods (Fattapposta, et al., 1996; Wasserman, 2006). Friedman ANOVA was calculated within groups during the experimental sessions, among the tests as dependent samples. The Wilcoxon test was used to compare two tests as dependent samples. Kruskal-Wallis analysis of Variance was calculated to compare groups as independent samples. The Mann-Whitney test was used to compare two tests as independent samples. Correlations were determined with the Spearman rank correlation test.

RESULTS

No association was found between the variables studied and the age or sex of the subjects. Results have been divided into two sections Reaction Times and MRBMs.

Reaction Times

Table 1 shows the distribution of the mean values of EMG activation latency (EMG) and reaction times (RT1, RT2 and RT3) recorded before and after training in Alert (A), Choice (CH) and Choice+No go (CHNG) groups. Comparisons among groups showed a significant difference between A and the other two groups (CH and CHNG) both for EMG and RTs (Kruskal-Wallis analysis of Variance, $p < 0.003$; Post-hoc comparisons, A vs CH and A vs CHNG, Mann-Whitney test, $p < 0.008$). No differences were observed between CH and

CHNG before and after training. Training did not change significantly EMG and RTs in the Alert group, while a significant reduction of reaction time was recorded after training in CH and CHNG groups. EMG activation was reduced significantly only in CHNG (table 1). A reduction of RT variability was observed after training (table 2). The mean values (msec) of the variability index (VI) of RTs were reduced in CH and CHNG groups, but no effects were observed in the Alert test (table 2).

Table 1. Mean values of EMG activation and Reaction Times (msec) before and after training during A, CH and CHNG

	EMG activation	RT1	RT2	RT3
Alert before	230.64±41.79	355.57±51.67	528.24±61.93	709.48±90.15
Alert after	215.09±52.20	337.41±79.67	505.39±91.82	693.11±120
*p<	n.s.	n.s.	n.s.	n.s.
Choice before	388.60±108.5	679.06±133.9	894.94±150.9	1098.58±177.5
Choice after	335.60±56.80	567.28±79.16	751.96±97.05	930.78±123.9
*p<	n.s.	0.007	0.005	0.005
Choice+No go before	424.00±81.12	667.52±58.18	866.08±63.08	1059.58±76.21
Choice+No go after	337.80±75.36	577.00±89.52	751.34±95.50	924.07±100.1
*p<	0.008	0.007	0.005	0.005

*Wilcoxon test
n. s.= not significant.

Table 2. Variability Index (VI) (mean value) of Reaction Time before and after training during A, CH and CHNG

	VI 1	VI 2	VI 3
Alert before	23.39	36.34	53.76
Alert after	19.80	30.39	54.25
*p<	n.s.	n.s.	n.s.
Choice before	91.70	139.73	181.34
Choice after	52.94	77.68	102.09
*p<	0.005	0.005	0.005
Choice+No go before	74.94	105.68	161.61
Choice+No go after	48.66	64.84	98.27
*p<	0.007	0.005	0.005

*Wilcoxon test
n.s.= not significant.

MRBMs

The profile of MRBMs shown in figure 1 could be recognized in those recorded during A, CH and CHNG tests, but differences could be observed among groups and between before and after training in each group.

BP was the wave recorded during the pre stimulus period. There were no significant differences among the three groups (A, CH, CHNG) for BP, however an effect of training could be observed. If we compare the last 200 msec amplitude mean value before the imperative stimulus (3800-4000 msec after the beginning of the trial) with the amplitude of a same period of 200 msec recorded 2 seconds before (1800-2000 msec after the beginning of the trial), Test 1 (before training) did not show any significant difference (only an increment of 16.3 mV was recorded), while in Test 2 (after training) there was an increment of 230 mV (Wilcoxon test, $p < 0.05$).

The period following the imperative stimulus (pre motor period) showed the pre-motor potential (PMP), the duration of which increased passing from A to CH, to CHNG tests. Training did not affect PMP duration in A and CH groups, but reduced it in CHNG group (figure 2). MCP duration was lower in A than in CH and CHNG both before and after training. Training reduced MCP duration in all groups (Fig. 3). Effects of training were also observed on the latency of N1, N2 and P2 peaks (table 3). A significant reduction of N1 and N2 latency was recorded after training in CHNG, while a reduction of P2 latency followed training in the CH group. Training influenced the Alert test reducing the latency of N2 peak (table 3).

SPP amplitude was not different in the three tests, comparing before and after training, SPP latency (msec) was significantly different only in the CHNG test (Before training: 2740.8±462.4; After training: 1946.4±876.9; Wilcoxon test, $p < 0.02$).

Table 3. Mean values of MCP peak latency before and after training during A, CH and CHNG

	N1 latency (msec)	N2 latency (msec)	P2 latency (msec)
Alert before	391.82±80.51	612.00±137.8	923.82±161.2
Alert after	366.18±162.7	500.36±196.9	871.82±157.13
*p<	n.s.	0.03	n.s.
Choice before	590.40±118.4	821.80±322.8	1589.60±225.1
Choice after	559.80±100.1	861.20±338.5	1351.20±147.9
*p<	n.s.	n.s.	0.009
Choice+no go before	753.80±199.4	1259.40±285.3	1683.40±387.3
Choice+no go after	590.80±161.8	909.40±365.9	1418.20±196.4
*p<	0.005	0.007	n.s.

*.Wilcoxon test

n. s.= not significant.

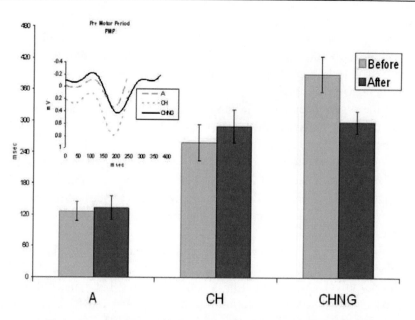

Figure 2. PMP duration before and after training. Comparisons among groups, before training: Kruskal-Wallis Analysis of Variance, H (2,31)= 19.39, p<0.0001. Post-hoc comparisons, Mann-Whitney Test, A vs CH, p<0.001; A vs CHNG, p<0.0002; CH vs CHNG, p<0.02. After training: Kruskal-Wallis Analysis of Variance, H (2,31)= 14.43, p<0.0007. Post-hoc comparisons, Mann-Whitney Test, A vs CH, p<0.001; A vs CHNG, p<0.001; CH vs CHNG, n. s.. Comparisons between Test 1 (before training) and Test 2 (after training) (Wilcoxon test), A: n. s., CH: n. s., CHNG: p< 0.01.

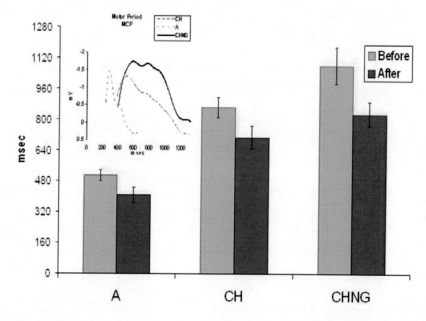

Figure 3. MCP duration before and after training. Comparisons among groups, before training: Kruskal-Wallis Analysis of Variance, H (2,31)= 20.65, p<0.0001. Post-hoc comparisons, Mann-Whitney Test, A vs CH, p<0.0001; A vs CHNG, p<0.0001; CH vs CHNG, n. s.. After training: Kruskal-Wallis Analysis of Variance, H (2,31)= 17.45, p<0.0002. Post-hoc comparisons, Mann-Whitney Test, A vs CH, p<0.001; A vs CHNG, p<0.0002; CH vs CHNG, n. s.. Comparisons between Test 1 (before training) and Test 2 (after training) (Wilcoxon test), A: p<0.04, CH: p<0.03, CHG: p< 0.03.

The above reported data have been obtained from Cz recordings. A comparison among Fz, Cz, C3 and C4 showed that some parameters such as N1 and P2 latency were not different. However, PMP and MCP duration were higher in Cz (mean values, PMP: 389.40 msec; MCP: 1080.20 msec) and lower in C4 (mean values, PMP: 159.20 msec; MCP: 676.40 msec) with intermediate values in Fz and C3 (Friedman ANOVA, PMP: $p < 0.0001$; MCP: $p < 0.0001$).

Table 4 shows the correlations existing between MRBMs recorded in the three tests (A, CH, CHNG) and reactivity (EMG, RT1). PMP duration is correlated with EMG activation, MCP duration, N1, P2 and SPP latency and RT1. The other parameters are correlated to the following until the correlation between P2 latency and RT1. These correlations occur before and after training.

**Table 4. Correlations (Spearman r) between MRBMs
and RT parameters before and after training**

		EMG start	MCP duration	N1 latency	P2 latency	SPP latency	RT 1
PMP duration	Before	0.800*	0.669*	0.906*	0.818*	0.630*	0.729*
	After	0.756*	0.490**	0.786*	0.651*	0.444***	0.737*
	EMG start	Before	0.773*	0.809*	0.806*	0.661*	0.908*
		After	0.634*	0.857*	0.738*	0.471***	0.823*
		MCP duration	Before	0.769*	0.843*	0.857*	0.745*
			After	0.441**	0.877*	0.637*	0.676*
			N1 latency	Before	0.841*	0.708*	0.762*
				After	0.607*	--	0.614*
				P2 latency	Before	0.707*	0.813*
					After	0.571**	0.766*

*p <0.001; ** p< 0.005; *** p< 0.01.

DISCUSSION

The main results of this experiment lead to the conclusion that a short lasting period of training of a motor action has not only effects on the execution of the movement but also on the neural structures involved in the motor action modifying MRBMs profiles. These effects seem to be more evident in complex tests such as Choice (CH) and Choice + No-go (CHNG). In particular, reaction times and their variability were reduced after training in both tests while no effects of training have been observed in the Alert test (A). The main effect of training on MRBMs has been recorded in the motor period on MCP duration which is reduced in A, CH and CHNG. The pre motor period showed a significant reduction of PMP duration only in the CHNG test.

The profiles of MRBMs recorded in the Alert test differed from CH and CHNG: peak latencies and wave durations occurred earlier in A. Differences between CH and CHNG, which require complex central signal processing and high mental effort, were less evident, occurred only in the pre motor period and disappeared after training.

The correlations existing between MRBMs recorded in the three tests (A, CH, CHNG) and reactivity (EMG, RT1) (Table 4) show that PMP duration is the first and the main parameter influencing not only EMG activation and RT1, but also MCP duration and the latency of N1, P2 and SPP peaks. These correlations point out that MRBMs waves are strictly related to the motor action and occur in a precise sequence.

The present results confirm the main effect of training in the tests involving central processing and analysis (Fontani, et al., 2007), particularly in test in which a go/no-go paradigm requires a strong cognitive engagement. In our experimental design, this test was associated with a motor action, consisting in the pressing of three keys, allowing the investigation of both reactivity and movement speed. This experimental procedure also allowed us to study cerebral waves related to movement (MRBMs) in more detail to determine the period of motor action in which the effects of training occurred.

That MRBMs are closely related to movement has been reported in several experiments in which MRBMs have been recognized during skilled performance tasks (Chiarenza, et al., 1983; Chiarenza, 1986) in trained and untrained subjects (Fattapposta, et al., 1996; Di Russo, et al., 2005) and have been also recorded during motor imagery (Fontani, et al., 2007). In the present experiment, the main effects of training on MRBMs occurred on the waves recorded after the presentation of the imperative stimulus, with a reduction of the latency of the peaks occurring during the pre-motor, motor and post-motor period. However, the amplitude of BP, a wave recorded before the imperative stimulus, was increased after training. This is in line with those studied which described an increase of BP amplitude after acquisition of a skilled motor task (Taylor, 1978). This could be due to an increase of attention (Grunewald & Grunewald-Zuberbier, 1983) or to a higher level of preparation for voluntary movements such as that induced by training (Papakostopoulos, 1978; Kristeva, 1984).

As for the waves occurring after the imperative stimulus, the PMP duration seems to be crucial in conditioning duration and latency of the following waves. This pre-motion positivity probably reflects stimulus processing and the development of motor strategies to react to the stimuli presented (Deecke, et al., 1969; Fontani, et al., 2007). If so, it could mean that training can reduce the time of central processing via a direct action on the central nervous system. This effect is shown by the reduction of PMP duration and is evident in CHNG test. This could mean that more complex is the stimulus processing required, more evident is the effect of training.

The variations of the waves that follow PMP seem to be linked to the variations of PMP duration (Table 4). It is known that MCP is linked to the motor action, is related to cortical activity and is affected by practice (Fattapposta, et al., 1996). Moreover, it has been shown that MCP is absent in subjects with learning disabilities (Chiarenza, Papakostopoulos, Guareschi Cazzullo, Giordana, & Giammari Alde, 1982).

In the present experiment we recorded a reduction of MCP duration after training in A, CH and CHNG. This shows an effect of training not only in tests involving a high central effort, but also in the simple Alert test.

On the basis of these results we may assume that training reduces the time of motor cortical engagement and quickens the transfer of motor action to muscles. This is confirmed by EMG activation and RT reduction and by other changes occurring in MRBMs after training: the N1 peak was recorded earlier after training, showing that faster stimulus processing (reduced PMP duration) was followed by faster motor activation. The latency of P2, recorded during the motor completion period and considered a somatosensory component (Chiarenza, 1991), was reduced after training as well as the latency of SPP, a peak which reflects the results of the control of a skilled performance and is higher when the accuracy of performance is greater (Fattapposta, et al., 1996; Papakostopoulos, Stamler & Newton, 1986). The latency of both peaks was reduced after training, but the amplitude was not affected. This could be interpreted as a prevalent effect of short lasting training on timing, while the quality of performance (probably requiring longer training periods) did not seem to be modified.

The results of the present experiment, showing a variation of cerebral waves related to movement, strengthen the hypothesis of a direct action of training on the central nervous system, probably influencing neuronal excitability mechanisms and fastening signal transduction. This seems to occur particularly when complex neural mechanisms are involved. The absence of an effect on simple reaction time could be explained by the good level of RT presented at the beginning of the experiment. Therefore, although the A RT latency tended to decrease after training, the reduction did not reach significance.

In conclusion, we may assume that short periods of training of a motor action can modify MRBMs profiles. These profiles have been modified particularly in their motor action period components such as MCP, but interesting effect can be observed also in the pre motor period in which information processing and the development of motor strategies play a crucial role in conditioning the performance of a motor action. Further studies are necessary to confirm these results and to clarify the effects of training on MRBMs recorded in simple or complex motor actions. Functional Magnetic Resonance Imaging studies could be very useful in this field, particularly to explain the MRBMs changes recorded during motor action. Moreover, other points remain to be clarified, such as the effects of short and long term training on MRBMs and the optimal amount and duration of training within an overall training programme to obtain MRBMs changes. These and other factors need to be investigated by more complete, long-term experiments to evaluate the possibility of an effective and suitable use of cortical recordings in motor training studies and practice.

REFERENCES

Brunia, C. H. (1988). Movement and stimulus preceding negativity. *Biol. Psychol.* 26, 165-178.

Chiarenza, G. A. (1986). Electrophysiology of skilled performances in children. *Ital. J. Neurol. Sci.* 5(Suppl.), 155-162.

Chiarenza, G. A. (1991). A critical review of physiological and clinical aspects of movement-related brain macropotentials in humans. *Ital. J. Neurol. Sci.* 12, 17-30.

Chiarenza, G. A., Papakostopoulos, D., Giordana, F., & Guareschi Cazzullo, A. (1983). Movement-related brain macropotentials during skilled performances: a developmental study. *Electroenceph. Clin. Neurophysiol.* 56, 373-383.

Chiarenza, G. A., Papakostopoulos, F., Guareschi Cazzullo, A., Giordana, F., & Giammari Alde, G. (1982). Movement-related brain macropotentials during skilled performance task in children with learning disabilities. In G. A. Chiarenza & D. Papakostopolous

(Eds.). Clinical application of cerebral evoked potentials in pediatric medicine. Amsterdam: *Excerpta Medica.* Pp. 259-292.

Deecke, L., Scheid, P., & Kornhuber, H. H. (1969). Distribution of readiness potential, pre-motion positivity, and motor potential of the human cerebral cortex preceding voluntary finger movements. *Exper. Brain Res.* 7, 58-168.

Di Russo, F., Pitzalis, S., Aprile, T., & Spinelli, D. (2005). Effect of practice on brain activity: an investigation in top-level rifle shooters. *Med. Sci. Sport Exer.* 37, 1586-1593.

Fattapposta, F., Amabile, G., Cordischi, M. V., Di Venezio, D., Foti, A., Pierelli, F., D'Alessio, C., Pigozzi, F., Parisi, A., & Morrocutti, C. (1996). Long-term practice effects on a new skilled motor learning: an electrophysiological study. *Electroenceph. Clin. Neurophysiol.* 99, 495-507.

Fontani, G; Maffei, D; Cameli, S & Polidori, F. (1999). Reactivity and event-related potentials during attentional tests in athletes. *Eur. J. Appl. Physiol.* 80, 308-317.

Fontani, G; Lodi, L; Felici, A; Corradeschi, F & Lupo C. (2004). Attentional, emotional and hormonal data in subjects of different ages. *Eur. J. Appl. Physiol.* 92, 452-461.

Fontani, G; Migliorini, S; Benocci, R; Facchini, A; Casini, M & Corradeschi, F. (2007). Effect of mental imagery on the development of skilled motor actions. *Percept. Motor Skills.* 105, 803-826.

Grunewald, G., & Grunewald-Zuberbier, E. (1983). Cerebral potentials during voluntary ramp movements in aiming tasks. In A. W. Gaillard & W. Ritter (Eds.), *Tutorial in ERP research: endogenous components.* Amsterdam: North Holland. Pp 311-327.

Kornhuber, H. H., & Deecke, L. (1965). Himpotentialanderungen bei Willkürbewegungen und passiven Bewegungen des Menschen: *Bereitschaftspotential und Reafferente Potential. Pflüg Archiv.* 284, 1-17.

Kristeva, R. (1977). Study of the motor potential during voluntary recurrent movement. *Electroenceph. Clin. Neurophysiol.* 42, 588.

Kristeva, R. (1984). Movement-related potentials with bilateral actions and with piano-playing. In R. Karrer, J. Cohen, & P. Tieting (Eds.), Brain and information: event-related potentials. *Ann. N. Y. Acad. Sci.* 425, 401-403.

Papakostopoulos, D. (1978). A precentral macropotential with short latency as a possible indicator of response and reafferent activity in man. *J. Physiology.* (London), 275, 72-73.

Papakostopoulos, D., Cooper, R. & Crow, H. J. (1975). Inhibition of cortical evoked potentials and sensation by self-initiated movement in man. *Nature.* 258, 321-324.

Papakostopoulos, D., & Crow, H. J. (1984). The precentral somatosensory evoked potential. In R. Karrer, J. Cohen, & P. Tieting (Eds.), Brain and information: event-related potentials. *Ann. N. Y. Acad. Sci.* 425, 256-261.

Papakostopoulos D, Stamler R & Newton P. (1986). Movement-related brain macropotentials during self-paced skilled performance with and without knowledge of results. In McCallum WC, Zappoli R, Denoth F (Eds): *"Cerebral psychophysiology: studies in event-related potentials".* (EEG Suppl. 38). Amsterdam: Elsevier, pp. 261-262.

Ranganathan, V; Siemionow, V; Liu, Z; Sahgal, V & Yue, G. (2004). From mental power to muscle power-gaining strength by using the mind. *Neuropsychologia.* 42, 944-956.

Shibasaki, H., Barret, G., Halliday, E., & Halliday, A. M. (1980). Components of the movement-related cortical potentials and their scalp topography. *Electroenceph. Clin. Neurophysiol.* 49, 213-226.

Solodkin, A., Hlustik, P., Chen, E. E., & Small, S. L. (2004). Fine modulation in network activation during motor execution and motor imagery. *Cereb. Cortex.* 14, 1246-1255.

Taylor, K. J. (1978). Bereitschaftspotential during the acquisition of a skilled motor task. *Electroenceph. Clin. Neurophysiol.* 45, 568-576.

van Boxtel, G., J., M., & Brunia, C. H. (1994). Motor and non-motor aspects of slow brain potentials. *Biol. Psychol.* 38, 37-51.

Wasserman, L. (2006). *All of nonparametric statistics.* New York: Springer.

Yan, J., & Dick, M. (2006). Practice effects on motor control in healthy seniors and patients with mild cognitive impairment and alzheimer's disease. *Neuropsychol. Dev. Cogn. B. Aging Neuropsychol. Cogn.* 13, 385-410.

Zimmermann, P & Fimm, B. (1992). Battery of tests for the study of attention (TAP). *Psytest,* Wűrselen, pp. 1-73.

In: Handbook of Motor Skills
Editor: Lucian T. Pelligrino

ISBN: 978-1-60741-811-5
© 2009 Nova Science Publishers, Inc.

Chapter 9

THE INFLUENCE OF OROMOTOR FUNCTIONS AND DIET CONSISTENCY ON CARIES EXPERIENCE AND GROWTH RATE IN CEREBRAL PALSIED INDIVIDUALS

Maria Teresa Botti Rodrigues Santos[1],
Maria Cristina Duarte Ferreira[2],
Paula Celiberti[3] and Renata Oliveira Guare[1]

[1] Discipline of Dentistry, Persons with Disabilities Division,
Post Graduation Professor, Universidade Cruzeiro do Sul, São Paulo, Brazil.
[2]. Universidade Paulista (UNIP), São Paulo, Brazil
[3] Department of Orthodontics and Pediatric Dentistry, School of Dentistry,
University of São Paulo (USP), São Paulo, Brazil

INTRODUCTION

Cerebral palsy (CP) describes a group of movement and posture development disorders attributed to non-progressive disturbances in the developing fetal or infant brain, causing activity limitations and being the most common cause of severe physical disability in childhood. The motor disorders of CP are often accompanied by disturbances of sensation, cognition, communication, perception, behavior, and seizure disorders.[1]

Oromotor dysfunction and oral-ingestive problems, as uncoordinated control mechanisms of orofacial and palatolingual musculatures[2], are often observed in CP individuals, and varies from mild to severe.[3] These disabilities are expressed by drooling, coughing, choking, rejection of solid food, food loss, and spillage during eating. Difficulties in spoon-feeding, biting, chewing, cup drinking, straw drinking, swallowing and clearing are also observed.[2]

Another nutritional issue to be considered is the common inability of severely oromotor impaired CP individuals to ingest solid food, which often leads to an exclusively liquid or semi-solid diet. In spite of contributing to some degree to growth and nutritional disturbances, especially at an early age, food consistency may also cause a significant impact on oral health. Therefore, a timely nutritional rehabilitation and preventive measures in oral health may significantly improve the quality of life of these individuals,[4-6] as well as prevent deleterious and noxious habits such as bottle feeding. Performing an adequate oral hygiene on CP individuals however, can be a very difficult task for the caregivers, due to the patient's persistent pathological biting reflex.[7]

Food consistency, sugared beverages, and long term oral medicines[4,8], associated with oromotor dysfunction and oral hygiene difficulties, may explain the high incidence of caries and periodontal diseases exhibited by the CP population.[9-13]

The influence of oromotor impairment in CP individuals as a risk factor in caries experience was not studied yet. Therefore, this study aimed at evaluating the influence of oral motricity and *diet consistency* on caries experience and growth rate in CP individuals.

MATERIAL AND METHODS

Subject's Selection

A group of 78 non-institutionalized CP individuals of both genders, aged 4 to 14 years old (9.5±2.3), living in Sao Paulo - Brazil (0.7 mg/L F^- in water supply), and attending the Special Children's Elementary School of Lar Escola São Francisco – Rehabilitation Center (Federal University of Sao Paulo, Brazil) were enrolled in this study. The main inclusion criterion was the CP medical diagnosis.

This study was approved by the Ethics in Human Research Committee of the Federal University of Sao Paulo School of Medicine, Brazil. After receiving detailed explanations about the study and agreeing to participate, a written consent for participation and publication of data was obtained from the adult responsible for each CP individual.

Patient medical records were reviewed for demographic and clinical data, including gender, age, type of movement disorder (spastic, dystonic, with athetosis or with ataxia, or a mixture of these disorders), clinical patterns of involvement (quadriplegia, diplegia, hemiplegia or double hemiplegia), and severity of CP. By means of Gross Motor Function Classification System (GMFCS), CP severity was measured and allocated in levels (I-V[14]), where each level indicates:

- level I: walking without restrictions, but with limitations in more advanced gross motor skills;
- level II: walking without assistive devices, but with limitations walking outdoors and in the community;
- level III: walking with assistive mobility devices, and with limitations walking outdoors and in the community;
- level IV: self-mobility with limitations. The patient is transported or uses a power mobility outdoors and in the community;
- level V: severely limited self-mobility, even with assistive technology.

OROFACIAL MOTOR FUNCTION ASSESSMENT

The assessment of individuals' orofacial motor functions was carried out by one examiner according to the Orofacial Motor Function Assessment Scale (OFMFAS).15 For OFMFAS assessment, individuals were positioned in the best sitting position, in a ventilated room, with trunk and pelvis aligned and without hip hyperextension. The shoulder girdle was kept forward, with abduction of the scapulae and the cervical spine elongated.

GUIDELINES OF THE OROFACIAL MOTOR FUNCTION ASSESSMENT SCALE

The oral motor evaluation involves assessment of oral posture and movements. The guidelines of the OFMFAS are consisted of 13 items considered important criteria for the assessment of oral-facial motor function in CP individuals. Each sub-item can be rated using a Likert scale ranging from 0 (unable to perform or determine, inconsistent) to 2 (adequately performed).

Table 1. Items of the OFMFAS

1. Jaw mobility   Subtotal:

a) voluntary jaw opening
- [ ] yes = 2   [ ] no = 0   [ ] unable to determine = 0

b) jaw opening
- [ ] midline = 2   [ ] right / left deviation = 1   [ ] inconsistent = 0

c) open against resistance
- [ ] normal / adequate = 2   [ ] weak = 1   [ ] unable to determine = 0

d) close against resistance
- [ ] normal / adequate = 2   [ ] weak = 1   [ ] unable to determine = 0

2. Voluntary jaw protrusion   Subtotal:

a) [ ] yes = 2   [ ] no = 0   [ ] unable to determine = 0
b) [ ] midline = 2   [ ] right / left deviation = 1   [ ] inconsistent = 0

3. Voluntary lateral jaw movements   Subtotal:

a) right
- [ ] yes = 2   [ ] no = 0   [ ] unable to determine = 0

b) left
- [ ] yes = 2   [ ] no = 0   [ ] unable to determine = 0

c) presence involuntary jaw movements during jaw lateral movements
- [ ] yes = 0   [ ] no = 2

4. Rapid coordinated jaw movements   Subtotal:

a) tooth tap
- [ ] present = 2   [ ] slow/ slows with time/ irregular/ erratic = 1   [ ] unable P/D = 0

b) excursion jaw lateral
- [ ] present = 2   [ ] slow/ slows with time/ irregular/ erratic = 1   [ ] unable P/D = 0

5. Voluntary facial movements   Subtotal:

a) show teeth
- [ ] symmetrical = 2   [ ] right/ left weakness = 1   [ ] unable P/D = 0

b) pucker lips
- [ ] symmetrical = 2   [ ] right/ left weakness = 1   [ ] unable P/D = 0

6. Lip muscle strength: puff-out cheeks/maintain pressure   Subtotal:

☐ present and strong = 2   ☐ present and weak = 1   ☐ unable P/D = 0

7. Rapid coordinated lip movements   Subtotal:

a) protrusion/retraction of lips
☐ present = 2   ☐ slow/ slows with time/ irregular/ erratic = 1   ☐ unable P/D = 0
b) pa-pa-pa-pa-pa-pa
☐ present = 2   ☐ slow/ slows with time/ irregular/ erratic = 1   ☐ unable P/D = 0

8. Glossopharyngeal and vagal motor activity   Subtotal:

ah!
☐ symmetrical = 2   ☐ right/ left weakness = 1   ☐ unable P/D= 0

9. Rapid coordinated palatal movements   Subtotal:

mm-bah, mm-bah
☐ adequate = 2   ☐ poor = 1   ☐ unable P/D= 0

10. Hypoglossal motor: voluntary tongue movements   Subtotal:

tongue protrusion
a) ☐ yes = 2   ☐ no = 0   ☐ unable to determine = 0
b) ☐ midline = 2   ☐ right/left deviation = 1 ☐ inconsistent = 0

11. Voluntary elevation and lateralization of tongue   Subtotal:

a) back incisors = ttt
☐ yes = 2   ☐ no = 0   ☐ unable to determine = 0
b) back soft palate = ing
☐ yes = 2   ☐ no = 0   ☐ unable to determine = 0
c) right corner mouth
☐ yes = 2   ☐ no = 0   ☐ unable to determine = 0
d) left corner mouth
☐ yes = 2   ☐ no = 0   ☐ unable to determine = 0

12. Rapid coordinated movements of tongue   Subtotal:

a) t-t-t-t-t
☐ present = 2   ☐ rhythm slows with time/ erratic = 1   ☐ unable P/D = 0
b) k-k-k-k-k

☐ present = 2   ☐ rhythm slows with time/ erratic = 1   ☐ unable P/D = 0

13. Oral abnormal reflexes   Subtotal:

a) suckle
☐ present = 0   ☐ absent = 2
a) tonic bite
☐ present = 0   ☐ absent = 2
a) gag
☐ present = 0   ☐ absent = 2
a) rooting
☐ present = 0   ☐ absent = 2

TOTAL:

* P/D = perform or determine

Items 1 to 12 assess voluntary movements, i.e., response to a verbal command. Item 13 involves the assessment of oral reflexes, such as suckle, tonic bite, gag, and rooting, which are stimulated by the examiner's forefinger. These items are presented in table 1.

During the assessment of all voluntary tasks, the examiner stimulated the individuals by performing all movements and showing the individuals how they should be performed. The examiner must be positioned opposite to the patient and should perform each movement at least three times, consecutively.

ITEM 1: JAW MOBILITY EVALUATION

In order to evaluate individuals' ability to coordinate the movements of their jaw, individuals are asked to voluntarily open their mouth (sub-item a). When the movement is performed adequately, score 2 is given to this sub-item (figure 1). When individuals are unable to perform the task, or when the examiner is unable to determine whether individuals do not understand the oral command (concerning a cognitive deficiency *or* mental retardation), the sub-item is marked with score 0. During jaw opening (sub-item b), the examiner must observe whether it is performed in the midline (score 2) or with right/left deviation (score 1).The score is recorded as inconsistent when lateral movements are made in an uncoordinated form during mouth opening, or when individuals are unable to perform the task.

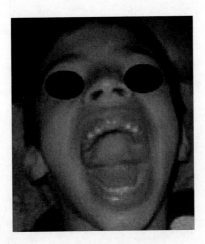

Figure 1. Evaluation of jaw mobility during opening movement.

In order to test the ability to open (sub-item c) and close (sub-item d) the mouth against resistance, the examiner position one hand on the top of the individual's head and the other hand is positioned with the thumb under the chin (open movement) or with the forefinger between the dental arches (close movement), creating a light resistance against the movement tested (figure 2). According to the individuals' ability to open and close the mouth, Score 2 is given when the movements against resistance is performed adequately, score 1 when it is performed weakly, and score 0 when it is difficult to know whether individuals do not understand the oral command or are unable to perform the task.

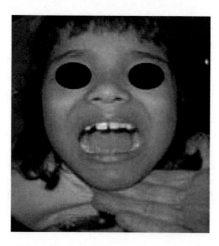

Figure 2. Evaluation of jaw mobility during opening against resistance.

ITEM 2: JAW PROTRUSION

Individuals are asked to make a protrusive jaw movement, (figure 3) (sub-item a). A light forefinger stimulus can be applied to the chin to encourage the individual to accomplish the movement. If the lower dental arch protrudes beyond upper dental arch, score 2 is given. When individuals cannot perform the protrusion, or when the examiner cannot determine whether individuals do not want to or do not know how to do perform the task (unable to determine), the score is recorded as 0. During the movement (sub-item b), it must be observed if the task is performed in the midline (score 2) or with right/left deviation (score 1). The task is recorded as inconsistent when individuals alternate midline and deviated jaw protrusive movements or are unable to perform them.

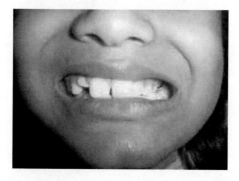

Figure 3. Evaluation of jaw mobility during protrusive movement.

ITEM 3: LATERAL JAW MOVEMENTS

Individuals are asked to move the jaw from the midline to the right (sub-item a) and back, and from the midline to the left and back (sub-item b) (figure 4). In order to encourage individuals, a light forefinger stimulus can be applied to the cheek, on the opposite side of the movement tested. Score 2 is registered when lower midline is deviated to the right (right jaw lateral movement) or the left (left jaw lateral movement). When individuals cannot perform lateral movements, or when the examiner cannot determine whether the patient does not want to or does not know how to do the task, score 0 is given. The observation of involuntary movements (sub-item c) during jaw lateral movements is scored as 0 (yes) or 2 (no).

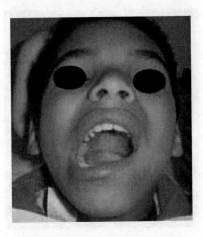

Figure 4. Evaluation of jaw mobility during lateral movements.

ITEM 4: RAPID COORDINATED JAW MOVEMENTS

To evaluate individuals ability to perform rapid and coordinated movements (sub-item a), the examiner must ask them to tap their teeth in rhythmic and coordinated movements for at least five seconds. When individuals are able to perform the movement, maintaining the rhythm, the score is recorded as 2. When, individuals are able to do only a few slow rhythmic taps before stopping, present a rhythm that slows with time, or if the taps are irregular, erratic, and without rhythm, the score is recorded as 1. The inability to determine whether individuals do not want to or do not know how to perform the task is scored as 0.

To evaluate the ability to perform excursion jaw lateral movements (item b), individuals are asked to perform side-to-side movements in a continuous way. The item is scored as 2 when the movements are adequately performed. When individuals are able to perform only a few slow rhythmic movements before stopping, with a rhythm that slows with time, or if the movements are irregular, erratic, or without rhythm, the item is scored as 1. The inability to determine whether individuals do not want to or do not know how to perform the task is scored as 0.

ITEM 5: VOLUNTARY FACIAL MOVEMENTS

The voluntary facial movements are tested by asking individuals to smile (figure 5), show the teeth as in a grin (sub item a), and pucker the lips as in sending kisses (sub item b) (figure 6). For both conditions, score 2 is registered when facial movements are symmetrical and score 1 when the movements observed present lateral deviation or have a weak result. The inability to determine whether individuals do not want to or do not know how to perform the task is scored as 0.

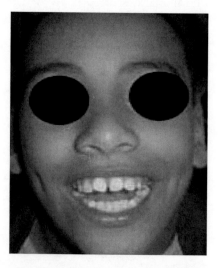

Figure 5. Evaluation of voluntary facial movements (showing the teeth).

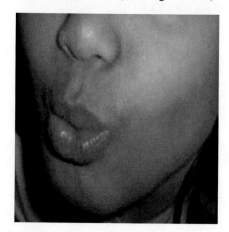

Figure 6. Evaluation during puckering the lips, as in sending kisses.

ITEM 6: LIP MUSCLE STRENGTH

In order to test lip muscle strength, individuals are asked to inflate the cheeks and keep the air inside the mouth with sealed lips for a few seconds (figure 7). The score is recorded as 2 when individuals are able to maintain cheeks inflated strongly, 1 when the task is performed weakly, and 0 when the examiner does not know whether individuals do not want to or do not know how to perform the task.

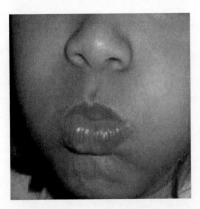

Figure 7. Evaluation of lip muscle strength by inflating cheeks and keeping the air inside the mouth with sealed lips.

ITEM 7: RAPID COORDINATED LIP MOVEMENTS

In this sub-item, individuals are asked to perform rapid coordinated lip movements, with a protrusion/retraction of lips, i.e. from smile to pucker, consecutively. Afterwards (sub-item b) individuals are asked to say "pa-pa-pa-pa". For both sub-items the scores are the same as described in item 4.

ITEM 8: GLOSSOPHARYNGEAL AND VAGAL MOTOR

Individuals are asked to say "ah" in order to verify glossopharyngeal and vagal motor movements (figure 8). Score 2 is registered when the examiner observes the soft palate elevation in a symmetrical way, score 1 when the elevation occurs in an asymmetrical or weak way, and 0 when the examiner is unable to know whether individuals do not want to or do not know how to perform the task.

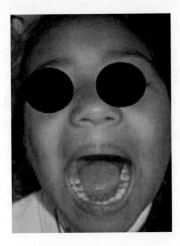

Figure 8. Evaluation of glossopharyngeal and vagal motor movements saying "ah".

ITEM 9: RAPID COORDINATED PALATAL MOVEMENTS

Individuals are asked to repeat the sounds "mm-bah" in a continuously way, in order to verify the ability to perform rapid coordinated palatal movements. Score 2 is registered when individuals are able to perform the task adequately, 1 when individuals are able to perform in a poor way (when it is not possible to distinguish the sounds clearly), and 0 when the examiner is unable to know whether individuals do not want to or do not know how to perform the task.

ITEM 10: HYPOGLOSSAL MOTOR: VOLUNTARY TONGUE MOVEMENTS

In order to test the ability to perform voluntary tongue movements, (sub-item a), individuals are asked to protrude the tongue (figure 9). If they are able to perform the movement adequately, score 2 is registered. The protrusion in the midline (sub-item b) receives score 2, when movement is performed with right/left deviation, score 1 is given. On both sub-items, score 0 is registered when the examiner is unable to know whether individuals do not want to or do not know how to perform the task

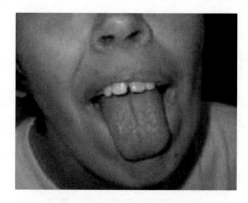

Figure 9. Evaluation of Hypoglossal motor voluntary tongue protrusive movements.

ITEM 11: VOLUNTARY ELEVATION AND LATERALIZATION OF TONGUE

Individuals' ability to voluntarily elevate and lateralize the tongue is evaluated by asking them to lift the tongue apex towards the palatal face of upper incisors (figure 10) saying "t-t-t-t" (sub-item a), to lift the tongue apex and position it rewards in the direction of the soft palate saying "ing" (sub-item b), to position the tongue apex on right corner of the mouth (figure 11a) (sub-item c) and finally to the left corner of the mouth (figure 11 b) (sub-item d). For all tasks in this item, score 2 is registered for able to perform, and 0 for not performed or unable to determine.

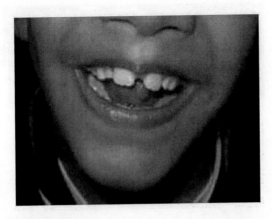

Figure 10. Evaluation of voluntary elevation of tongue.

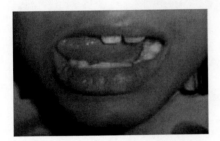
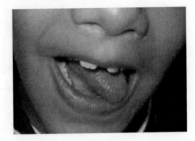

Figure 11. Evaluation of voluntary lateralization of tongue to the right (11a) and left (11b).

ITEM 12: RAPID COORDINATED MOVEMENTS OF TONGUE

Individuals are asked to perform rapid and coordinated tongue movements performing the sounds "t-t-t-t" (sub-item a) and "k-k-k-k" (sub-item b) in a continuously and rhythmic way. Scores are the same as described for item 4.

ITEM 13: ABNORMAL ORAL REFLEXES

The evaluation of the presence or absence of oral reflexes is achieved by observing the individuals' reaction to stimuli. The rooting reflex is evaluated after a touch stimulus made by the examiner's forefinger above the upper lip, below the lower lip, and on labial comissura. The presence of this reflex is observed when the patient rotates the head towards the stimulus direction (figure 12). For the suckle-swallow reflex, the forefinger is gently placed on the tongue apex. Its presence is confirmed when backward-forward tongue movements, such as suction movements, are observed (figure 13). Biting is assessed by touching the buccal gum, near lower molars. An upward jaw movement into a strongly clenched posture is observed when the reflex is present, making it difficult for the patient to open the mouth (figure 14). The gagging reflex is tested through a touch that begins on the tongue apex moving rearward up to the tongue anterior 2/3. This reflex is present when the contraction of the oropharyngeal muscles is observed (figure 15).

The individual's OFMFAS final score was obtained by adding all sub-item values. Individuals were then classified as severely impaired (1st quartile: score ≤19), moderately impaired (2nd quartile: score between 20 and 31), slightly impaired (3rd quartile: score between 32 and 41) or very slightly impaired (4th quartile: score ≥ 42).

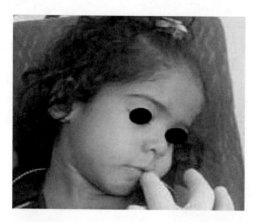

Figure 12. Evaluation of the rooting reflex.

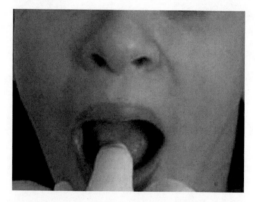

Figure 13. Evaluation of the suckle-swallow reflex.

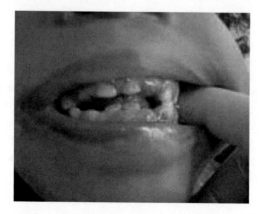

Figure 14. Evaluation of the biting reflex.

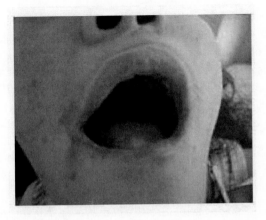

Figure 15. Evaluation of the gagging reflex.

ORAL HEALTH AND CARIES EXPERIENCE ASSESSMENT

After receiving a new tooth brush and dentifrice, the caregivers were instructed how to perform oral hygiene correctly. Then, under supervision, each CP individual had their teeth brushed by the respective caregiver.

Afterwards, the air-dried teeth were submitted to visual and tactile examinations on a dental unit, under artificial illumination, with the use of a plane intra-oral mirror and a round-ended dental probe.

Oral health status assessment was performed by a trained and calibrated single examiner, according to standard procedures.[16] Caries experience was assessed using the DMFT/dmft index, for permanent and primary dentition, respectively (figure 16). For children with mixed dentition, dmft and DMFT were recorded. Decayed teeth were assessed only at cavity threshold. Teeth exhibiting white spot lesions were, therefore, considered sound.

In order to evaluate the intra-examiner reproducibility, 10 random children were submitted to two subsequent examinations with a 7 day interval between them, and with no assess or knowledge of the CP individuals previous oral health status (Kappa=0.89). No radiographic examination was carried out.

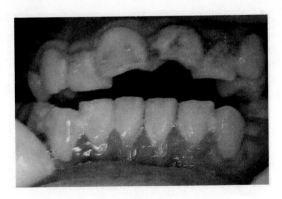

Figure 16. Intra-oral aspects of an individual with cerebral palsy.

DIET CONSISTENCY ASSESSMENT

CP individuals enrolled in this study were periodically controlled by speech therapists (Lar Escola São Francisco). These professionals, beyond other orientations to the caregivers, also prescribed the adequate diet consistency for each individual, *based on their feeding difficulties, with the objective to avoid choking and food aspiration. Diet consistency was divided in 3 groups, as follows:*

- *Solid food: This food consistency is one normally offered to individuals with no severe oromotor dysfunction, and consisted of food in pieces, which needed to be chewed (figure 17).*
- *Semi-solid food: Food with a paste-like consistency, but still presenting pieces of the smashed, kneaded or triturated foods. Cereals, vegetables, cookies or bread smashed with milk and triturated or finely pulled meat are examples of semi-solid food. (figure 18).*
- *Liquid food:* Food has to be homogeneous, smooth and without pieces. *This consistency is obtained through* mixing, beating, or blending food with the use of a mixer. Fruits, soups, and cooked vegetables and meat can be prepared like this, but afterwards, they have to be strained. Custards and yogurts are also *indicated (figure 19).*
-

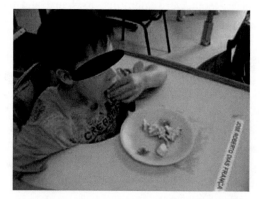

Figure 17. Solid food.

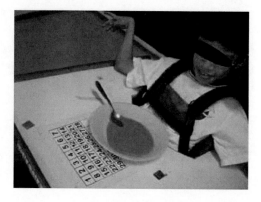

Figure 18. Semi-solid food.

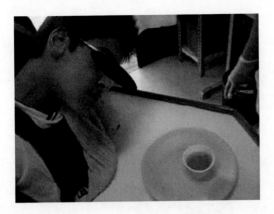

Figure 19. Liquid food.

In order to assess the consistency of the CP individuals diet, the caregivers were asked which of the 3 consistencies were prescribed by the speech therapist and if they were in accordance to the real dietary habits of these individuals.

GROWTH RATE

Growth rate was assessed through the measurement of weight and height. Individuals were weighted on a digital scale in a thin layer of clothing and dry diaper or underwear (figure 20).

Due to CP individuals' difficulties on standing straight, height was measured through the knee segment length *KH* (figure 21) and the estimation of stature (S) were determined from segmental measures in the equation:

Knee height (KH in cm) → *S = 2.69 x (KH) + 24.2cm*[17]

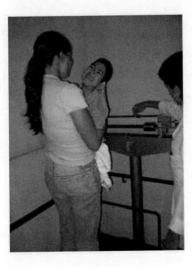

Figure 20. **W**eight measured with the CP individual being carried by the caregiver.

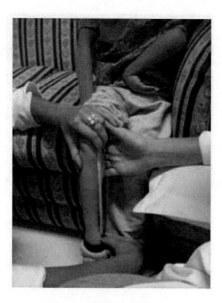

Figure 21. Height measured using the knee segment length.

The results were compared to CP growth curves[18] on the P10, P25, P50, P75, and P90 percentiles for height and weight, according to age and gender (figures 22, 23, 24 and 25).

For statistical analyses Chi square, Fisher exact, Kruskall-Wallis and Dunn tests were used. The significance level was set at p<0.05.

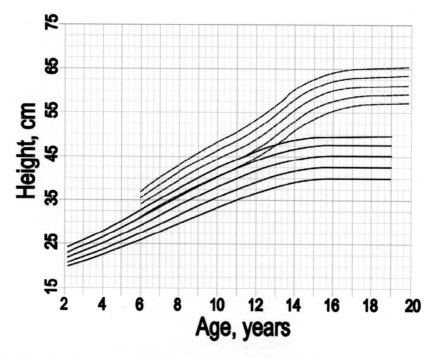

Figure 22. Height for CP girls (-) and healthy girls (-------), according to Stevenson et al.[17]

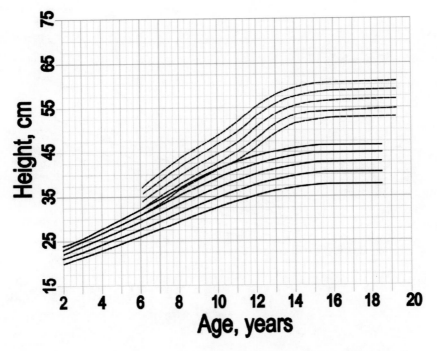

Figure 23. Height for CP boys (-) and healthy boys (-------), according to Stevenson et al.[17]

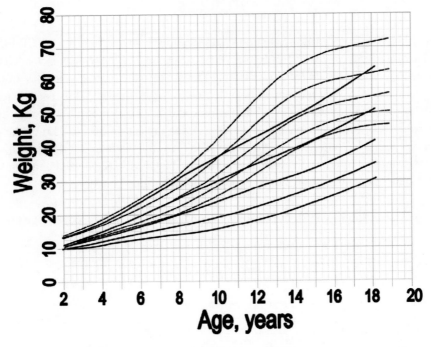

Figure 24. Weight for CP girls (-) and healthy girls (-------), according to Stevenson et al.[17]

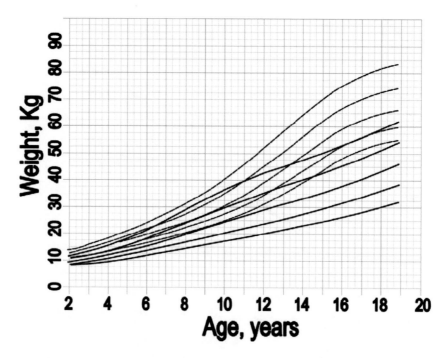

Figure 25. Weight for CP boys (-) and healthy boys (-------), according to Stevenson et al. [17]

RESULTS

Regarding the Gross Motor Function Classification System, from the 78 CP individuals enrolled in this study, 4 (5.1%) presented GMFCS level I, 2 (2.6%) presented level II, 6 (7.7%) presented level III, 44 (56.4%) presented level IV, and 22 (28.2%) level V of GMFCS.

Concerning the type of movement disorder, 64 individuals (82.1%) presented spastic CP, 13 (16.6%) presented dystonic CP with athetosis and 1 (1.3%) presented ataxia. About the clinical patterns of involvement, quadriplegic CP was present in 36 (46.2%) of the patients, diplegia was found in 25 (32.1%) of the patients and hemiplegia in 3 (3.8%) of them.

The distribution of CP individuals, according to the OFMFAS, age and gender are shown in table 2. The sample was shown to be homogenous regarding gender (p=0.701).

Table 2. Distribution of CP 78 individuals according to OFMFAS scores, age and gender

OFMFAS	Female			Male			Total		
	n	%	Age (mean ±SD)	n	%	Age (mean ±SD)	n	%	Age (mean ±SD)
I	8	23.5	9.4±2.3	17	38.6	9.6±2.7	25	32.1	9.5±2.5
II	16	47.1	9.5±2.2	15	34.1	8.3±2.0	31	39.7	8.9±2.1
III	9	26.5	9.3±2.1	9	20.5	10.1±2.4	18	23.1	9.7±2.2
IV	1	2.9	12.0±.0	3	6.8	12.0±1.7	4	5.1	12.0 ±1.4
Total	34	100.0	9.5±2.1	44	100.0	9.4±2.5	78	100.0	9.5±2.3

Considering oromotor function and gender, 23.5% of female (F) individuals and 38.6% of male (M) were found to be severely impaired, 47.1%F and 34.1%M moderately impaired, 26.5%F and 20.5%M slightly impaired, and 2.9%F and 6.8%M very slightly impaired.

The distribution of CP individuals, according to the OFMFAS scores, weight and height are shown in table 3.

Oromotor function was found to be a statistically significant factor on CP individuals' weight and height (p<0.05) when compared to CP growth curves[18] on the P10, P25, P50, P75, and P90 percentiles. Severely and moderately impaired individuals exhibited the P10 and P25 percentiles more frequently than slightly and very slightly impaired ones.

Table 3. Distribution of 78 CP individuals according to OFMFAS scores, weight and height

OFMFAS	Female				Male			
	n	%	Weight	Height	n	%	Weight	Height
I	8	23.5	18.4 ± 4.6	1.1±0.1	17	38.6	17.0±4.4	1.1±0.1
II	16	47.1	20.0±5.7	1.2±0.1	15	34.1	19.8±6.9	1.1±0.1
III	9	26.5	25.7±4.8	1.2±0.1	9	20.5	25.6±6.1	1.2±0.1
IV	1	2.9	35.6±0.0	1.5±0.0	3	6.8	36.9±14.5	1.3±0.1
Total	34	100.0	21.6±6.2	1.2±0.1	44	100.0	21.1±8.2	1.1±0.1

The distribution of the CP individuals according to diet consistency and DMFT index is shown in table 4.

Table 4. Mean scores [± SD] of DMF-T index and diet consistence of the 78 CP individuals

Diet consistency	n	DMFT (mean ±SD	P
Solid food	21	1.5±1.9 [a]	0.0053*
Semi-solid food	23	2.9±2.4 [b]	
Liquid food	34	3.6±2.2 [c]	

The data was compared by the Kruskal-Wallis test *P<0.05. Dunn test showed that [a] differs significantly from [b] and [c].

The Kruskal-Wallis test demonstrated a statistically significant difference on total DMFT values (p=0.0053) and diet consistency (table 4). The Dunn test verified that individuals on solid food diet intake presented statistically significantly the lowest DMFT (p<0.05) compared to the ones on a semi-solid and a liquid food diet intake.

Oral motricity was shown to be significantly associated with weight and stature in both genders (p<0.05), presenting the severely and moderately impaired groups a greater number of cases on the P10 and P25 percentiles, when compared with the CP growth curves[18] on the P10, P25, P50, P75 and P90 percentiles for height and weight, according to age and gender.

DISCUSSION

Understanding the impact of oromotor dysfunction, and its consequences, on oral health status, may be helpful in identifying individuals at high risk of developing dental caries and for planning preventive strategies and dental treatment for these individuals.

The sample of this study included CP individuals of both genders, attending the Special Children's Elementary School of Lar Escola São Francisco – Rehabilitation Center, and aged 4 to 14 years old (9.5±2.3). The eligibility criterion for students was that they should not have a cognitive deficit higher than 3 years of their chronological age, independently of global motor deficit. According to chronological limits established by the school, the students up to 4 years old were not evaluated.

In relation to gender, the male/female ratio found was of 1.3:1. Similar results were observed by Kiely et al.[19], in which the ratio found was of 1.4:1. Despite the greater prevalence of male gender observed in this study, when OFMFAS was considered, severely and moderately impaired individuals (I and II) were found similarly in both genders (72.7% e 70.6%).

It was observed for both genders that individuals with OFMFAS I and II presented the lower corporal weight values. This data suggests that the severity observed in OFMFAS evaluation may be helpful in reflecting the low weight in relation to age. This information can be of great value when patients need to be medicated according to their corporal weight, as when local anesthesia, antibiotics, analgesics and anti-inflammatories are needed. In severely compromised CP children, this must be respected in order to achieve an adequate dosage in these patients.

The direct measures of the stature are not possible in the majority of CP individuals due to the presence of contractions, articular deformities, scoliosis and involuntary movements.[20] The use of the shinbone (tibia) length may result in overestimated values with greater standard error of estimation (1.4 cm), when compared with a knee height of 1.1cm.[17]

Generally, the corporal mass rate is not an adequate screening for malnutrition, being a better indicator of acute malnutrition than for the chronic.[21] The CP child generally experiences long periods of malnutrition, being considered chronic cases.

The knee height was used as an alternative stature measure in individuals with impaired mobility, as an accurate, reliable and affordable substitute for assessing length in this type of individual.[17]

In relation to the height, it was observed that the female gender presented lightly superior values when compared with male gender, what is similar to that observed in no neurological impaired children.[22]

Oromotor dysfunctions at an early age disturb both growth and nutritional status and, therefore, CP children must receive early rehabilitation interventions.[4-5]

This study observed that CP individuals who were fed with a liquid diet presented total-DMF significantly higher than those who were fed semi-solid and solid diets. The individuals with severe oromotor impairment were unable to ingest solid food and the harmful role of a liquid diet consumed at an early age should be taken into account.[4,8,23] Probably these factors must be considered in relation to growth and development of CP individuals that presented minor weight/height rates in both genders as well.

High caries prevalence in CP individuals has been reported in the literature.[9-13] Food consistency, the number of carbohydrate exposures per day[4,8,23], the difficulty found in mastication due to the biting reflex [7], reduced salivary flow[24], long-term liquid oral medication[25], extremely high dental treatment needs[26] and problems related to dental management[27] are some of the points described in the literature. However, none of the studies took into account oromotor impairment in CP individuals as a risk factor.

Severely orofacial motor impaired individuals (score range ≤19 – OFMFAS I) were those fed on a liquid diet and presented the highest total-DMF. In view of the fact that the presence of caries in deciduous teeth exposes the individuals to high risk in permanent teeth[28], it is a fundamental requirement that these individuals begin to receive early preventive measures and, as part of this program, their caregivers should receive proper instruction, training and motivation regarding the realization of adequate oral hygiene, plaque control, dental floss use and fluoride therapy, as well as promoting adequate diet consistency; thus preventing deleterious and noxious habits such as bottle feeding.

The severity of the neurological damage is reflected, in a direct way, in the oral cavity through the oral motricity impairment, being directly associated with growth patterns in those individuals.

CONCLUSION

Oromotor dysfunction in children with CP is associated with poor growth and increased caries experience

ACKNOWLEDGMENTS

This study was approved by the Ethics Committee of the Federal University of Sao Paulo School of Medicine, Brazil, under the protocol number 0425/03.

REFERENCES

[1]   Bax M, Goldstein M, Rosenbaum P, Leviton A, Paneth N, Dan B, Jacobsson B, Damiano D; Executive Committee for the Definition of Cerebral Palsy. Proposed definition and classification of cerebral palsy. *Dev. Med. Child Neurol.* 2005; 47:571-6.

[2]   Meningaud JP, Pitak-Arnnop P, Chikhani L, Bertrand JC. Drooling of saliva: a review of the etiology and management options. *Oral Surg. Oral Med. Oral Pathol. Oral Radiol. Endod.* 2006; 101:48-57.

[3]   Yilmaz S, Basar P, Gisel EG. Assessment of feeding performance in patients with cerebral palsy. *Int. J. Rehabil. Res.* 2004; 27:325-9.

[4]   Gangil A, Patwari AK, Aneja S, Ahuja B, Anand VK. Feeding problems in children with cerebral palsy. *Indian Pediatr.* 2001; 38:839-46.

[5]   Sonis A, Castle J, Duggan C. Infant nutrition: implication for somatic growth, adult onset diseases, and oral health. *Curr. Opin. Pediatr.* 1997; 9:289-97.

[6]   Sullivan PB, Lambert B, Rose M, Ford-Adams M, Johnson A, Griffiths P. Prevalence and severity of feeding and nutritional problems in children with neurological impairment: Oxford Feeding Study. *Dev. Med. Child Neurol.* 2000; 42:674-80.

[7]   Dos Santos MT, Nogueira ML. Infantile reflexes and their effects on dental caries and oral hygiene in cerebral palsy individuals. *J. Oral Rehabil.* 2005; 32:880-5.

[8]   Hou M, Fu P, Zhao JH, Lan K, Zhang H. Oral motor dysfunction, feeding problems and nutritional status in children with cerebral palsy. *Zhonghua Er. Ke Za Zhi.* 2004; 42:765-8.

[9]   Gupta DP, Chowdhury R, Sarkar S. Prevalence of dental caries in handicapped children of Calcutta. *J. Indian Soc. Pedod. Prev. Dent.* 1993;11:23-7.

[10]   Bhavsar JP, Damle SG. Dental caries and oral hygiene amongst 12-14 years old handicapped children of Bombay, *India. J. Indian Soc. Pedod. Prev. Dent.* 1995; 13:1-3.

[11]   dos Santos MT, Masiero D, Simionato MRL. Risk factors for dental caries in children with cerebral palsy. *Spec. Care Dentist.* 2002; 22:103-7.

[12]   Rodríguez Vázquez C, Garcillan R, Rioboo R, Bratos E. Prevalence of dental caries in an adult population with mental disabilities in Spain. *Spec. Care Dentist.* 2002; 22:65-9.

[13]   Guare R. de O, Ciamponi AL. Dental caries prevalence in the primary dentition of cerebral palsied children. *J. Clin. Pediatr. Dent.* 2003; 27:287-92.

[14]   Wood E, Rosenbaum P. The gross motor function classification system for cerebral palsy: a study of reliability and stability over time. *Dev. Med. Child Neurol.* 2000;42:292-6.

[15]   Santos MT, Manzano FS, Ferreira MC, Masiero D. Development of a novel orofacial motor function assessment scale for children with cerebral palsy. *J. Dent. Child. (Chic.)* 2005; 72:113-8.

[16]   World Health Organization. Oral health surveys: basic methods, 4th edn. Geneva: WHO; 1997.

[17]   Stevenson RD. Use of segmental measures to estimate stature in children with cerebral palsy. *Archives of Pediatric and Adolescent Medicine.* 1995; 149: 658-62.

[18]   Stevenson RD, Conaway M,Chumlia WC, Rosembaum P, Fung EB, Henderson RC, Worley G. Growth and health in children with moderate-to-severe cerebral palsy. *Pediatrics.* 2006; 118: 1010-8.

[19]   Kiely M, Lubin R, Kiely J. Descriptive epidemiology of cerebral palsy. *Public Health Review.* 1984; 12: 79-101.

[20]   Patrick J, Boland M, Stolski D, Murray GE. Rapid correction of wasting in children with cerebral palsy. *Dev. Med. Child Neurol.* 1986; 28:734-9.

[21]   Radheshyam B. A comparison of five anthropometric indices for identifying factors of malnutrition. *American Journal of Epidemiology.* 1987; 126:258-67.

[22]   Day SM, Strauss DJ, Vachon PJ, Rosenbloom L, Shavelle RM, Wu YW. Growth patterns in a population of children and adolescents with cerebral palsy. *Dev. Med. Child Neurol.* 2007; 49:167-71.

[23]   Haschke F. The nutrition commission of the Austrian Society of Pediatrics and Adolescent Medicine. Prevention of caries. *Padiatr. Padol.* 1992; 27:109-11.

[24]   Santos MT, Siqueira WL, Nicolau J. Flow rate, pH and buffer capacity in saliva of adolescents with cerebral palsy. *J. Disabil. Oral Health.* 2006; 7:185-8.

[25] Sahgal J, Sood PB, Raju OS. A comparison of oral hygiene status and dental caries in children on long term liquid oral medications to those not administered with such medications. *J. Indian Soc. Pedod. Prev. Dent.* 2002; 20:144-51.

[26] Mitsea AG, Karidis AG, Donta-Bakoyianni C, Spyropoulos ND. Oral health status in Greek children and teenagers, with disabilities. *J. Clin. Pediatr. Dent.* 2001; 26:111-8

[27] Dicks JL. Outpatient dental services for individuals with mental illness: a program description. *Spec. Care Dentist.* 1995; 15:239-42.

[28] Skeie MS, Raadal M, Strand GV, Espelid I. The relationship between caries in the primary dentition at 5 years of age and permanent dentition at 10 years of age - a longitudinal study. *Int. J. Paediatr. Dent.* 2006; 16:152-60.

In: Handbook of Motor Skills
Editor: Lucian T. Pelligrino

ISBN: 978-1-60741-811-5
© 2009 Nova Science Publishers, Inc.

Chapter 10

A CASE STUDY OF CAPACITIES AND LIMITATIONS RELATED TO ARTHROGRYPOSIS MULTIPLEX CONGENITA AND COMPUTER INTERFACES

Wayne Shebilske and Jennifer Border
Wright State University, Dayton, OH, USA

ABSTRACT

We describe Arthrogryposis Multiplex Congenita (AMC), the presence of multiple joint contractures at birth, and we analyze the capacities and limitations of the second author, Jennifer Border, who has this condition. In AMC, the joints (arthro) of hands, wrists, elbows, shoulders, hips, feet, and knees are often fixed in a curved (gryp) position. Characteristically, the thumbs are pinned in the palms, and the hands are bent toward the arms, which are turned toward the body. Range of motion is limited by these joint contractures and often by muscle weakness. The purpose of analyzing capacities and limitations is to lay a foundation for human-centered assistive technologies especially computer interfaces. Determining an optimal interface for Jennifer is timely because her physicians have asked her to stop using a stylus held in her mouth, which has been her main interface with computer keyboards. Jennifer developed a repetitive motion injury in her shoulders from frequent use of this interface throughout grade school, high school, college, and her current first year in a Human Factors Psychology graduate program. This injury is affecting not only her interface with computers, but also other important tasks such as preparing and eating meals for which she is heavily reliant on her shoulder muscles. To prepare meals, for example, she holds containers in her mouth and pours by tilting her head and shoulders. In order to maintain these essential abilities, she must find an alternative computer interface and work station. Alternative interfaces under consideration are voice, eye movements, and EMG signals from facial muscles. Preliminary evaluations of these alternatives and their combinations will be made, but the present focus will be on analyzing Jennifer's capacities and limitations as a step toward a human-centered final choice.

BACKGROUND

A general description of AMC and repetitive motion injury will provide a background for our case study.

ARTHROGRYPOSIS MULTIPLEX CONGENITA (AMC)

AMC is the presence of multiple joint contractures at birth. A contracture is a limitation in the range of motion of a joint. The joints affected can vary from a few to nearly all joints in the individual's body (Hall, Jaffe, Paholke, & Staheli, 1998). The cause of AMC is relatively unknown; however, there are a few theories (Hall & Staheli, 2002). One of the most accepted theories is that the fetus did not have sufficient room to move in the mother's womb for normal movement. This lack in movement may cause the joint contractures. Restricted movement enables the development of extra connective tissue around the affected joints. The extra tissue then fixes the joint in place and limits more movement. The tendons around the affected joint may not have stretched to their normal length, which inhibits muscle growth and additional joint movement. Another accepted theory is that muscular atrophy occurs (Hall, Jaffe, Paholke, & Staheli, 1998). Specific causes of the atrophy are unknown, but suspected causes include muscle diseases (for example, congenital muscular dystrophies), maternal fever during pregnancy, and viruses. A third theory is that tendons, bones, joints, or joint linings may develop abnormally (Hall, Jaffe, Paholke, & Staheli, 1998). For example, tendons may not be connected to the proper place in a joint. The last two theories are believed to be genetic.

There are a variety of different types of AMC and the two most popular ones are Amyoplasia and distal.

Amyoplasia is considered "classical Arthrogryposis". It literally means no, "a", muscular, "myo", growth, "plasia" (Hall & Staheli, 2002). The joints typically affected are hands, wrists, elbows, shoulders, hips, feet, and knees and are symmetrical. Normally the elbows are stuck in a straight position, the arms are twisted toward the body, the wrists are flexed, and the thumbs are trapped in the palms (Hall & Staheli, 2002). The legs are usually more affected. The hips may be dislocated and the knees are either stuck in flexion or extension. The feet are severely equinovarus (clubbed; feet go down and inward (Hall, Jaffe, Paholke, & Staheli, 1998). Due to the fixed joints, in childbirth, the baby often is born with broken bones. Other characteristics in addition to the affected joints in Amyoplasia are absent muscle tissue that is replaced by fat and fibrous tissue, midfacial haemengioma, and normal intelligence. (Hall, Jaffe, Paholke, & Staheli, 1998).

Distal only affects an individual's limbs. The hands are usually clenched with overlapping fingers. The feet are also stuck in an equinovarus position. In addition, it is inherited through an autosomal dominant trait, chromosome 9. Intelligence is usually normal. (Hall, Jaffe, Paholke, & Staheli, 1998).

REPETITIVE MOTION INJURY

A repetitive motion injury (RMI) is described as a muscular condition that is developed from repeated motions that occur during a normal day (National Institute of Arthritis and Musculoskeletal and Skin Diseases NIAMS, 2006). It is caused by numerous uninterrupted or unnatural repetitions in an activity or over exertion of one's muscles (NIAMS, 2006). In a person's shoulder, an injury involves the tendons, ligaments, and muscles that hold the shoulder joint in place during motion (NIAMS, 2006). Injuries often occur in the rotator's cuff in athletes or people who lift heavy objects over their head daily. A rotator cuff is in the shoulder and comprises of four muscles and tendons that surround the ball of the shoulder joint that is connected the top of the arm (American Academy of Orthopedic Surgeons, 2007). Injuries are also caused by the degeneration of tendons over extended periods of time. The tendons in these individuals become irritated, inflamed, and may wear down, causing injuries.

CASE STUDY

Jennifer Border has Amyoplasia and a repetitive motion injury. Although she likes her current computer work station and interface, they are putting her health at risk. We are committed to putting her needs at the center of our search for an alternative work station and interface. Achieving this commitment was not as easy as it might sound. On the one hand, Jennifer was uncomfortable with it, because she usually overcomes challenges created by her condition as opposed to asking others to accommodate her. On the other hand, her major professor and senior author on this article was not comfortable violating a fundamental principle of human-centered design, which is to adapt technology to individuals as opposed to asking individuals to adapt to technology (e.g. Norman, 1988; Shebilske et al, 2007). The conflict between these opposing perspectives was resolved in discussions that recognized the value of Jennifer's can-do attitude, which serves her well in all that she does including this project, and the value of human-centered design, which must take into account her amyoplasia, her adaptive skills with her current work station and interface, as well as her repetitive motion injury.

Jennifer continually demonstrates her self reliance, persistence, and skill in overcoming limitations imposed by her amyoplasia. For example, while sitting between the senior author and another professor at a recent seminar, Jennifer suddenly swiveled in her chair like a ballerina turning toward the wall behind her. She then nudged her glasses against the wall, turn backed to look through them, repeated the sequence two more times, and announced to the astonished professors next to her that she had just adjusted her glasses against the wall. Jennifer's habit of self reliance is valuable because it enables her to care for her needs when others are not around. However, this habit made it difficult for Jennifer to embrace the goal of adapting an interface and workstation to her needs.

Embracing a Jennifer-centered designed became easier for Jennifer when we discussed the potential for follow-up research that would extend lessons learned from the present research to others. The others will include those who have AMC as well as those who have different medical or practical reasons for needing a computer interface other than their hands. Jennifer was more receptive, not only to the idea that a Jennifer-centered approach would be valuable, but also to the idea that a successful outcome would depend in large part on her contributions. Furthermore, her contributions would be enabled by her self reliance, persistence, skills, intelligence, and training in Human Factors Psychology.

AMYOPLASIA

Amyoplasia affects all of Jennifer's limbs. Her arms are similar to the background description except for her elbows. Her elbows are bent and fused at a 120 degree angle. Many muscles in her arms are smaller or nonexistent and were replaced by extra connective tissue and fat. This limits her range of motion. She is unable to lift her arm above her waist unless she uses a prop. Then she still cannot reach her head or neck. Her hands have weak muscle strength. Her thumbs are folded into her palm. This makes grasping things like pens, books, utensils difficult, but she is able to do it with adaptations.

Her knees are fused straight and her ankles are fused in a 90 degree angle. Her hips have full range of motion, but are rotated laterally out, which makes it difficult to sit with her legs together. To adjust to her legs, she sits with her legs apart, hips rotated out, and her feet in the air. Her height is 4' 8".

Her jaw is slightly affected, but through physical and speech therapy as a child, it is unnoticeable. Her speech is very clear. Her torso was affected only in the stomach. Some muscles are missing, but she has learned to compensate by using her back.

To compensate, she's learned to use her unaffected body parts and use the muscles that are normal. Her back, neck, head, shoulders, and jaw are all used for most activities that usually require use of one's arms. For example, to cook meals, she uses her chin to open the freezer/fridge. She also uses her jaw to open packages, stir, and pour ingredients.

ADAPTIVE SKILLS WITH THE CURRENT WORKSTATION AND INTERFACE

Her school work station is on her bed. She lays on her stomach with her arms propped underneath her. She uses a tablet pc that is propped up on a pillow and book for the right height. She types and does all cursor control with a stylus in her mouth. Her typing speed is ~30 WPMs. She is able to type more slowly (14 WPMs) with her hands. When a cd or flash drive is needed, she uses her mouth to place them in their respective slots.

When she needs a book or article, she prefers to read it on her Kindle. A Kindle is an electronic book reader that was developed by Amazon.com. It is very small and lightweight. To turn pages, she only has to press next page and the screen will change. She reads one of the many books or articles that are not in a kindle format by placing the book on her pillow with her jaw. She then opens and turns pages with her face. This method is especially difficult when reading very thick books whose pages did not lay open easily. She then props the book open with her chin or a weight and moves the item when she reaches the words it covers.

REPETITIVE MOTION

Throughout all of these activities, Jennifer is resting on her elbows with her arms crossed. To move on the bed, she rotates her shoulders to the necessary place. The rotation of her shoulders is the target area for the repetitive motion injury that is motivating the search for a new interface. Central to this search, therefore, will be a new work station that removes the cause of her injury and enables effective use of the new interface. She has tried positioning herself sitting up at a desk workstation. She is capable of doing it, but it produces more strain on her back and the front of her arms than the laying position.

Jennifer's current work station and computer interface are working effectively, but they are causing a repetitive motion injury in her shoulders that is of concern to her specialized orthopedist. She is specifically worried about her rotator's cuff in both shoulders. In March 2008, Jennifer injured her rotator's cuff. It is believed the cause of the injury was due to the repetitive motion when using her computer to type papers. She had two large research term papers (total pgs. 28) due within 4 days of each other. The motion that is of concern is when Jennifer rocks back and forth on her crossed arms, which rotates her shoulder joints. This motion occurs when Jennifer is reaching across her tablet PC screen and when reaching for papers nearby with her mouth. Jennifer's orthopedist stated that accessing her computer with the current methods was ruining her rotators cuff and in the future would cause a tear. A tear would immobilize her shoulder, resulting in more range of motion restriction than she already has. In addition to the current injury, in the past, Jennifer has fractured both arms a total of four times due to falls. One of her fractures was located at the top of her right arm directly below her rotators cuff. Based on her history and current condition, Jennifer's orthopedist estimates that we have no more than about two years to complete the transition to a new work station and interface safely.

ALTERNATIVE WORKSTATION AND INTERFACE

When searching for an alternative work station and interface, advantages and disadvantages of the current interface needs to be examined. Advantages of the current system are the user's efficiency, knowledge, and personal familiarity with the methods. She has used modified versions of this system for the past twelve years and has developed many adaptations to work with it. Disadvantages are its strain on Jennifer's shoulders and its immobility. For Jennifer's busy lifestyle as a graduate student and future educator, using the computer at work would be an advantage, but her current interface limits her to using her computer in her apartment. Can we modify Jennifer's present system to preserve the advantages and to overcome the disadvantages? Or will Jennifer have to switch to a qualitatively different system to overcome the disadvantages?

Modifying the Present System

We plan to consult an ergonomics specialist about modifying Jennifer's present system. Since mobility is a goal and since Jennifer's motorized wheel chair provides her best mobility, we will ask the specialist to evaluate whether Jennifer's present system could be transitioned safely to her motorized wheel chair. That is, could Jennifer, while seated in her wheel chair, type with a mouth-held stylus and perform the other related functions as fast as or faster than she does now without straining her shoulders or other body parts? The modified system would have to include holders for her notebook pc, her Kindle, and her other reading materials. The holders would have to be easy for Jennifer to use, and they would have to be positioned so that Jennifer could work efficiently and effectively without straining her body. The last requirement may prove to be impossible for the repetitive motion required to type with a mouth-held stylus. For example, even though Jennifer's neck muscles are strong, experts might conclude that typing with a mouth-held stylus will eventually put Jennifer's neck at risk regardless of the workstation design. In this case, Jennifer will have to consider switching to a qualitatively different interface. If typing with a mouth-held stylus can be made safe through workstation design, we will evaluate their desirability relative to qualitatively different interfaces. Ergonomic holders and supports for Jennifer's body will be critical for all systems, and they will be adapted to the interface that is best for Jennifer now and in the future.

Switching to a Qualitatively Different Interface

We are seeking qualitatively different interfaces that have the potential to be as efficient as and as effective as her current system without straining her body and without requiring much training. Alternatives under consideration are voice, eye movements, and EMG interfaces.

Voice Interface

Jennifer gave up on past voice interfaces because they made too many errors. Relative to her mouth-held stylus system, voice interface errors resulted in a net loss in efficiency and effectiveness. Recent improvements, however, have motivated Jennifer to try voice interfaces again. Specifically, she will try Dragon NaturallySpeaking 9. This interface is designed to type words on a computer screen with 99% accuracy for normal speech rates. It recognizes voices without training and continually improves as an individual uses it. Since normal speech rates are over 120 words per minute and typing rates are often less than 40 words per minute, this interface could help many of us whether or not we have a disability. In addition to typing, this interface controls other computer functions such as starting programs, using menus, controlling the mouse, and surfing the web (*www.NuanceStore.com*).

Why is research needed? Although Dragon Naturally Speaking 9 is rated as the best voice interface, it is not perfect (reviews.cnet.com/voice-recognition/dragon-naturally-speaking-10/4505-3528_7-33227363.html). For example, CNET reviewers found success with about four out of five spoken words. Research will be designed to determine whether or not this success rate yields a net gain over Jennifer's current system, which will depend in part on the efficacy of error recovery procedures. If Dragon Naturally Speaking 9 works for Jennifer today, it is likely to work better in the future, because the potentially large market should drive future improvements.

Eye Movement Interface

Jennifer will also try an eye movement interface. Specifically, she will try The EyeTech TM2, which replaces a mouse (http://www.enablemart.com/Catalog/Head-Eye-Controlled-Input/Quick-Glance-3). With this system, Jennifer would move the mouse pointer by looking at the desired location. TM2 can be used with Windows software and it can be combined with an on-screen keyboard or with DynaVox communication software (http://video.aol.com/video-detail/using-dynavox-with-the-eyetech-tm3/78865354). Jennifer might be able to transfer her proficiency using a keyboard with a mouth-held stylus to using it with TM2. A camera mounted below a computer monitor focuses on one eye or both eyes while TM2 software computes where the eye is looking and moves the cursor accordingly. Calibration is achieved quickly and can be carried to a new session or updated. Research would be required to determine which of several click options would be best for Jennifer. The options include eye blink and a hardware switch that Jennifer might be able to operate with her hand. Research would also be required to determine whether the limited allowable head movement fits Jennifer's needs.

Electromyography (EMG)/ Electrooculography (EOG) Interface

Another possibility is an EMG/EOG interface. Jennifer has already explored one such interface, Brian Fingers (http://www.brainfingers.com/). With this system, Jennifer wears a headband which detects electrical signals from her facial muscles (EMG) and eye movements (EOG). Brainfingers also has the potential to measure brainwaves, electroencephalographic (EEG), but Jennifer did not use this potential. The software decodes these signals to control mouse and keyboard events. Jennifer used EMG signals from her jaw to control vertical movements and a variety of high amplitude EMG thresholds were paired with different types of clicking (left, right, and timed clicks). Shifts in EOG signals produced right horizontal movements. However, if the signals were stable, the cursor would drift automatically to the left. BrainFingers interfaces with powerful software, such as DynaVox, and Windows.

Jennifer tested two typing programs with Brainfingers. One program was WiViK, which is an on-screen keyboard that is set up similar to a standard keyboard with the exception of an extra line of keys that have predictive text. The other typing program was Gaze Talk, which is a predictive text entry system that has a restricted on-screen keyboard. The keyboard's layout consists of 8 different boxes that contain the next predicted word or character.

WiViK's interface allowed the user to select from a full standard keyboard. The full keyboard had the potential advantage of transferring skills from Jennifer's current system, but this potential was not realized. The main reason was that Jennifer did not develop enough control with Brainfingers to hit each small key reliably when the whole keyboard was displayed. More practice might enable Jennifer to overcome this limitation.

Gaze Talk's interface worked the most efficiently with Brainfingers for Jennifer. There were only 8 very large key selections to choose from which enabled accurate selections. However, the small quantity of selections also slowed down the typing speed. Frequently, the user had to choose characters that were not predicted by Gaze Talk. The predictive text, which was a useful feature in Gaze Talk for casual conversation, was not as useful for transcribing a scientific article. Researchers may want to look into producing a variety of different word dictionaries relative to the needed vocabulary.

Combining Interfaces

After learning more about the strengths and weakness of voice, eye movement, and EMG/EOG interfaces for Jennifer, we will consider combining systems that are best for specific functions. For example, one system might work best for typing papers and another might work best for sending and receiving email or for surfing the internet. Ideally, research will show that one system is best for all of these applications, but we will be open to the possibility of combining them. A facilitating factor for combinations is the fact that a small workstation could easily accommodate all three of the interfaces that are under consideration. A limiting factor is the fact combinations would require practice on each system and on their combinations.

TESTING ALTERNATIVES

Making definitive comparisons among the complex alternatives will require systematic assessment tools and methods that are guided by a theory that is well-matched with such complexity.

Usability Proficiency Assessment Tool (UPAT) for the Web and Windows

We will adapt a UPAT prototype that was built to test ability to use tables, headings, forms, images, links, and combinations of these web features in the context of a simulated web site (Shebilske et al., 2009). The simulation was design to be representative of typical commercial web sites on which people make purchases. The UPAT tasks, which are shown in table 1, required participants to perform the kinds of operations that are typical in such web sites.

The UPAT tasks are performed in the order presented in Table 1. Each task has time limits so that the UPAT testing will end after a fixed time whether or not participants completes all tasks. Pilot observations have guided the setting of time limits that enables each participant to complete enough to assess their strengths and weaknesses on each task. All tasks are assessed in about 30 minutes. The order in which alternative interfaces will be tested with the UPAT task will be appropriately counterbalanced. The counterbalancing will be similar to small-N design methods that previous research in our lab has used (Levchuk, Shebilske, and Freeman, in press).

We will extend UPAT to test Windows applications. For example, Word usage will be tested with the transcription task that was designed to test Jennifer's ability to use Brainfingers. Jennifer transcribed text from an empirical psychology journal article in 15 minute intervals over a three month period. Other texts, such as less formal emails, will also be added. These texts are different from each other in vocabulary and structure, and both are relevant to Jennifer's career. We have already seen that the predictive feature of Gaze Talk worked well for casual conversation but not for the journal article. With an extended UPAT, we will test whether this limitation occurs in the predictive features of other systems such as Dragon NaturallySpeaking 9.

Table 1. UPAT tasks

Task ID	Task Description	Task Objective
Search a Table	Participant is required to search a TABLE for the lowest "total cost" of a book and to add the lowest cost book to their shopping cart.	Test skill of navigating through table elements.
Find Headings	Participant is required to search for a CD under the heading, "Symphonies."	Test skill of finding headings on page.
Complete a Form	Fill a form that consists of different elements such as text box, combo box, radio buttons and check boxes.	Test skill in filling form fields.
Click Image	Click on the image hyperlinked as " THE PHANTOM OF THE OPERA."	Test skill in identifying image objects and interacting with them.
Find Links	Identify specific links and click on them.	Test skill in identifying links on page.
Comprehensive Evaluation	Navigate on a simulated entertainment information web site. Read specific items and interact with them.	Test skill in interacting on a complete web site by searching for information, navigating to and from different pages, filling out forms and exiting from the web site.

COMPLEX ALTERNATIVES AND DYNAMICAL SYSTEMS THEORY

Dynamical Systems theory, which is a framework for understanding complex systems (e.g. Barabasi, 2002; Clark, 1997; Johnson, 2001; Juarrero, 1999; and West, 2006), seems well matched to the complexity of the systems to be investigated in the planned research. These systems will include Jennifer, her computer, their interface, and the workstation. Much of the research will be aimed at description, which is at the heart of Dynamical Systems theory.

Juarrero (1999) explains that Dynamical Systems theory restored rigorous description back to the highest ranks of formal reasoning. Aristotle had put it there as the formal cause, which is used to explain phenomenon. Formal cause is "that which makes anything that sort of thing and no other" (Juarrero, 1999, p.2). Newtonian science excluded formal cause in favor of efficient cause, the "push-pull impact of external forces on inert matter" (Juarrero, 1999, p.2). The restoration of formal cause to science depended on Dynamical Systems theory's fundamental ideas, which many scholars have described. For example, some fundamental ideas are describing state spaces, and using mathematics to describe trajectories through state spaces (Clark, 1997). The coordinates of a state space frame possible relationships among variables in a complex dynamical system. The trajectories are coordinated relationships that reflect the systems formal cause.

Studies of state space trajectories led to a) the realization that complex systems have order in their variability, b) mathematics to describe this order, and c) the insight that much can be learned by studying this order in variability, which is called fractal variability. West (2006) reviews this insight with respect to physiological systems. For example, order in the variability of heart rate comes from systematic influences of the sympathetic and parasympathetic nervous systems. Congestive heart failure is characterized by loss of these influences and by a corresponding loss of heart rate variability. In the extreme, congestive heart failure causes completely regular heart rate after which death soon follows. Similarly, fibrillation, a completely random heart rate, also causes death. Accordingly, our life depends on fractal variability in our heart rate, and studying this ordered variability gives insights into how our health depends on complex interactions among the parts of our body.

West (2006) presents a computational procedure for determining whether a series of heart beats is a fractal time series as opposed to a completely regular or completely random series. He also presents computational procedures for specifying trajectories through state spaces for fractal time series. He then applies both procedures to illustrate fractal variability in other time series including healthy breath rate and gate rate. He shows further that pathologies in the heart, breath, or gate systems are accompanied by changes in the output of these procedures. Finally, he emphasizes that such changes indicate that something is wrong as opposed to specifying what is wrong.

Jennifer generates time series when she types. Although we could compute Jennifer's time series in many ways, we plan to start by computing intervals between responses. Following West's (2006) lead, we anticipate that this procedure will show that Jennifer's typing generates fractal time series and that changes in fractal variability will reflect strengths and weakness in the alternative interfaces. Our goal is for changes in these descriptive statistics to guide us in tracking down specific strengths and weakness. A feel for how this goal might be achieved can be gained by thinking of components in Jennifer's typing systems as interacting components in a network and by comparing distributions for random processes and fractal processes in networks. A completely random process has a normal distribution, but fractal processes have a power law distribution. For example, a normal distribution describes well the number of national highways that serve cities, with a typical number for most cities and some random increase or decrease in that number for some cities. In contrast, a power law distribution describes an air traffic system in which many small air ports are connected through a few hub airports. A normal distribution also describes a fibrillating heart rate. In contrast, a power law distribution describes a healthy heart rate and many other complex systems. Barabasi (2002) argues that the power law is as ubiquitous as it is because it stems from the adaptive function of systematically grouping parts such as grouping together parts that use similar information. Such systematic influences change as a complex system interacts with its complex environment. If Jennifer changes fractal variability when she changes her interfaces, we will seek to understand how the interfaces facilitate or inhibit expedient interactions among system components.

We will be especially watchful for qualitative changes in fractal variability indicative of a system transitioning from one defined state to another. Such transitions are called "phase transitions." Our initial analysis of them will be done by West's (2006) method of plotting the values obtained on trial N+1 as a function of trial N. Johnson (2001) illustrated phase transitions with two examples. One is temperature causing water to transition from ice, to liquid, and to gas. Another example is a seed sprouting as a function of mathematically specifiable relationships among temperature, water, and light. The same variables influence the plant after it sprouts, but the influences are described by different functional relationships. This example illustrates that knowing how to predict effects of variables on one side of a phase transition, does not enable one to predict effects on the other side of a phase transition.

The inability to predict across phase transitions is a general principle of dynamical systems theory, and it has important implications for the present project. We anticipate that the complex system of Jennifer interacting with her computer will go through phase transitions as she switches from one interface and workstation to another and as she acquires skills with each. Accordingly, we will study each interface and workstation as opposed to trying to choose a new system based on what we know about her current system. We anticipate further that systems that yield completely regular response rates or randomly varied response rates will be less effective than ones that have fractal variability. Finally, we anticipate that describing the order in the variability will inform our understanding of the systems including their strengths and weaknesses.

HUMAN-CENTERED CRITERIA FOR PRIORITIZING ALTERNATIVE INTERFACES

Although we do not have enough information to make a final choice among the alternative interfaces, we know enough to specify human-centered criteria for prioritizing them. The criteria will take into account what we know about Jennifer and the alternatives. The criteria will be designed to guide the proposed research and the final choices.

We have summarized much about Jennifer's history and current needs. The parts that will be taken into account include:

- Jennifer's career goals favor a mobile workstation that she can use at home, work, and other professional environments.
- Jennifer has achieved a high proficiency level using a mouth-held stylus for keyboard inputs. However, this interface in her current workstation is putting her at risk of further repetitive motion injuries.
- Positive transfer from her current skills to her new system is important. Ideally, the alternative that has the most positive transfer will also have the best long-term potential. If not, however, the immediate benefits of building on current skills could be outweighed by the potential long-term benefits that might be gained by acquiring new skills. For example, a voice system would build the least on Jennifer's current skills, and it would require improving error correction skills, but we will evaluate whether it has the best potential for meeting all her needs in the long-term.
- The potential for skill acquisition to cause phase transitions implies that meaningful comparisons will require Jennifer to practice extensively with each system.
- Jennifer has the intelligence, self reliance, persistence, and motivation to do the research that will be needed to build an empirical foundation for choosing the best interface and work station for her.

We anticipate that the data base will also have general implications for others, but the goal of moving forward with potential benefits for others will be secondary to choosing the best interface and work station for Jennifer.

REFERENCES

American Academy of Orthopaedic Surgeons. (2007). *Rotator cuff tears and treatment options*. Retrieved October 10, 2008, from http://orthoinfo.aaos.org/ topic.cfm? topic=A00406

Barabasi, Albert-Laszio (2002). *Linked: How everything is connected to everything else and what it means for business, science, and everyday life.* New York: Penguin Books.

Clark, Andy (1997). Being there: Putting brain, body, and world together again. Cambridge, MA: MIT Press.

Lynn T. Staheli, Judith G. Hall, Kenneth M. Jaffe, Diane O. Paholke (1998). *Arthrogryposis: A Text Atlas.* Cambridge, MA: Cambridge University Press.

Hall, J. G. & Staheli, L. T.(2002). *Arthrogryposis Multiplex Congenita: what it is and how it is treated.* [Brochure]. Portland, OR.

Johnson, Steven (2001). *Emergence: The connected lives of ants, brains, cities, and software.* New York: Scribner.

Juarrero, Alicia (1999). *Dynamics in action: Intentional behavior as a complex system.* Cambridge, MA: Bradford Books.

Levchuk, G. Shebilske, W. and Freeman (in press). A model driven instructional strategy: The benchmarked experiential system for training (BEST). *Journal of Mathematical Psychology.*

National Institute of Arthritis and Musculoskeletal and Skin Diseases NIAMS/National Institutes of Health

Norman, D.A. (1988). *The psychology of everyday things.* New York: Basic Books.

Shebilske, W., Narakesari, S., Alakke, G., and Kegley, J. (2007). Software Helping Military Troops and Persons With Disabilities Help One Another. *Proceedings of the First International Conference on Technology-based Learning with Disability.*

Shebilske, W., Narakesari, S., Alakke, G., Douglass, R. and Faulkner, E. (2009). Web Usability and Screen Readers. *Proceedings of the annual CSUN Conference, March16-21,2009.*

Staheli, L.T., Hall, J. G., Jaffe, K. M., & Paholke, D. O. (1998). *Arthrogryposis a text atlas.* New York, NY.: Cambridge University Press.

West, Bruce. (2006). *Where medicine went wrong: Rediscovering the path to complexity.* New Jersey: World Scientific Publishing Co.

In: Handbook of Motor Skills
Editor: Lucian T. Pelligrino

ISBN: 978-1-60741-811-5
© 2009 Nova Science Publishers, Inc.

Chapter 11

COMPARATIVE STUDY ON THE DEVELOPMENT OF MANIPULATIVE SKILLS IN CHIMPANZEES AND HUMANS

Misato Hayashi[*][1] *and Hideko Takeshita*[2]

[1] Primate Research Institute, Kyoto University, Japan
[2] University of Shiga Prefecture, Hikone City, Shiga, Japan

ABSTRACT

Manipulative activity is based on both manual motor skills and cognitive development. Humans and chimpanzees, the closest living relatives of human beings, share manual dexterity in manipulating objects in their daily lives. Chimpanzees are also known to use tools in their natural habitat to achieve a variety of goals. This chapter reports the findings gained by assigning tasks using identical objects conducted in a face-to-face situation for chimpanzees and human children. Manipulative skills in both species were analyzed as a non-verbal scale for direct comparison by focusing on their manipulative patterns. Tasks using blocks of different shapes were designed to test physical understanding involved in making a vertical stack. The subjects were required to selectively use appropriate orientation of differently-shaped blocks in order to stack them efficiently. The subjects acquired the solution of manually changing the orientation of the blocks to the appropriate one. The results illuminated a fundamental similarity between chimpanzees and humans. Tasks using nesting cups were originally designed to assess cognitive development in human children by analyzing the behavioral strategies of combining multiple cups into a nesting structure. The manipulation of nesting cups was described in a form of sequential codes in both chimpanzees and humans to illuminate the patterns of making a hierarchical combination among objects. Some of the subjects from both species succeeded in making a nesting structure with nine cups. The subjects tried to solve the task by reducing the number of cup units and by combining cups in an appropriate order. In sum, manipulative behavior revealed high levels of physical intelligence shared by chimpanzees and humans.

---

[*] Contact address: E-mail: misato@pri.kyoto-u.ac.jp. Section of Language and Intelligence, Primate Research Institute, Kyoto University, 41 Kanrin, Inuyama, Aichi, Japan 484-8506. Tel.: +81-568-630548; Fax: +81-568-622428

INTRODUCTION

Comparative studies among primates can be a way of investigating the unique characteristics of human evolution and development (Takeshita, Myowa-Yamakoshi and Hirata, 2009). Primates, including humans, share a motor skill of manipulating objects using hands [Crast et al., 2009], which are evolved as an adaptation to their arboreal life for grabbing branches in the forest. The skill of object manipulation is applied in various kinds of situations in their daily lives to efficiently change the surrounding environment. In this sense, the skill of object manipulation is fundamental to physical intelligence. Manipulative activity is based on both manual motor skills and cognitive development. Chimpanzees, the closest living relatives of human beings, share manual dexterity in manipulating objects and are also known to use tools in their natural habitat to achieve a variety of goals.

Tool use requires both manual motor skills and high levels of cognitive ability. Thus, people had believed that humans comprise the only species that can manufacture and use tools. In 1964, the first evidence of tool use was reported in a wild chimpanzee community [Goodall 1964]. Up to now, tool use has been reported in three other species of great apes (bonobos, gorillas and orangutans), long-tailed macaques and capuchin monkeys [McGrew and Marchant, 1997; Breuer, Ndoundou-Hockemba and Fishlock, 2005; Malaivijitnond et al., 2007; Watanabe, Urasopon and Malaivijitnond, 2007]. Among the list of tool-using species, both chimpanzees and humans are known to be proficient tool users, in part due to their remarkable manual dexterity.

By using tools, chimpanzees are able to access food items that would otherwise be inaccessible. For example, a chimpanzee uses a stick to fish termites within subterranean mounds [Lonsdorf, 2005; Sanz, Morgan and Gulick, 2004], while an anteater has specifically evolved a long and sticky tongue for the same purpose. The high level of material intelligence of chimpanzees therefore enables them to surmount physical constraints by effectively changing the environment with the aid of the tools.

One precursor of tool-using behavior is called "combinatory manipulation." whereby an individual relates a manipulating object to something else (including substrates or other objects) [see review in Hayashi, Takeshita and Matsuzawa, 2006]. Torigoe (1985) compared the repertoire of object manipulation in 74 species of primates using wooden cubes as a manipulanda. The result showed that combinatory manipulation (referred as secondary manipulation) was rarely seen in primates. They had a tendency to focus on manipulating one object and rarely combined it with another object.

In human developmental studies, combinatory manipulation can be used as a milestone in assessing cognitive development in infancy and childhood. For example, humans start to insert a rod into a hole on a box and to stack up blocks at around one year of age. Humans also start to insert a cup into a larger cup and the number of cups successfully combined into a nesting structure increases as their age develops. This chapter reports the findings gained by tasks using identical objects conducted in a face-to-face situation for chimpanzees and human children. Manipulative skills in both species were analyzed as a non-verbal scale for direct comparison by focusing on their manipulative patterns (figure 1). The chimpanzee subjects were kept at Primate Research Institute, Kyoto University, Japan in an enriched enclosure with other group members. The long-term research is continuing in a variety of study settings including a face-to-face paradigm [reviewed in Matsuzawa, 2003; Matsuzawa, Tomonaga and

Tanaka, 2006]. Human subjects (aged one to four years) were the participants in the "Umikaze" Infant Laboratory of the University of Shiga Prefecture.

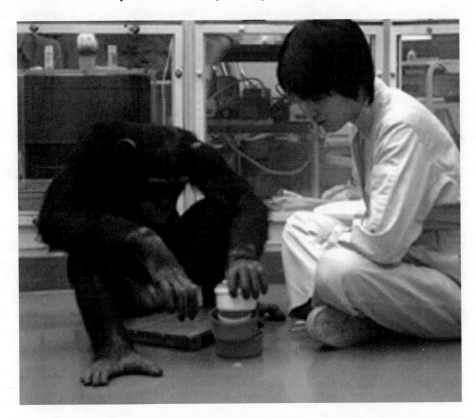

Figure 1. A chimpanzee subject (Ayumu) trying to combine cups in a face-to-face situation.

EMERGENCE OF STACKING-BLOCK BEHAVIOR

In order to stack blocks, a manipulated block should be appropriately oriented in relation to another block. An individual has to finely control the location of where to place a block and also the timing of releasing the block from the hand on top of a tower of blocks. Block-stacking play is a common activity in human children, but it is rarely observed in non-human primates: so far, only four species of great apes (chimpanzee, bonobo, gorilla and orangutan) are known to stack up blocks. The other primates may manipulate a block by manually holding it or by trying to break it with their teeth. If you imagine the natural life of primates in the wild, this manipulative tendency might be reasonable. Stacking objects in the wild may not produce any meaningful result for survival. In contrast, an individual may find hidden edible items by breaking off branches or nuts.

Stacking-block behavior is categorized as an example of combinatory manipulation. Hayashi and Matsuzawa (2003) reported early cognitive development in mother-reared infant chimpanzees. The study showed that chimpanzee infants spontaneously started to insert an object into a hole, but the development of stacking blocks was delayed in chimpanzees. On the contrary, humans start to show the two types of combinatory manipulation at around the same time, at one year of age [Ikuzawa 2000]. The study setting for chimpanzees was simple: the infant chimpanzees observed their mother exhibiting the combinatory manipulation (Hayashi et al., 2009) in order to reveal the spontaneous pattern of object-manipulation development under a natural learning situation for chimpanzees. Human experimenters did not assist the infants in stacking blocks during the first three years after birth.

Only one female chimpanzee, named Pal, spontaneously started stacking blocks when she was two years and seven months of age, indicating that simple observation of the mother's stacking model was enough to develop the stacking-block behavior in at least one out of three infant chimpanzees. Without any reinforcement, Pal continued stacking blocks and successfully made a tower of seven blocks when she was two years and eight months old. Pal sometimes showed excitement after a successful stacking of many blocks by jumping above the tower of blocks with smile on her face. In contrast to human mothers, the chimpanzee mother did not show active teaching or active encouragement while the infant was manipulating the blocks.

The other two infant chimpanzees never showed any sign of stacking blocks for three years after birth, although the testing situation was identical to the successful individual. Moreover, even the successful individual stopped stacking after several months of practice by herself, which resulted in no direct reward.

When the three infants reached three years and one month of age, the human experimenter started actively teaching by using a food reward. One of the three infants, Ayumu, had no difficulty in orienting a manipulated block towards another block following the guidance of the human experimenter such as pointing to another block on the floor. When he successfully stacked the block onto another, the human experimenter gave him a food reward such as a slice of apple or orange. Pal, the first chimpanzee infant to spontaneously stack blocks, restarted stacking when she realized that she could receive a food reward by stacking.

One remaining chimpanzee, Cleo, did not understand the intention of the human guidance and tried to give the block back to the experimenter's hand. She did not pay attention to the block on the floor. Thus, two or three blocks were glued together to enhance the height of block tower. Moreover, the human experimenter put his hand close to the top of the tower so that Cleo inevitably oriented the block towards the tower as a result of trying to give it back to the experimenter. If Cleo oriented or actually touched a manipulated block to the glued tower of blocks, the behavior was rewarded with food. With this repetition, Cleo gradually learned to stack blocks by orienting a block in hand to the glued tower and releasing the block from the hand onto the tower. Once she learned that the stacking behavior was rewarded, she continued to stack blocks the same way as the other two infants.

Interestingly, the species difference appeared not only in the age of onset in stacking behavior but also in the pattern of development after the first success. Ikuzawa (2000) reported that 50% of the humans stack one block at the age of one year and two months. At one year and eight months of age, 50% of humans stack five blocks successively, resulting in a tower of six blocks. Thus, it takes humans six months from the first success in stacking a block to the success of making a tower of six blocks. Humans easily orient a block in hand to another block on the floor, but fine adjustment for the place and timing of releasing the block seems difficult for human infants and children. All three chimpanzee subjects succeeded in making a tower of six blocks within one month after their first success. It indicated that the motor skills in chimpanzees were already developed before their first success in stacking.

Following the motor-skill development, cognitive ability of perceiving or understanding a goal of stacking blocks developed in chimpanzees. In the human case, both abilities may develop at around the same time or the motor skills may develop later, leading to a gradual increase following their manipulative development.

STACKING BLOCKS OF DIFFERENT SHAPES

During the previous training phase, cube-shaped blocks were used exclusively. In the new task, blocks of cylindrical shape were first introduced to the chimpanzees who already had the ability to stack cubic blocks. Tasks using blocks of different shapes were designed to test physical understanding involved in making a vertical stack (Hayashi and Takeshita, in press) . In the case of cubic blocks, if blocks are stacked with enough overlap between them, a base block can support an upper block. By using blocks of different shape, the subjects were required to selectively use the appropriate orientation for stacking. If the orientation was inappropriate, the subjects were required to actively change the orientation of the blocks in order to stack them efficiently. The interaction between the subject and the objects was important in the solving process.

Povinelli (2000) focused on chimpanzee's intelligence in physical domain using a variety of tasks that mainly ask their understanding on the tool properties. Povinelli and Dunphy-Lelii (2001) further examined physical understanding in a task of making an oblong block stand on a platform. In this task, the reaction to failure (such as visually inspecting bottom of malfunctioning block) was the main variable analyzed to infer to the causal understanding. The present study, however, allowed the subjects to freely manipulate blocks to actively solve the problem in the process of manual activity. If the orientation of a block is not appropriate for stacking, the subject is required to actively change the orientation to an appropriate one. This active manipulative solution may thus directly reveal the physical intelligence of the subject in a problem-solving situation. It might also be informative in helping us understand how chimpanzee relate object property to function, a capacity which chimpanzees demonstrate in the wild when manufacturing and modifying tools for given purposes [Sanz and Morgan, 2006].

The task required the subject to stack up four blocks (two cubic blocks, one cylindrical block in appropriate orientation, and one cylindrical block in inappropriate orientation). When the subject stacked all four blocks, he/she received a relatively large piece of food reward. One session consisted of five trials and was conducted once a day. Among the three infants, only the individual who spontaneously started to stack cubic blocks (Pal) succeeded in stacking cylindrical blocks efficiently from the beginning. Among three adults, the two with the most experience with staking cubic blocks succeeded from the first session.

The remaining two infants and one adult with less experience in stacking cubic blocks failed to selectively use the appropriate orientation of cylindrical blocks at the beginning. They frequently tried to stack a cylinder in inappropriate orientation. As a result, they had difficulties in staking all four blocks. After the blocks would fall, however, the orientation of the block was sometimes changed accidentally to the appropriate one and the chimpanzees took that opportunity to stack all four blocks. In other cases, they put a cylinder in inappropriate orientation as the last block in the tower of four blocks, thus completing the task, although the orientation of the last block did not generate a stable tower. However, after accumulating experiences in manipulating cylinders, even the unsuccessful individuals gradually started to change the orientation of blocks. Finally, all six chimpanzees became proficient in stacking up all four blocks including two cylinders [more precise data are reported in Hayashi (2007a)].

A triangular block was then introduced to the subjects who mastered the skill of stacking cylindrical blocks efficiently. A triangular block has three types of placement on the floor and only one of them is suitable for stacking. The other two orientations cannot support another block since the top surface is slanted. In order to stack the next block on a triangular block, a subject should carefully ensure that both the bottom and top orientations of the stacked block are horizontal.

The new task setting was almost identical to the previous one: the only difference was that the cylindrical blocks were replaced by triangular blocks. However, all the six subjects (including the three infants at four years of age and three adults) who were successful at stacking cylindrical blocks failed to stack the new triangular blocks efficiently in their first session. They showed many errors such as trying to stack a next block on the slanted surface of triangular blocks. They even released their hands on the slanted surface and it inevitable resulted in the fall of the released block. It might be hard for them to recognize the difference in orientation of triangular blocks since all the surfaces are flat and stackable. This might be related to an effect of "affordance" [Lockman, 2000]. The shape of cylinder might be more salient in allowing them to discriminate differences in orientation while the orientation of triangular shapes cannot so readily be distinguished.

We continued to test the three infants with triangular blocks to chart the development of their understanding of the task. After an accumulation of experience, all three juvenile chimpanzees finally succeeded in stacking triangular blocks although the speed of acquisition varied among the three individuals. They showed less contact with inappropriate orientation in the later period. They also started to actively change the inappropriate orientation to an appropriate one. Although it took them a long time to master this task, the chimpanzees were able to eventually learn how to stack triangular blocks successfully.

There were several ways to change the orientation of blocks. The successful infant chimpanzee at the beginning of cylindrical-block stacking (Pal) changed the orientation of blocks with using both hands. Pal picked up blocks of inappropriate orientation from the floor using a hand and manually rotated it few times with using both hands. The other two infant chimpanzees frequently changed the orientation of blocks with using a hand and mouth. They picked up blocks from the floor using a hand and used their mouth for the support during rotation (figure 2). One chimpanzee, Cleo, gradually shifted to change the orientation of blocks using a hand and rotate it on the floor.

The stacking-block tasks were conducted in human children (aged one to four years) in an identical test situation in a face-to-face paradigm. Humans who had the ability of stacking cubic blocks spontaneously changed the orientation of cylindrical blocks from the beginning. However, the stacking of triangular blocks was difficult for human children during the age of one year. Humans started to succeed in stacking triangular blocks efficiently after they reached two years.

In sum, the subjects acquired the solution of manually change the orientation of blocks into appropriate one during the stacking task of differently shaped blocks. The result illuminated fundamental similarity between chimpanzees and humans in the domain of physical intelligence.

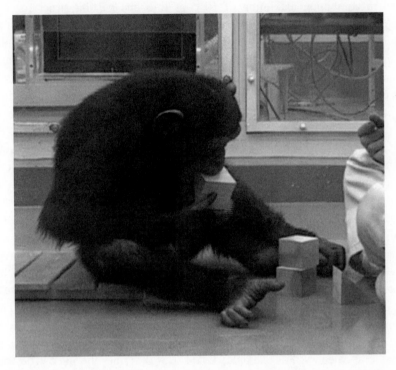

Figure 2. A chimpanzee subject (Ayumu) changing orientation of a cylindrical block with the support of the mouth.

NESTING CUP TASK

The nesting cup task was originally designed to show the existence of consistent strategies in the naturally occurring manipulative play in human children [Greenfield, Nelson and Saltzman, 1972]. The task requires the subject to make a nesting structure by combining multiple round cups of different diameter. The first paper reported that there was developmental shift of combining strategies in human children. First, they made the combination of only two cups and did not combine more cups into the structure (pairing method). This type of combination was dominant for children at around one year of age. Second, the human subjects made the combination of three or more cups by successively moving one cup at a time (pot method). This type of combination reached its peak at 20 months old. Third, the human subjects made the combination of three or more cups by moving multiple cups as a unit (subassembly method). This type of combination became dominant for children at three years of age. The authors claimed children's use of consistent strategies in combining cups was parallel to some grammatical structure in language acquisition.

The nesting cup task was further applied to studies in non-human primates [Matsuzawa, 1991; Johnson-Pynn et al., 1999] and for different analyzing paradigm such as focusing on error-correction strategies [DeLoache, Sugarman and Brown 1985]. The previous studies illustrated that subassembly method, the most advanced strategy in human development, was observed in both chimpanzees and capuchin monkeys. Moreover, chimpanzees and capuchins succeeded in combining maximum of 10 cups into one nesting structure. Thus, the three category of combining strategy did not show the species specificity. In addition, there has been discussion on the necessary requisite for the nesting skill. Johnson-Pynn and Fragaszy (2001) argued that perceptual-motor learning is more important factor in the nesting task rather than conceptions of reversible relationship (an intermediate cup is smaller than previous cup and larger than subsequent cup) or linguistic capacities. The nesting task may be a good paradigm to assess and discuss about primates' skill in both cognitive and motor domain.

Hayashi (2007b) designed a new method of describing the whole sequence of cup manipulation in a form of sequential codes. The aim of the new notation system was to gain more precise information on sequential structures which may lead to the systematic analysis on grammatical rules exist in motor activity. In the new notation system, a segment of cup manipulation was denoted as a code consisting of a combination of two set of numbers and one letter: in a form of n_1Xn_2. The first number refers to the "object", i.e., *what* was manipulated by the subject. The letter code refers to the "action" involved in the manipulation, i.e., *how* the object was manipulated. The second number refers to "location" in an object-object combination if any, i.e., where the manipulated object was related to. Each segment of behavior is separated from those before and after it by slashes. Thus, the entire flow of manipulation was described in the form of sequential codes. In the nesting cup task, the cups were numbered from 1 to 5 (smallest to largest) and the letter codes were given to each behavioral category. For example, 1N2/12N3/ describes the most efficient combination of three cups: the subject *inserted the smallest cup into the second largest cup* and *moved the two-cup combination as a unit into the largest cup*. If the number before a letter code was plural (like the second manipulation in the above example), it corresponds to the subassembly strategy in a segment level.

Hayashi (2007b) also utilized "state transition analysis" which focused on the efficiency of reaching the goal of making a nesting structure. The state of the cups was defined by two parameters: "number of unit" and "contiguity". Number of unit indicated how many structures or individual cups exist in a static condition. At the beginning of each trial, the number of unit corresponded to the number of cups given to the subject scattered separately on the floor. The score for a full nesting structure was 1, the goal of each trial where all the cups were nested in one structure. The second parameter, contiguity, indicated how many pairs of cups were seriated in a successive order. For example, if a subject inserted cup-2 into cup-3, contiguity increases because cups 2 and 3 are combined without any intermediate cup or a gap between them. On the contrary, if a subject inserted cup-2 into cup-5, contiguity doesn't change due to the gap (absence of cups 3 and 4) between 2 and 5.

This chapter reports the manipulation of nine cups in chimpanzees and humans of different ages. They succeeded in nesting five cups and were successively given nine cups for the first time in their life. Among three chimpanzees and three humans reported in this chapter, one chimpanzee and two humans successfully made one nesting structure at the end of trial. Table 1 showed the basic information for the participants and the overall results. However, even in the successful individual, the cup manipulation was not straightforward to the direction of the goal.

There were many progression and regression in each trial. We applied "state transition analysis" to illuminate their pattern of making a hierarchical combination among objects. The efficiency of combination can be plotted in a two-dimensional plane (figure 3). In the case of trial with nine cups, the starting point is the right-down corner of the plane (9, 0) where all the nine cups were separately placed on the floor and no contiguous pair of cups. The goal of a trial is the left-up corner (1, 8) where the nine cups were seriated in one nesting structure and eight contiguous pairs of cups. The most efficient way of combining nine cups can be shown as a straight line connecting the right-down and the left-up corner of the plane.

Table 1. List of subjects who participated in the nesting of nine cups

	Name	Sex	Age	Success
Chimpanzee	Ai	Female	15 years (adult)	Yes
Chimpanzee	Ayumu	Male	6 years 6 months (juvenile)	No
Chimpanzee	Pal	Female	6 years 3 months (juvenile)	No
Human 1	IO	Female	3 years 4 months	Yes
Human 2	YS	Female	2 years 3 months	Yes
Human 3	HS	Female	2 years 3 months	No

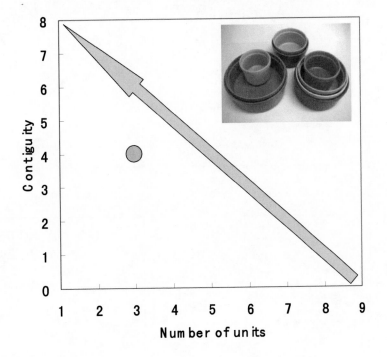

Figure 3. Scheme of state transition analysis. A line arrow indicates the most efficient way of combining nine cups. A point on the two-dimensional plane (3, 4) is an example shown in the picture: three units and four contiguous pairs.

Figure 4 illustrated the efficiency of cup manipulation by three chimpanzees and three human children. Three subjects reached the left-up corner of the plane, indicating there success in making a full-nesting structure. The other three subjects stopped manipulation without completing a nesting structure. One chimpanzee subject, Ayumu, piled up units of cups into one structure but the cups were not neatly paired. Another chimpanzee, Pal, combined eight cups appropriately but the fifth cup was left aside. Pal finally reversed the fifth cup and piled it on the eight-cup structure. One human of age two years and three months stopped manipulation after making three cup-structure with low contiguity.

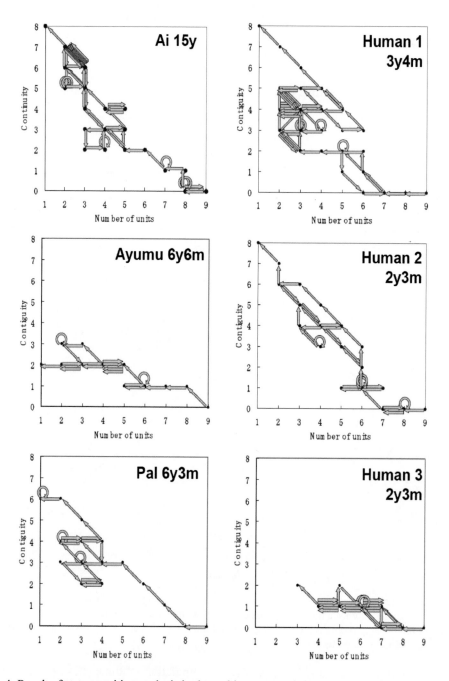

Figure 4. Result of state transition analysis in three chimpanzees (left column) and three humans (right column) during the first attempt in nesting nine cups.

Even successful subjects of both species showed many trial-and-error in making the final nesting structure. Each arrow in figure 4 indicated the type of cup-state transition. The most efficient type is directed to left-up showing that a cup was combined appropriately: resulted in the decrease of unit number and the increase of contiguity. This type of efficient transition occurred in 23–28% among the total occurrence of cup-state transition for the three successful subjects and 32% for Pal, who reached close to the goal. However, the occurrence of efficient transition was 14% for the other two unsuccessful subjects. Unsuccessful subjects did not show the transition which increased only contiguity, shown in straight-up arrow, except one case by the third human subjects. Successful subjects showed this type of transition in 23–28% of the total occurrence of cup-state transition. This type of transition was made by removing a cup (or a cup-unit) from not-contiguous unit, and inserted into other cup or unit in appropriate order without any gap between them.

There might be two possible strategies in achieving the goal of full-nesting structure. One is to reduce the number of cup-unit exist on the floor, to the left direction in figure 4. Another is to increase the contiguity by making more contiguous pairs, in other words, by avoiding a gap between cups. The present analysis revealed that unsuccessful subjects had strong tendency to reduce the number of unit on the floor but they pay less attention to increase the contiguity of the cup combination.

The present data of the first attempt in nesting nine cups showed comparable manipulation patterns in chimpanzees and human children. The further study should deal with more comprehensive information from more number of individuals and from different ages. The internal rule exhibited in the process of cup manipulation will be illuminated by using the precise notation system. This approach can shed light on the evolution and development of intelligence embedded in motor skills.

CONCLUSION

This chapter reported the direct comparison between chimpanzees and humans in two kinds of cognitive tasks. The tasks involved objects to be manipulated by the subjects. The first task focused on their understanding of physical rules by using differently shaped blocks. The second task focused on the behavioral strategies shown in the process of making a hierarchical nesting structure. In both tasks, chimpanzees and human children showed similar patterns of manipulation.

The present tasks revealed that both chimpanzees and humans were capable of actively manipulating objects to achieve the goal of the tasks. The present task required the subject to apply existing motor skills and underlying cognitive abilities in order to complete a trial under new task settings. Subjects acquired the understanding of how a block serves as a supporting surface to the next block and the skill of actively changing the orientation of the block to the appropriate one. Facing nine cups, the subjects tried to make a full nesting structure by successively combining multiple cups and reducing the number of units. Chimpanzees and human children share the flexible physical intelligence and the manual motor skills that enable real action in the surrounding environment.

ACKNOWLEDGMENTS

The study reported in this chapter was supported by grants from JSPS and the Ministry of Education, Science, and Culture in Japan (#19700245 to Misato Hayashi, #16203034 to Hideko Takeshita, and #20002001 to Tetsuro Matsuzawa) and from the Benesse Corporation. Special thanks are due to Tetsuro Matsuzawa, Masaki Tomonaga, Masayuki Tanaka, Sana Inoue, Tomoko Takashima, Etsuko Nogami, Kiyonori Kumazaki, Norihiko Maeda, Shohei Watanabe, Juri Suzuki, Takako Miyabe, Akino Watanabe and Akihisa Kaneko for their great advice and support in conducting the daily work and care of chimpanzees at the Primate Research Institute, Kyoto University. The human data was collected in collaboration with Masako Myowa-Yamakoshi, Ari Ueno, Keiko Yuri and Aya Saito with the support of mothers and children participating in the "Umikaze" Infant Laboratory of the University of Shiga Prefecture.

REFERENCES

Breuer, T., Ndoundou-Hockemba, M., Fishlock, V. (2005) First observation of tool use in wild gorillas. *PLoS Biology.* 3, e380 2041-2043.

Crast, J., Fragaszy, D., Hayashi, M., Matsuzawa, T. (2009) Dynamic in-hand movements in adult and young juvenile chimpanzees (*Pan troglodytes*). *American Journal of Physical Anthropology.* 138, 274-285.

DeLoache, J. S., Sugarman, S., Brown, A. L. (1985) The development of error correction strategies in young children's manipulative play. *Child Development.* 56, 928-939.

Goodall, J. (1964) Tool-using and aimed throwing in a community of free-living chimpanzees. *Nature.* 201, 1264-1266.

Greenfield, P. M., Nelson, K., Saltzman, E. (1972) The development of rule-bound strategies for manipulating seriated cups: a parallel between action and grammar. *Cognitive Psychology.* 3, 291-310.

Hayashi, M. (2007a) Stacking of blocks by chimpanzees: developmental processes and physical understanding. *Animal Cognition.* 10, 89-103.

Hayashi M (2007b) A new notation system of object manipulation in the nesting-cup task for chimpanzees and humans. *Cortex.* 43, 308-318.

Hayashi, M., Matsuzawa, T. (2003) Cognitive development in object manipulation by infant chimpanzees. *Animal Cognition.* 6, 225-233.

Hayashi, M., Sekine, S., Tanaka, M., Takeshita, H. (2009) Copying a model stack of colored blocks by chimpanzees and humans. *Interaction Studies.* 10, 130-149.

Hayashi, M., Takeshita, H. (in press) Stacking of irregularly shaped blocks in chimpanzees (*Pan troglodytes*) and young humans (*Homo sapiens*). *Animal Cognition.*

Hayashi, M., Takeshita, H., Matsuzawa, T. (2006) Cognitive development in apes and humans assessed by object manipulation. In T. Matsuzawa, M. Tomonaga, M. Tanaka (Eds.) *Cognitive Development in Chimpanzees.* (pp. 395-410). Tokyo: Springer.

Ikuzawa, M. (2000) Developmental diagnostic tests for children, 2nd edn. (in Japanese). Kyoto: Nakanishiya.

Johnson-Pynn, J., Fragaszy, D. M. (2001) Do apes and monkeys rely upon conceptual reversibility? A review of studies using seriated nesting cups in children and nonhuman primates. *Animal Cognition.* 4, 315-324.

Johnson-Pynn, J., Fragaszy, D. M., Hirsh, E. M., Brakke, K. E., Greenfield, P. M. (1999) Strategies used to combine seriated cups by chimpanzees (*Pan troglodytes*), bonobos (*Pan paniscus*), and capuchins (*Cebus apella*). *Journal of Comparative Psychology.* 113, 137-148.

Lockman J. J. (2000) A perception-action perspective on tool use development. *Child Development.* 71, 137-144.

Lonsdorf, E. V. (2005) Sex differences in the development of termite-fishing skills in the wild chimpanzees, Pan troglodytes schweinfurthii, of Gombe National Park, Tanzania. *Animal Behaviour.* 70, 673-683.

Malaivijitnond, S., Lekprayoon, C., Tendavanittj, N., Panha S., Cheewatham, C., Hamada, Y. (2007) Stone-tool usage by long-tailed macaques (*Macaca fascicularis*). *American Journal of Primatology.* 69, 227-233.

Matsuzawa, T. (1991) Nesting cups and metatools in chimpanzees. *Behavioral and Brain Sciences.* 14, 570-571.

Matsuzawa, T. (2003) The Ai Project: historical and ecological contexts. *Animal Cognition.* 6, 199-211.

Matsuzawa, T., Tomonaga, M., Tanaka, M. (2006) Cognitive Development in Chimpanzees. Tokyo: Springer.

McGrew, W. C., Marchant, L. F. (1997) Using tools at hand: manual laterality and elementary technology in Cebus spp. and Pan spp. *International Journal of Primatology.* 18, 787-810.

Povinelli, D. J. (2000) Folk physics for apes: the chimpanzee's theory of how the world works. Oxford: Oxford University Press.

Povinelli, D. J., Dunphy-Lelii, S. (2001) Do chimpanzees seek explanations? Preliminary comparative investigations. *Canadian Journal of Experimental Psychology.* 55, 187-195.

Sanz, C. M., Morgan, D. B. (2006) Chimpanzee tool technology in the Goualougo Triangle, Republic of Congo. *Journal of Human Evolution.* 52, 420-433.

Sanz, C., Morgan, D., Gulick, S. (2004) New insights into chimpanzees, tools, and termites from the Congo Basin. *The American Naturalist.* 164, 567-581.

Takeshita, H., Myowa-Yamakoshi, M., Hirata, S. (2009) The supine position of postnatal human infants –Implication for the development of cognitive intelligence. *Interaction Studies.* 10, 252-269.

Torigoe, T. (1985) Comparison of object manipulation among 74 species of non-human primates. *Primates.* 26, 182-194.

Watanabe, K., Urasopon, N., Malaivijitnond, S. (2007) Long-tailed macaques use human hair as dental floss. *American Journal of Primatology.* 69, 940-944.

In: Handbook of Motor Skills
Editor: Lucian T. Pelligrino

ISBN: 978-1-60741-811-5
© 2009 Nova Science Publishers, Inc.

Chapter 12

TRADITIONAL MIRROR THERAPY (TMT) IN THE PHYSICAL THERAPY MANAGEMENT OF MOVEMENT AND POSTURAL CONTROL PROBLEMS

Martin J. Watson

School of Allied Health Professions (AHP) & Health and Social Sciences
Research Institute, Faculty of Health,
University of East Anglia (UEA), Norwich NR4 7TJ, UK

INTRODUCTION

Mirrors have a long history as an 'essential' piece of rehabilitation equipment, and can be found in many physical therapy treatment areas. Traditionally one of their main uses is to provide patients with a reflected body image of themselves, usually as (a component of) a therapeutic strategy aimed at retraining movement control and posture. For example, when as a result of central nervous system (CNS) damage such as stroke, people have impaired postural control, then therapists might provide them with a reflected mirror image of themselves to deliver augmented visual feedback during treatment sessions where motor training is occurring.

There has recently been much interest in the therapeutic use of mirrors placed perpendicular to the patient's coronal plane; i.e mirrors able to reflect an image of one limb onto the limb of the opposite body side. Recent works by researchers such as Ramachandran [1-4], and Sutbeyaz and Yavuzer [5, 6], have indicated that this may be a useful therapeutic strategy in instances where CNS pathology has resulted in unilateral instances of paresis, neglect or phantom pain. So for example, a mirror might be used to reflect the left (sound) arm onto the right (paralysed) arm following a stroke, as part of a therapeutic strategy aiming to rehabilitate movement on the affected side. One proposed mechanism is that reflection creates an illusion of normal movement/sensation on the affected side of the body, thus facilitating voluntary production of movement and/or normal sensory processing on that side.

Whilst this newer work, now often referred to as 'mirror therapy', is advancing, the original more traditional and (possibly) simpler therapeutic use of mirrors described at the start appears to be being somewhat overlooked and neglected. In this more traditional context (hereafter referred to as 'Traditional Mirror Therapy' or TMT), a full length body mirror is typically placed in front of the person (i.e. parallel to their coronal plane), thus providing them with a full frontal image of their body and its movements. In this way the person is provided with augmented (visual) feedback of their postural alignment and/or bodily movement. This might typically be carried out in conjunction with corrective instructions from the therapist.

One of the puzzles regarding TMT is the apparent absence of any evidence base or instructional advice for what is in effect a fairly simple and straightforward training strategy with a seemingly long history. The notion of therapist/educator-provided augmented feedback during (motor) learning is a well established one; in a recent narrative review for example, van Vliet and Wulf identified a reasonably substantial (albeit nascent) evidence base for this general strategy for motor skills training following stroke [7]. They identified verbal, visual, video and kinematic feedback strategies as the main ones which have been used and evaluated by therapists working with this very common patient group. Interestingly however, this overview did not identify any literature relating to TMT. Similarly, if one accesses key physical therapy instructional texts, there is usually a very limited amount of information on TMT. For example, in a fairly seminal UK text, Howe and Oldham [8] state that *"Full length mirrors are frequently used in physiotherapy departments to make patients more aware of their static posture either in sitting or standing and dynamic posture during movement. Mirrors are also employed in gait retraining..."* (p.237). Howevere no further details are provided.

It is perhaps not difficult to explain this dearth of information regarding TMT. Despite its longstanding presence in the physical therapist's armamentarium, it is easily conceivable that the approach has yet to receive the level of investigation and exploration which it deserves. The physical therapy evidence base is still in its relative infancy and the majority of existing therapeutic strategies await appropriate formal evaluation; TMT is probably no exception in this respect.

The aim of this chapter is to provide an overview of several aspects of TMT. Specifically, the chapter covers 3 topics, these being:

- Literature: what is known about TMT from published peer-reviewed reports of formal investigations of this strategy
- Recent research: an overview of 3 pilot projects conducted by the author and colleagues which each evaluate an aspect of TMT
- Clinical perspectives: a report of a pilot evaluation of how practising UK clinicians utilise TMT

WHAT IS KNOWN ABOUT TMT: EXISTING SCIENTIFIC STUDIES

As stated in the introduction to this chapter, there appears to be a dearth of evaluative studies into the effectiveness of TMT in motor skill acquisition training. The author is currently undertaking a systematic review of the literature, and this has so far identified a (limited) number of studies of this topic. Of those published in peer-reviewed English language journals, the following are amonst the main studies which have so far been identified and stand out as representative examples of this limited knowledge base. These studies identify that there is in fact an evidence base in existence, although this does so far appear to be fairly limited.

Ross et al's 1991 study [9] was an evaluation of the use of mirror feedback as a component of treatment for long-standing facial nerve palsy. Subjects were engaged in daily practice of facial muscle exercises, using their reflected mirror image to obtain feedback during this process. The wider remit of this project was to evaluate whether electromyographic feedback, in combination with a mirror-based facial exercise regime, was any more advantageous than mirror-based exercises alone. A third group of subjects who received neither form of intervention acted as controls. Overall, treatment of either form appeared to confer benefits on subjects in terms of improvements in facial muscle control, facial symmetry and electrical measurements of facial nerve responses, in comparison with control subjects who received no therapy. There were no differences in outcome between the two intervention groups.

Gauthier-Gagnon et al's 1986 study [10] compared the effects of two different forms of training in the rehabilitation of standing postural control in two groups of unilateral below-knee amputees. The "traditional approach" treatment group received weight-shifting and balance exercises, combined with therapist provided verbal instructions and manual correction, but also utilising visual feedback via mirror. The experimental group received this same training, but augmented by the addition of auditory feedback generated and delivered by a pressure sensitive Limb Load Monitor placed beneath the prosthetic limb. The study reported that "both treatment modalities were shown to be equally effective in the early retraining of stance" (p.137); i.e. outcomes were comparable in both groups. This study clearly does not permit an evaluation of the effects of mirror feedback in isolation, although it might be argued that it suggests that this modality cannot be 'bettered' by the addition of augmented auditory feedback. it is also interesting to note from the graphical displays of some of the results that the 'mirror only' group appeared to demonstrate a higher level of postural control post-treatment.

Sewall et al's 1988 study [11] analysed the use of concurrent mirror feedback in a sports performance context, namely when young men learn a weightlifting technique (the 'power clean movement'). Eighteen college students participated in this study. Half of the group practised the technique with the use of mirrors whilst the other half did this without, both groups having first received standardised training in the specific weightlifting method via an instructional videotape. All subjects were assessed at the start and end of the study according to quality of technique, using a recognised weightlifting scoring system administered by a blinded assessor. Both groups showed improvements in technique by the end of the trial (p<0.01), but there were also differences in performance between the two in favour of mirror use (p<0.05). Whilst this study appears to support mirror feedback, the researchers made the significant point that they may have provided demonstration of the axiom that "subjects perform best under the condition in which they practice" (p.717), insofar as the best post-test results were obtained when subjects were assessed whilst using a mirror. It was apparent however that even without mirror feedback at assessment, the group which had used reflected body image to learn the technique were better performers by the end of the trial.

Radell et al's 2003 study [12] attempted to evaluate the effects of mirror feedback when female dance students were learning new ballet skills. One group of 14 students learned without the use of mirrors whilst another group of 13 students used mirrors. When students were assessed at the end of the semester it was found that dancers who had not used mirror feedback generally achieved better scores than those who had. Therefore in this instance mirror feedback appeared to have had a deleterious effect on motor skill acquisition. The authors reflect on how, in this specific context, such a result might come about because "the use of the mirror was distracting and inhibited the dancers' ability to focus more internally on the performance" (p.963). In other words, this is a group whose members have the potential to become overly focused on the aesthetics of personal body form and function, and that mirror use might potentially aggravate this effect, to the detriment of skill acquisition.

Vaillant et al's 2004 study [13] looked at the effects of simple mirror feedback on standing postural stability in healthy elderly people. A group consisting of 11 subjects with a mean age of approximately 70 years had their postural sway assessed whilst stood on a force platform. Subjects were assessed in two separate conditions: with and without mirror feedback. Perhaps unsurprisingly their postural sway appeared to be reduced when mirror feedback was available to subjects. The nature of the evaluation system permitted a somewhat more complex analysis: medio-lateral postural sway (i.e. side-to-side movement) was more significantly reduced when using the mirror than was antero-posterior (backwards-forwards) movement. This finding was attributed to the fact that subjects' sensory systems were better able to detect the latter than the former whilst viewing their reflected body image.

With the exception of Radell's work, all of the preceding studies appear to provide some support for the notion that TMT can contribute to the control and/or training of movement and posture. Two of the five studies appeared to find in clear favour of mirror useage [11, 13], with a third being cautiously favourable when results were looked at in more detail [10]; a fourth study could be interpreted as showing that the benefits conferred by mirror useage could not be improved upon when augmented by additional EMG-based input [10]. The study by Radell et al [12] could perhaps be considered as a special case, looking at a healthy subject group (dancers) for whom mirror use is apparently counter-productive. Three of these five studies were of course looking at normal as opposed to impaired study groups, hence having limited implications for neurological rehabilitation. Conversely the Ross et al study at least concerned a peripheral nervous lesion, whilst Gauthier-Gagnon et al provide some sense of the intervention's worth in a scenario of potentially gross postural/control problems; i.e. unilateral loss of structural and sensory integrity following limb amputation. Furthermore the Vaillant study indicates this therapy's potential worth in a predominantly aging population. Overall therefore the existing evidence base, whilst somewhat limited in amount and nature, does provide some support for the effectiveness of TMT in a skill (re)learning context.

THREE RECENT PROJECTS

UK undergraduate students on honours degree courses typically undertake final year projects which may involve carrying out small scale empirical research. There is debate in some quarters regarding the extent to which work of this sort can contribute significantly to an existing evidence base – such projects are after all intended primarily as an opportunity for students to develop their skills of enquiry. Nonetheless useful work can be and is sometimes undertaken by pre-registration undergraduate physical therapy students which is worthy of dissemination. In this section a brief overview of 3 pertinent student projects is provided, each of which was supervised by the writer. All of these studies aimed to identify the extent to which a reflected body image provides useful visual feedback during some form of movement/postural control.

Study 1: The Effect of Simple Mirror Feedback on Limb Position Sense

This study set out to evaluate the effects of mirror feedback on the abilities of subjects to replicate joint angles [14]. The premise of this study was that a reflected body image confers on subjects an enhanced awareness of limb/body spatial positioning. Eighteen healthy subjects were each asked to replicate 3 pre-determined angles of shoulder joint abduction (50°, 110° and 140°), the precise amplitudes of which they were blind to. Each angle was first passively demonstrated to the subject, following which the arm was lowered, and then the subject was asked to actively replicate the initial limb position. Accuracy of joint angle replication was measured by the experimenter using a plurimeter, according to standardised criteria. Order of testing for the 3 pre-determined joint angles was counterbalanced across subjects, as were the conditions of testing, these being 1) visual feedback via mirror only, 2) visual feedback via direct sight of arm only, and 3) visual feedback by mirror and direct sight of arm. For condition 1, a cardboard blinker was used to prevent subjects from seeing sideways, thus preventing direct (lateral) sight of arm whilst permitting straight-ahead view of a reflected image of the limb. For the mirror conditions (1 and 3), subjects were presented with a frontal body image reflection, provided using a full length mirror placed directly in front of them. Data on accuracy of joint angle replication were analysed using a one factor within subjects ANOVA test. This identified that any differences occurring between the conditions did not reach statistical significance (F=0.444, p=0.590). The 95% confidence intervals for accuracy of replication did however suggest that condition 1 showed the best results, with condition 2 showing the worst. These results therefore suggested some support for the notion that mirror reflection confers benefits rearding limb position awareness.

Study 2: The Effect of Simple Mirror Feedback on Sitting Postural Control

This study aimed to evaluate how providing subjects with their reflected body image influences their sitting postural control [15]. This is a pertinent context for physical therapists, who might for example use mirrors to help patients to relearn their sitting postural control abilities when these are impaired say following stroke. Eighteen healthy female undergraduate students (mean age 20.8 years) had their postural sway evaluated in two standardised experimental conditions; with and without mirror feedback. Subjects were tested three times under each condition (hence 6 tests in total), with a mean performance value for each of the two conditions then being derived. Order of testing across the 6 tests was varied for each subject using a Latin Square procedure, to control for a learning effect. As these were subjects with intact neuromuscular systems, they were asked to maintain a complex (standardised) sitting position during each test, thus challenging their postural control abiliites. (Subjects were asked to perform balanced sitting, with knees extended so that their legs were held out straight in front of them; both arms were held out to their sides.) Subjects were evaluated by requiring them to sit on the seat plate sensor of a Balance Performance Monitor (BPM) [16, 17]. This was used to generate values for the amount of postural sway occurring, measured as length of sway path (mm) during a 30 second sampling period. Group mean sway path with mirror feedback was lower (i.e. better) than without, with values of 165.72mm [SD 40.52mm] versus 244.74mm [SD 68.48mm]. This difference was statistically significant (related t test, t = 4.873, p<0.001, 95% CI 44.80mm – 113.23mm). This suggested that mirror feedback had an immediate effect on postural control ability, with subjects apparently being more stable when able to view their reflected body image when adopting a complex sitting position.

Study 3: The Effect of Simple Mirror Feedback on Standing Postural Control

A similar study to the previous one was undertaken, but evaluating the extent to which the availability of a reflected image influences *standing* postural control [18]. Twenty healthy subjects were used in this evaluation. A similar protocol to the previously described study was used, wherein all subjects were tested under two conditions; i.e. standing 1) *with* and 2) *without* the availability of a reflected body image. As with the previous study, subjects were tested 3 times in each of the two conditions, with order of testing across these 6 trials being varied between subjects to control for systematic bias due to a learning effect. To make the test position more challenging for these healthy young subjects, they were each asked to maintain a standardised one-legged balanced standing position during all tests. Postural stability was ascertained by evaluating subjects whilst stood on a single foot plate sensor connected to a BPM, monitoring postural sway (sway path, measured in mm). Group mean sway path with mirror feedback was lower (i.e. better) than without, with values of 178.67mm [SD 41.13mm] versus 229.04mm [SD 38.21mm]. This difference was statistically significant (related t test, t = 7.350, p<0.001, 95% CI 36.02mm – 64.71mm). This suggested that mirror feedback had an immediate effect on standing postural control ability, with subjects apparently being more stable when able to view their reflected body image.

Overall, all 3 of these studies appeared to find support for the notion that, in normal subjects, a simple reflected mirror image enables improved postural control. Two of these studies presented statistically significant results, suggesting perhaps a relatively strong effect, albeit in a sample of healthy subjects. All of these studies had positive finding regarding the *immediate* effect of mirror feedback, suggesting that once subjects have a mirror image available then there is an instant alteration in control abilities. The mechanisms of this effect, and its ability to carry over during a movement training situation, requires investigation. Finally, the extent to (and means by) which the effects revealed in these studies are transferable to a patient population needs to be elaborated.

ASSAYING UK CLINICIANS' VIEWPOINTS
AND PERCEPTIONS REGARDING TMT

What do physiotherapists actually do with mirrors during routine clinical practice? Most UK physiotherapy departments appear to own a mirror. Furthermore the author observes that, when asked, most clinicians working in relevant clinical areas will profess to using mirrors during clinical practice. Yet it seems difficult to pinpoint what it is that therapists actually do with them. As indicated earlier, there is a shortage of texts discussing specifically how TMT should be carried out, and investigative research still appears to be in its relative infancy. An additional source of confusion is that anecdotally some clinicians appear to dislike TMT, claiming that it is counterproductive, unuseful, or indeed contra-indicated.

A strategy recently adopted by the author has been to undertake a preliminary assessment of how UK clinicians typically using TMT in everyday clinical practice. This is in preparation for a more substantial and formal survey of national practice. The recent evolution of internet-based information sharing brought about by Web 2.0 innovations has begun to impinge positively on physiotherapy practice [19], and in the UK this has occurred primarily by way of the Chartered Society of Physiotherapy's (CSP's) Interactive CSP (iCSP) initiative. This facility enables practicing clinicians, as well as physiotherapy academics and researchers, to pose questions online to all registered CSP colleagues. In March 2008 a query regarding TMT was posed by the author to the neurology section of iCSP. After first explaining that comments were being saught regarding the more traditional form of mirror usage, the 'question' posed was as follows:

To inform some ongoing research work, I am very keen to gauge clinicians' opinions of the usefulness or otherwise of this therapeutic strategy. Have you had some positive experiences of the use of mirror feedback for postural/movement training? Are you aware of situations where it is unwise to use this form of training feedback? Do you feel that this is an outdated or useless strategy? I would be very interested to see colleagues' comments, whilst hopefully also encouraging a discussion of the topic.

A small number of responses were initially received regarding this query, albeit similar in number to those shared for other queries posed to this site. (Busy clinicians are perhaps still somewhat reluctant to engage in web initiatives like this, except in instances where the queries being posed/discussed are of very specific and immediate relevance to contributors/respondents.) A reminder was posted after several weeks, to attempt to ensure that an extensive as possible online discussion had been undertaken on the topic. Eleven experienced clinicians eventually participated in this electronic forum. This relatively small group appeared to offer a rich diversity of views and contributions. Some of their responses appeared either explicitly or implicitly related to movement relabilitation following stroke, although some broader views were also shared. An attempt was made to theme and sub-categorise all of the contributions, and this resulted in the following summary of findings. (All of these appeared to relate to situations where the subject looks ahead into a mirror placed directly in front of them, unless otherwise stated.)

- Specific strategies. A number of successful strategies were specifically identified, including:
    - The 'cover my body' strategy, where, to encourage normal postural control in sitting, the therapist sits behind the subject and encourages him/her to align themselves in the mirror so that their reflected body image 'covers' the reflected body image of the therapist who is sat behind them;
    - Using the mirror to simply provide a 'snap-shot' of progress for the patient; i.e. showing them their reflected body image, as occasional feedback regarding success during postural control training. The mirror is taken away again once it has been used for this purpose. (It was suggested that mirror feedback is something which some of us are accustomed to using anyway for certain everyday functional tasks, but that it is otherwise confusing if used to excess and out of personal context);
    - Placing the mirror behind the patient. This reputably enables the therapist (who is in front of the patient, giving administering postural/movement training) to gain an 'all round' picture of the patient's postural alignment whilst they are providing them with therapy.
- Specific scenarios where mirror use is found to be useful and successful. These scenarios included:
    - Working with patients with so called 'pusher' syndrome. This is a situation where subjects with stroke have problems recognising that they are actively moving away from midline, pushing themselves excessively towards the affected side when either sat or stood, in an erroneous effort to self-correct their postural alignment [20]. A mirror image apparently enables some people with this problem to identify what it is they are doing wrong and thus helps them to correct the problem;
    - Subjects who require help to find their midline alignment. (This includes the above 'pusher' type patients, but appeared to extend beyond that group also);
    - As a therapeutic adjunct when encouraging patients to hold their heads up; i.e. facilitation of active neck/cervical extension/retraction and head elevation in instances where poor head/neck control results in the head falling forward onto the chest. A corrective effect apparently occurs when the subject is asked to "look up and look at yourself in the mirror";
    - Walking training, in instances where there is poor side-to-side weight transfer; i.e. subjects are encouraged to move their body (image) from side to side whilst walking "so that it touches each lateral edge of the mirror";
    - Patients with good problem-solving abilities, but who have impaired sensation/proprioception, who are instantly able to perceive (via reflected body image) the deficiencies of their postural

alignment/control and are hence able to do something actively about this;

o During dressing training, particularly where this is occurring in the bathroom and there are bathroom mirrors available. This was presumed by respondents to be helpful as this is a natural environment and setting for such activity (and for mirrors to be present) for some patients.

- Specific reflections and advice on mirror use. This included:

o To progress with mirror usage during movement/posture training by later working without a mirror; i.e. its use should be withdrawn as movement control improves;

o To always ask the patient first before using a mirror in therapy, primarily in case patients are concerned regarding seeing their own image;

o That mirror use can be useful to restore self-esteem, providing subjects with the opportunity to see how successful therapy has been;

o That therapists will often know instantly whether mirror feedback is going to be useful or not with a particular patient, as soon as it is tried with a particular individual;

o That there may be specific time-limited periods during rehabilitation where mirror use appears to be useful, before/after which this strategy does not work as well.

- Adverse effects of mirror use. The following suggestions were made:

o That right/left reversal seen in the reflected body image is simply too confusing for some people (including sometimes therapists too) and that clinicians therefore need to be on the lookout for this. It was noted that mirrors can sometimes exaccerbate or cause left/right confusion;

o That some people do not like/wish to see themselves in a mirror. One therapist reported an extreme adverse reaction following mirror use, when a patient was very shocked to see how they looked as a result of illness, and became incapacitated for several days as a result;

o That some of the stroke patients who have cognitive attentional/ neglect problems don't respond well to mirror use because they cannot attend properly to a reflected mirror image.

Overall this preliminary survey, undertaken via an internet based resource, provided relatively rich feedback regarding TMT, giving a strong sense of some of the contexts for its optimal use. Future more extensive survey (and possibly structured interview and observational) work might enable elaboration regarding the general procedures adopted by therapists when carrying out TMT. There is obviously a need to identify the frequency of this strategy's use, as well as the specific clinical diagnoses and functional problems for which it is optimally useful for. Finally the notion that there are circumstances where TMT might be contra-indicated requries further exploration. The views and insights of the recipients of TMT, as well its users, obviously need to be taken into account.

CONCLUDING COMMENTS

Traditional mirror therapy (TMT) does appear to have a significant role to play in providing augmented feedback during the remediation of movement and postural control problems. Physical therapists have probably been aware of the benefits of this strategy since the very early days of the profession, although evaluations and elaborations of its utilisation have so far had limited presence. Formal scientific studies of this strategy are limited in number, although some useful evaluations nonetheless exist. These provide pointers for the types of clinical/educational roles which mirrors might provide, as well as giving some indications of the further research which needs to be conducted. The writer has facilitated pertinent small scale student research projects which also identify how a simple reflected image may immediately enhance the movement and postural control abilities of subjects. Whilst these projects have all involved normal healthy subjects, they all suggest that mirror reflections can easily improve subjects' motor abilities. Finally, although only preliminary in nature, a survey of clinicians has produced some very useful insights into the probable uses (and limitations) of this therapeutic strategy. As with many of the therapeutic modalities currently used by physical therapists, there therefore appears to be much to support the continued and extended use of this approach, pending further evaluations and evaluations.

REFERENCES

[1]   Ramachandran, V.S. and D. Rogers-Ramachandran, *Synaesthesia in phantom limbs induced with mirrors. Proc. Biol. Sci.* 1996. 263(1369): p. 377-86.

[2]   Ramachandran, V.S., E.L. Altschuler, and S. Hillyer, *Mirror agnosia. Proc. Biol. Sci.,* 1997. 264(1382): p. 645-647.

[3]   Ramachandran, V.S., et al., Can mirrors alleviate visual hemineglect? Med. Hypotheses. 1999. 52(4): p. 303-305.

[4]   Altschuler, E.L., et al., Rehabilitation of hemiparesis after stroke with a mirror. Lancet. 1999. 353(9169): p. 2035-6.

[5]   Sutbeyaz, S., et al., Mirror therapy enhances lower-extremity motor recovery and motor functioning after stroke: a randomized controlled trial. Archives of Physical Medicine and Rehabilitation. 2007. 88(5): p. 555-9.

[6]   Yavuzer, G., et al., Mirror Therapy Improves Hand Function in Subacute Stroke: A Randomized Controlled Trial. Archives of Physical Medicine and Rehabilitation. 2008. 89(3): p. 393-398.

[7]   van Vliet, P.M. and G. Wulf, Extrinsic feedback for motor learning after stroke: what is the evidence? Disability & Rehabilitation. 2006. 28(13-14): p. 831-840.

[8]   Howe, T. and J. Oldham, *Posture and balance*, in *Human movement: an introductory text*, M. Trew and T. Everett, Editors. 2001, Churchill Livingstone: Edinburgh. p. 225-239.

[9]   Ross, B., J.M. Nedzelski, and J.A. McLean, Efficacy of feedback training in long-standing facial nerve paresis. Laryngoscope. 1991. 101(7 Pt 1): p. 744-50.

[10] Gauthier-Gagnon, C., et al., Augmented sensory feedback in the early training of standing balance of below-knee amputees. Physiotherapy Canada, 1986. 38(3): p. 137-142.

[11] Sewall, L.P., T.G. Reeve, and R.A. Day, Effect of concurrent visual feedback on acquisition of a weightlifting skill. Perceptual and Motor Skills. 1988. 67: p. 715-718.

[12] Radell, S.A., D.D. Adame, and S.P. Cole, Effect of teaching with mirrors on ballet dance performance. Perceptual and Motor Skills. 2003. 97(3 Pt 1): p. 960-4.

[13] Vaillant, J., et al., Mirror versus stationary cross feedback in controlling the center of foot pressure displacement in quiet standing in elderly subjects. Archives of Physical Medicine and Rehabilitation. 2004. 85(12): p. 1962-5.

[14] Tuff, N. and M.J. Watson, The effect of visual feedback via mirror on immediate performance of an upper limb positioning task. Physiotherapy. 2005. 91(1): p. 56.

[15] Watson, M.J., Peck, M., A pilot study investigating the immediate effects of mirror feedback on sitting postural control in normal healthy adults. Physiotherapy Research International, 2008. 13(4): p. 204.

[16] Haas, B.M. and T.E. Whitmarsh, Inter- and intra-tester reliability of the Balance Performance Monitor in a non-patient population. Physiotherapy Research International. 1998. 3(2): p. 135-147.

[17] Haas, B.M. and A.M. Burden, Validity of weight distribution and sway measurements of the Balance Performance Monitor. Physiotherapy Reearch International. 2000. 5(1): p. 19-32.

[18] Watson, M.J. and May, A., An investigation of the immediate effects of mirror feedback on standing postural control in normal healthy adults. Clinical Rehabilitation. (in press)

[19] Barsky, E. and D. Giustini, Web 2.0 in physical therapy: a practical overview. Physiotherapy Canada, 2008. 60(3): p. 207-210.

[20] Perennou, D.A., et al., Lateropulsion, pushing and verticality perception in hemisphere stroke: a causal relationship? Brain. 2008. 131(Pt 9): p. 2401-13.

In: Handbook of Motor Skills
Editor: Lucian T. Pelligrino

ISBN: 978-1-60741-811-5
© 2009 Nova Science Publishers, Inc.

Chapter 13

EFFECT OF MULTI-MODAL IMAGERY INTERVENTION ON PRE-COMPETITIVE ANXIETY AND STRESS LEVELS IN ELITE TENNIS PLAYERS

Ricardo Weigert Coelho, Flavia Justus,
Birgit Keller and Bubens Tempski
Federal University of Parana State, Brazil

ABSTRACT

This study investigated the effect of multi-modal imagery on anxiety and perceived stress levels in tennis players. The quasi-experimental design included pre- and post-treatment test subjects and a control group. Male tennis players (n=49) ranging in age from 16 to 18 years old (M=16.96, SD= 0.82) were divided into two groups: (1) a treatment imagery group and (2) a placebo imagery group used as the control group. The 27-item Competitive State Anxiety Inventory (CSAI-2) was used to assess anxiety and the Perceived Stress Scale (PSS10) to assess stress. The results showed a significant multivariate difference ($p < .05$) between the treatment imagery and control groups in terms of cognitive anxiety, self-confidence and perceived stress. The findings suggest that imagery is a powerful mental tool for overcoming some specific types of anxiety and stress.

Keywords: sports, coaching, healthcare, adolescence, sports psychology.

INTRODUCTION

Sports play an important part in the lives of many athletes, but the search for physical perfection and an incredible desire for success, allied with the economic and political interests involved, have brought sports to a level that requires participants to expend a great deal of effort and involvement, thus leading to anxiety and stress. It is evident that the search for successful athletic results and an over-competitive ethic have become dominant forces that strongly influence a player's anxiety and stress levels. Perhaps the most frequent concern of sports psychologists is whether athletes can withstand the psychological stress of intense competition. In this regard, consistent information about methods that can lessen the impact of anxiety and stress on the lives of these athletes is very valuable. One of these methods is imagery which, according to Williams (1994), is a mental process that programs the mind to react optimally. It is the use of senses to mentally reconstruct an experience.

The use of imagery as a psychological tool seems to be an effective method to promote self-efficacy (Beauchamp, Bray, & Albinson, 2002), self-confidence (Carter & Kelly, 1997) and improve athletic performance and learning (Feltz & Landers, 1993; Gammage, Hall, & Rodgers, 2000; Martin, Moritz, & Hall, 1999; Paivio, 1985; Taylor & Shaw, 2002).

Imagery is also widely used as an intervention method in medicine to help motor reorganization in hemiplegic stroke patients (Scott & Frey, 2004), to control pre-surgical anxiety (McCaffrey & Taylor, 2005), to help healing of injuries and post-traumatic stress disorder (Holmes, Grey, & Young, 2005), to control post-surgical stress (Sloman, 2002; Richardson, 2003) and to reduce pain (Ackerman & Turkoski, 2000).

However, as Morris, Spittle, and Watt (2005) pointed out:

Not all imagery has a positive impact; in some cases, imagery can stop fully recovered athletes from reproducing their pre-injury form because they repeatedly image themselves breaking down at the point of maximum effort. What we can imagine can make us anxious or confident, determine our focus during play, motivate us to extra effort, or convince us that all is lost (p. 5).

If this is true, use of a suitable imagery method is crucial to successful building of self-confidence and control of competitive emotional pressure, which should lower anxiety and stress levels.

Many mental imagery methods and models have been suggested. Pavio's planned model identified two primary functions of imagery—motivation and cognitive—which work on specific and general levels. These functions are cognitive specific, cognitive general, motivation specific and motivation general. Motivation general refers to confidence, stress, anxiety and arousal. Motivation specific refers to applying various emotions and mental aspects to specific situations. Cognitive general incorporates strategies and general concepts of games, while cognitive specific addresses the technical mechanics and details of performing specific task.

Hall, Mack, Paivio, and Hausenblas (1998), using the original imagery model of Paivio suggested a multidimensional model connecting stress and imagery. They introduced two more aspects in Paivio's model, which they called motivational general-arousal (MGA, imaging physiological and emotional arousal) and motivational general-mastery (MGM, imagining being confident).

An important issue related to imagery is an athlete's ability to use the technique. This ability depends upon the quality of their visual and kinesthetic perceptions. Visual imagery is the ability to clearly see specified images, whereas kinesthetic imagery is the ability to feel images as they are portrayed (Cherie, Fry, Li, & Relyea, 2002). Martin et al. identified imagery ability as a potential moderating variable in their applied model. They stated that the relationship between different types of imagery and athletes' cognitive, affective and behavioral responses may be influenced by the degree to which they can utilize visual and kinesthetic imagery effectively. Results of studies related to this assumption indicate that elite athletes who utilize imagery possess well-developed imagery ability (Orlick & Partington, 1988; Barr & Hall, 1992).

Many studies have revealed that imagery used for anxiety regulation purposes have a strong positive effect on developing confidence (Carter & Kelly, 1997; White & Hardy, 1998; Callow & Hardy, 2001; Manassis & Doganis, 2004). However, Martin et al. suggested that a prerequisite for imagery intervention is a good understanding of the impact that different types of imagery have on various cognitive, affective and behavioral responses in sports situations.

Besides imagery content, other important issues considered in the present study were anxiety and stress. Anxiety and stress as psychopathological entities are interrelated and sometimes even confusing. Thus, it is imperative that these terms are operationally defined for clarity.

Stress, as defined by Selye (1956), is the result when situational demands are perceived to exceed available coping resources. Stressful situations are not sufficient causes of pathology and illness behavior. Instead, stress is a potential for event-elicited health risk. Stress also depends on a transaction between the person and the environment, assuming that individuals actively interact with their environment (Lazarus & Folkman, 1984). Stressful events are assumed to increase when they are appraised as threatening or demanding, and when coping resources are judged as insufficient to address that threat or demand (Cohen, Karmack, & Mermelstein, 1983).

Anxiety is defined here as a component and possibly a result of stress that is characterized by a state of conditioned activation in which thoughts and feelings of worry, concern and uncertainty dominate (Martens, Vealey, & Burton, 1990). Anxiety is divided into state (relatively transient and context-specific) and trait (enduring, general and dispositional) dimensions (Spielberger, Gorsush, & Lushene, 1970). However, understanding how behavior truly interacts with cognition and emotion seems to be very complex and cannot be analyzed in one-dimensional model and theories. A more complex conceptual structure describing how these constructs are interconnected has been advocated by Hardy (1996) and Hardy and Parfitt (1991) in the model of cusp catastrophe, and by Eysenck and Calvo (1992) in their processing efficiency theory. A more comprehensive debate of these multidimensional models is beyond the scope of this paper.

The assumption at this point is that improvement of an athlete's confidence using imagery has a diminishing effect on anxiety and stress levels, making athletes less inclined to perceive themselves in a threatening situation, thus enhancing their performance.

The purpose of this study was to examine the effect of a multi-modal and motivational general-mastery imagery intervention method (MGM) in increasing self-confidence to self-regulate the athletes anxiety and stress levels.

Self-confidence is the key theoretical issue in the present study, because (MGM) type of imagery can be used to build an athlete's confidence, which we suppose is inversely related to anxiety and stress, so we use the proposal of Martin et al. that imagery intervention is a key strategy for overcoming competitive stress and anxiety in building an athlete's confidence toward competition.

Based on the assumption that self-confidence diminishes the perception of threat and consequently lowers stress and anxiety levels, it was hypothesized that the multi-modal imagery treatment group would demonstrate higher levels of self-confidence and lower levels of anxiety and stress in the post-treatment test compared to the control group.

METHODS

Before data collection, the proposed study was submitted and approved by the ethics committee of the Federal University of Paraná State, Brazil.

The approach used was a quasi-experimental design with pre- and post-treatment test subjects and a control group (Isaac & Michael, 1983). Initially, a sample of 64 male volunteers who were elite tennis players registered with the Paraná Tennis Federation, Brazil was recruited. The players were involved in regional and national tournaments and practiced 4 h/day, 5 days/week during the three-month pre-season. Subjects were randomly assigned to either the treatment or control group using a matching method considering ability, practice time and experience of high competition levels.

The first data (pre-treatment test) were collected 15–5 min before warm-up for a first-round game during the classification phase of a national tournament, which was selected to guarantee the participation of all subjects. After nine weeks of imagery treatment, a second test (post-treatment test) was administered 15–5 min before warm-up for a first-round game during the classification phase of another national tournament.

Withdrawal by some subjects led to a decrease and mismatch in group size, with 23 subjects in the treatment group and 26 in the control group, ranging in age from 16 to 18 years (M=16.96, SD= 0.82). Among the 15 subjects who withdrew from the study, four players had physical injuries, six cited personal reasons and five withdrew for unknown reasons. To assess pre-competitive anxiety state, the 27-item Competitive State Anxiety Inventory (CSAI-2; Martens et al., 1990) was used to measure the subjects' somatic anxiety, cognitive anxiety and self-confidence. Somatic anxiety refers to physiological arousal, whereas cognitive anxiety refers to worry and negative thoughts that are experienced before a competition and self-confidence refers to emotional and performance confidence. The CSAI-2 has 27 items overall, with nine items for each of three sub-scales: cognitive anxiety, somatic anxiety and self-confidence. All items are rated on a four-point Likert scale varying from 1 (not at all) to 4 (very much). The scale demonstrates a high degree of internal consistency (0.79–0.90) and constructs validity (Martens, et al.). In the present study, we used scores for the three subscales independently as dependent variables (cognitive anxiety, somatic anxiety and self-confidence).

Stress was assessed using the Perceived Stress Scale (Cohen et al., 1983). The original scale contained 14 items. The 10-item version of the scale (PSS10) has also been validated. According to Cohen et al. the PSS10 allows assessment of perceived stress without any loss of psychometric quality (actually a slight gain) over the longer PSS14. The PSS questionnaire addresses general feelings and thoughts. PSS10 scores are obtained for negative and positive responses using a Likert-type scale that varies from 0 (never) to 4 (very often).

All subjects performed pre- and post-treatment tests, which consisted of answering both the CSAI-2 and PSS10 questionnaires. For both tests (pre- and post-treatment) the players were told to answer the questions according to how they felt at that moment, that is, before competition. They were given no other instructions or comments.

The treatment involved a multi-modal (relaxation, imagery and behavior modeling video) intervention conducted three times per week for 25 minutes after ordinary technical and physical practice for a period of nine weeks between tournaments. Close to 70% (30 players) of the 49 subjects attended at least 90% of the treatment or placebo intervention sessions and all subjects attended at least 75% of the sessions.

During the treatment phase, all the subjects from both groups met with their coaches and the researcher in a quiet place. In the first session, a lecture on imagery technique was delivered to all subjects in both groups. The subjects were then randomly divided into the control and treatment groups. The treatment group was taught how to use imagery to promote self-confidence and positive feedback on their skills performance and then practiced the technique.

The treatment group was exposed to multi-modal imagery intervention at each session as follows: after a 10-min relaxation procedure (using a progressive method of relaxation), the subjects were directed to visualize themselves successfully playing a game. They had been taught how to generate positive thoughts and behavior regarding their abilities and how to overcome negative thoughts before and during games and to imagine a positive outcome. In five of the sessions, a 10-min video tape showing professional winning athletes playing games, focusing on their posture, behavior, decision-making processes and body language strategies, was played.

Placebo imagery intervention was delivered to the control group. This involved imaging self-perception, remembering good moments experienced in the past, and imagining being on the beach and in the countryside.

A 2×2 multifactor analysis of variance (MANOVA; pre- and post-treatment, control and experimental groups) was used to analyze the main effect among variables at a significance level of $p < .05$.

RESULTS

We tried to control the random limitation of the study by matching the individual differences in ability level, practice time and experience of high competition levels, and then randomly assign them to either group. However, the withdrawal of 15 subjects violated the assumption of homogeneity of variance, so Levene's test for equality of variance was conducted for pre-treatment scores to assess homogeneity between groups. Levene's test demonstrated no significant main effect between the control and experimental groups in terms of perceived stress, cognitive anxiety, confidence and somatic anxiety. These findings satisfied the assumption of homogeneity of variance between groups.

Kolmagorov-Smirnov tests were also used to assess the normality of the group scores. The results revealed that all scores were normally distributed.

Multifactor analysis of variance testing of perceived stress and anxiety subscales showed a main effect for control vs. experimental, Wilks' $\lambda = 1.63$, $F(4, 91) = 37.051$, $p < .01$, pre- vs. post-treatment, Wilks' $\lambda = 1.26$, $F(4, 91) = 28.65$, $p < .01$, and interaction between control vs. experimental and pre- vs. post-treatment groups Wilks' $\lambda = 1.44$, $F(4, 91) = 32.68$, $p < .01$.

Univariate analysis revealed a significant main effect for perceived stress, cognitive anxiety and self-confidence at $p < .05$. There was no significant effect for somatic anxiety (table 1). ANOVA also revealed significant interaction effects for perceived stress $F(1, 94) = 6.87$, $p < .05$, cognitive anxiety $F(1, 94) = 4.42$, $p < .05$, and self-confidence $F(1, 94) = 5.07$,

$p < .05$. However, the interaction was not significant for somatic anxiety $F(1, 94) = 0.78$, $p > .05$.

Table 1. Mean scores and standard deviations for measures of anxiety and stress in the study groups

Group	Perceived stress		Cognitive anxiety		Somatic anxiety		Self-confidence	
	M	SD	M	SD	M	SD	M	SD
Pre-treatment								
Control	15.19	5.72	21.92	6.27	22.38	6.89	22.58	6.50
Experimental	16.87	6.72	19.96	7.22	21.74	5.65	20.96	7.22
Post-treatment								
Control	15.81	3.91	21.27	5.85	22.65	6.42	21.50	5.66
Experimental	12.17*	4.34	13.83*	4.01	24.39	5.10	24.91*	6.29

Note: * indicates comparisons in which the difference is significant ($p < .05$).

CONCLUSION

Before addressing any conclusion, some limitations in this study must be considered. First, imagery ability differs from athlete to athlete. However, this limitation was somehow controlled by the kind of sample used (elite athletes), which according to Orlick and Partington, and Barr and Hall, elite athletes possess well-developed imagery ability; they do not differ much in their imagery ability. Second, the intervention used was multi-modal (relaxation, behavior modeling video and MGM imagery) and not by imagery itself.

The purpose of this study was to investigate whether multi-modal imagery intervention affects perceived stress, cognitive anxiety, somatic anxiety and confidence levels in tennis athletes. The results partially support the study hypothesis that building an athlete's self-confidence through multi-modal imagery intervention (MGM) would lower pre-competitive anxiety and stress levels. The findings demonstrate a positive outcome for the imagery intervention group compared to the control subjects.

The results for stress and two anxiety subscales (cognitive anxiety and self-confidence) indicate that multi-modal imagery intervention for nine weeks represents a useful tool to build self-confidence and to lower cognitive anxiety and perceived stress levels in tennis athletes. These findings are in accordance with previous studies (Sloman; Richardson; Scott & Frey; Holmes et al.; McCaffrey & Taylor) in the area of physiotherapy and medicine that concluded that imagery is an efficient psychological intervention to control anxiety and stress in many disturbing situations.

Another important finding is that the specificity of the situation must be considered when using imagery. The psychological benefits conferred by imagery must be heading for specific situation. Imagery cannot be viewed in a general manner and not all imagery intervention is a reliable method for every situation or psychological demand, which is the case for somatic anxiety, where the player must be aware of and perceive the physiological response to anxiety. They seem confounding to be stressed or anxious in being tired. This is consistent with Martin et al. who suggested that a prerequisite for the use of imagery intervention is a greater understanding of the impact that a specific type of imagery has on various cognitive, affective, and behavioral responses in sport situations. The most important factors related to performance for most sports are self-confidence, intensity, arousal regulation and concentration. However, the importance of any one of them differs according to the specific demands of each sport (Taylor & Shaw).

The results are also corroborated by Defrancesco and Burke (1997), who pointed out that some sports such as tennis, which requires fine and accurate movements, are relatively long in duration with many short bursts. This means that building and maintaining self-confidence is the primary goal for intervention in tennis. In fact, imagery interventions can result in improvements in an athlete'sport confidence levels over time (Carter & Kelly). This finding is also in accordance with Hanton, Mellalieu, and Hall (2004), who reported the effects of high and low levels of self-confidence on symptoms associated with competitive anxiety. High self-confidence increases the intensity of thoughts and feelings of total control over the situation and the experiences of positive thoughts and images regarding forthcoming performance-lowering anxiety levels.

The results of this study lead to some useful conclusions. The study demonstrates that an athlete under competitive pressure is likely to be influenced by tendencies to perceive himself in a threatening situation, leading to anxiety and stress. As a result, self-confidence is threatened and coping mechanisms such as multi-modal imagery proposed by this study could be employed. Another conclusion is that low self-confidence can cause negative thoughts and thus increase anxiety levels. On the other hand, when self-confidence is high, it controls anxiety and stress and maintains concentration and focus, which are major tenets for enhancing performance.

Our findings indicate that cognitive strategies such as multi-modal imagery build high self-confidence, which protects against debilitating mental interpretation associated with competitive anxiety in stressful situations. However, the athlete's inability to recognize symptoms of anxiety and stress must be considered in the future. Therefore, specific imagery intervention is recommended to lower somatic anxiety. We suggest a more appropriate intervention for the athletes to develop more facilitative interpretation of the symptoms associated with their pre-competitive anxiety and stress. This might include the MGA part of the Hall, Mack, Paivio, and Hausenblas model. In practice, coaches and psychologists should be aware of specific demands in sports (Martin et al.). They should understand the principles and effectiveness of specific coping behaviors or situations before using appropriate intervention. For future research, a more efficient and specific imagery method for overcoming somatic anxiety should be investigated. A method that teaches players to feel and identify somatic symptoms of anxiety and stress and to control them would be appropriate. Use of a direct measure of anxiety and stress, such as salivary cortisol, could also be considered. Participation in an imagery program with a specific objective and proper intervention seems to decrease anxiety and stress in many stressful situations. Our results indicate that negative perception of a threatening event is a state of mind that can be controlled by mental practices such as multi-modal imagery.

REFERENCES

Ackerman, C., & Turkoski, B. (2000). Using guided imagery to reduce pain and anxiety. *The Journal for the Home Care and Hospital Profession. 19*, 524-530.

Barr, K., & Hall, C. (1992). The use of imagery by rowers. *International Journal of Sport Psychology. 23*, 243–261.

Beauchamp, M.R., Bray, S.R., & Albinson, J.G. (2002). Pre-competition imagery, self-efficacy and performance in collegiate golfers. *Journal of Sports Sciences. 20*, 697-705.

Callow, N., & Hardy, L. (2001). Types of imagery associated with sport confidence in netball players of varied skill levels. *Journal of Applied Sport Psychology. 13*, 1-17.

Carter, J.E., & Kelly, A.E. (1997). Using traditional and paradoxical imagery interventions with reactant intramural athletes. *The Sport Psychologist. 11*, 175-189.

Cherie, L.A., Fry, M.D., Li, Y., & Relyea, G. (2002). Differences in imagery content and imagery ability between high and low confident track and field athletes. *Journal of Applied Sport Psychology. 14*, 67–75.

Cohen, S., Karmack, T., & Mermelstein, R. (1983). A global measure of perceived stress. *Journal of Health and Social Behavior. 24*, 4, 385-396.

Defrancesco, C., & Burke, K. (1997). Performance enhancement strategies used in a professional tennis tournament. *International Journal of Sport Psychology. 28*, 185-195.

Eysenck, M.W., & Calvo M.G. (1992). Anxiety and performance: the processing efficiency theory. *The Cognition and Emotion. 6*, 409-434.

Felz, D.L., & Landers D.M. (1993). The effects of mental practice on motor skill learning and performance: A meta-analysis. *Journal of Sport Psychology. 5*, 25-57.

Gammage, K.L., Hall C.R., & Rodgers, W.M. (2000). More about exercise imagery. *The Sport Psychologist. 14*, 348-359.

Hall, C., Mack., D.E., Paivio, A., & Hausenblas, H.(1998). Imagery use by athletes: Development of the sport imagery questionnaire. *International Journal of Sport Psychology. 29*, 73-89.

Hanton, S., Mellalieu, S.D., & Hall, R. (2004). Self-confidence and anxiety interpretation: A qualitative investigation. *Psychology of Sport & Exercise. 5*, 477-495.

Hardy, L. (1996). A test of catastrophe models of anxiety and sports performance against multidimensional theory models using the method of dynamic differences. *Anxiety Stress and Coping: An international Journal. 9*, 69-86.

Hardy, L., & Parfitt, G. (1991). A catastrophe model of anxiety and performance. *British Journal of Psychology. 82*, 163-178.

Holmes, E.A., Grey, N., & Young, K.A..D. (2005). Intrusive images and hotspots of trauma memories in posttraumatic stress disorder: an exploratory investigation of emotions and cognitive themes. *Journal of Behavior Therapy and experimental Psychology. 36*, 3-17.

Isaac, S., & Michael, W.B. (1983). *Handbook in Research and Evaluation*. San Diego, California: Edits Publishers.

Lazarus, R,S., & Folkman, S. (1984). *Stress appraisal and coping*. New York: Springer.

Manassis, G., & Doganis, G. (2004). The effects of mental training program on juniors pre-competitive anxiety, self-confidence and tennis performance. *Journal of Applied Sport Psychology. 16*, 118-137.

Martens, R., Vealey, R.S., & Burton, D. (1990). *Competitive Anxiety in Sports*. Champaign, Il: Human Kinetics.

Martin, K.A., Moritz, S.E., & Hall, C.R. (1999). Imagery use in sport: A literature review and applied model. *The Sport Psychologist. 13*, 245–268.

McCaffrey, R., & Taylor, N. (2005). Effective anxiety treatment prior to diagnostic cardiac catheterization. *The Science of Health and Healing. 19*, 70-73.

Morris, T., Spittle, M., & Watt, A.P. (2005). *Imagery In Sport*. Champaign, Il: Human Kinetics. pp. 3-11.

Orlick, T., & Partington, J. Mental links to excellence. (1988). *The Sport Psychologist. 2*, 105-130.

Paivio, A. (1985). Cognitive and motivational functions of imagery in human performance. *Canadian Journal of Applied Sport Sciences. 10*, 22-28.

Richardson, S. (2003). Effects of relaxation and imagery on the sleep of critically ill adults. *Dimensions of Critical Care Nursing. 22*, 182-190.

Scott, H., & Frey, J. (2004). Stimulation through simulation? Motor imagery and functional reorganization in hemiplegic stroke patients. *Brain and Cognition. 55*, 328-331.

Selye, H. (1956). *The Stress of Life*. New York: McGraw-Hill.

Sloman, R. (2002). Relaxation and imagery for anxiety and depression control in community patients with advanced cancer. *Cancer Nursing: An International Journal for Cancer Care. 25*, 432-435.

Spielberger, C.D., Gorsush, R.L., & Lushene, R.E. (1970). *Manual for the State-Trait Anxiety Inventory*. Palo Alto, CA: Consulting Psychologists Press.

Taylor, J.A., & Shaw, D.F. (2002). The effect of outcome imagery on golf putting performance. *Journal of Sports Science. 20*, 607-613.

White, A., & Hardy, L. (1998). An in-depth analysis of the uses of imagery by high-level slalom canoeists and artistic gymnasts. *The Sport Psychologist. 12*, 387-403.

Williams, J.M. (1994). *Applied sport psychology: person growth to peak performance*. Mountain View, CA: Mayfield.

In: Handbook of Motor Skills
Editor: Lucian T. Pelligrino

ISBN: 978-1-60741-811-5
© 2009 Nova Science Publishers, Inc.

Chapter 14

A DEVELOPMENTAL SYSTEMS APPROACH TO THE STUDY OF MOTOR DEVELOPMENT

Carl Gabbard[*]

Texas A&M University, USA

ABSTRACT

Motor development research has experienced greater frequency in top-tier science journals over the past 25 years. While some dialogue has been of environmental factors, to a much greater extent, discussions of motor development have focused on the biological, psychological, cognitive, or movement aspects of change. Few would disagree that to truly understand the mechanisms and processes associated with change in human form and level of motor behavior, a more comprehensive and integrated approach is needed – one that links biological and environmental theory. One such approach and the focus of this chapter is the *Developmental Systems Perspective*.

INTRODUCTION

Motor development is the study of *change* in motor behavior as influenced by biological and environmental factors (Gabbard, 2008). Change in this context typically means the observation of growth (change in size) and development (change in level of functioning) over time. Over last 25 years, there has been a substantial increase in the presence of motor development research in top tier journals of human development, psychology and neuroscience. This attraction is due in large part to acknowledgement that level of motor development is a critical factor in child behavior. Additional evidence of this emergence is the observation that aspects of motor development are mentioned with increasing frequency in broad-based theoretical treatises within the fields of cognitive psychology, developmental

---

[*] Address: Carl Gabbard; TAMU 4243; College Station, TX 77843-4243; (979) 845-1277; Fax-847-8987; E-mail c-gabbard@tamu.edu

neuropsychology, developmental psychobiology, and neuroscience (e.g., Johnson, Spencer, & Schöner, 2008; Michel, 2001; Thelen, Schöner, & Scheier, 2001).

Although some mention is given to environmental factors, to a much greater extent, discussions of motor development have focused on *dynamic systems theory* (e.g., Adolph, 2008; Fischer & Pare'-Blagoev, 2000; Lewis, 2000; Schöner & Thelen, 2006; Thelen & Smith, 2006). I wish to underscore that the term of focus here is '*developmental systems*,' not dynamical systems; with the latter being a sub set of the former. My intent with this chapter is to point out the potential advantages of using a broader perspective (framework) for the study and understanding of motor development - the *Developmental Systems Perspective.*

As a general framework, the *Developmental Systems Perspective* advocates the notion that human development is the product of changing relations between the developing person and his or her changing multilevel environmental contexts (Gottlieb, 2000; Lerner, 2002). This approach recognizes that a person is a dynamic, self-organizing unit consisting of several systems (e.g., neurological, muscular, skeletal, and cognitive) with multilevels within each system (e.g., Lewis, 2000; Thelen, 1995). From this perspective, contemporary theory such as *dynamic systems theory* is a sub set of the more general developmental systems view. Inherent with this approach is recognition of the reciprocal interactions between our biological characteristics and the environment, which produce change in human form and behavior. This reciprocity has done much to close the long debated issue surrounding the idea that human behavior is the product of nature or nurture (de Waal, 1999; Thelen, 1995). Most contemporary scientists view these two forces as fundamentally intertwined and inseparable, and part of a complex developmental system (de Waal, 1999; Gottlieb, 2000).

From the developmental systems perspective, change in human and motor behavior may be described with theories associated with *Environmental Contexts* and *Biological Systems.* What follows is a sample (certainly not an exhaustive list) of theories with ties to the developmental systems perspective. That is, theories that may be used to gain a more comprehensive understanding of the complex story associated with change in motor behavior. Although a multitude of developmental questions may be relevant, arguably, the most common contemporary line of inquiry deals with the explanation of mechanisms and processes associated with the acquisition of motor skills – commonly referred to as the study of *Perception to Action.*

ENVIRONMENTAL CONTEXTS

The term environmental context is associated with the circumstances, objects, or conditions by which one is surrounded. Also known as ecological systems in the field of ecological psychology, examples include the home, school, culture, and social influences within (e.g., family, peers, and coaches); all of which have shown to influence motor development. Among the noted ecological models, *Bronfenbrenner's Ecological Systems* theory and *Gibson's Ecological Perspective*, have close relevance to the study of motor development.

Bronfenbrenner's Ecological Systems Theory

This model represents one of the most extensive frameworks in the ecological systems theory (Bronfenbrenner, 1986, 2000); one that has enormous potential for studying environmental influence on motor development. This perspective emphasizes the broad range of situations and contexts individuals may encounter as described by five distinct systems: the microsystem, mesosystem, exosystem, macrosystem, and chronosystem. In brief, these systems represent the environmental settings and relationship ranging from the home, to the community, and to the culture in which one lives. Aside from the more obvious influence of the home, a relevant example is city government (parks), which is responsible for the quality of play and recreational opportunities, such as youth sports, playgrounds, and swimming facilities. Also included in this framework are sociohistorical contexts. For example, females of today are much more likely to participate in athletic endeavors than they were 20 years ago. As will be discussed in a subsequent section, settings and events within systems represent "affordances"; opportunities for developing and maintaining motor skill.

This theory looks at a child's development within the context of the system of relationships that form his or her environment. The theory defines complex "layers" of the environment, each having a potential effect on a child's development. A more recent update of the model highlights the child's own biology as a primary environment al agent. The interaction between factors in the child's maturing biology, his immediate family / community environment, and the societal landscape fuels and guides development. Change or conflict in any one layer may cause a ripple effect on other layers. To study a child's development, we must look not only at the child and her immediate environment, but also at the interaction of the larger environmental context. Bronfenbrenner's Process-Person-Context-Time (PPCT) construct has been used effectively to study various relations between the individual and multileveled context. This model accounts for the influences of individuals (person), their interactions with the environment and the responses they provoke from the environment (process), their interactions within immediate settings (context), and changing sociocultural influences on development (time). The results of a dissertation topic internet search via ProQuest, indicated that in 2007, 23 dissertations used Bronfenbrenner's model.

For example, Tudge and colleagues (2003) used the PPCT to focus on the relations between school-relevant activities (including play) of preschool-aged children and teachers' subsequent perception of the children's competence once they had entered school. They observed 3-year-olds' engagement in everyday activities (Process) and their initiation of those activities (Person) over a period covering the equivalent of an entire waking day. Children were drawn from two social classes (Context). The preschool observations were followed by two consecutive years of teacher reports of academic competence following entry into elementary school (Time). Of more direct relevance to the movement domain, Salmon and Timperio (2007) studied child and adolescent behavior (physical activity) as influenced by select characteristics of the neighborhood social and physical environment (e.g., peer relations, family interaction, urban design, access, safety concerns, peer relations).

Gibson's Ecological Perspective

This popular view provides insight into an important question in motor development: How do individuals perceive and act on information in the environment? Proposed by Eleanor and James Gibson (1979, 1988, 2001), this view contends that infants can directly perceive information in the environment and act with a reasonable response. This is in contrast to the traditional constructivist notion suggesting that past experience is critical in order to act on information in a meaningful manner. In the Gibsonian perspective, perceiving is experiencing. The infant is an active explorer in this process where perception and motor action are coupled. That is, we cannot study perception independent of movement. The environment, cast in the ecological settings noted in Bronfenbrenner's systems, for example, provides affordances that invite and challenge the child to perceive and act on information. In addition to the more obvious set of affordances such as toys, materials, apparatus, and availability of space, stimulation and nurturing by parents (and others) provide the additional component of events. The notion of affordances emphasizes that there is an ecological fit between the individual and the situation. The study of affordances in perception and as agents for change has been given considerable attention in the motor development and ecological psychology literature (e.g., Clark & Uzzell, 2002; Rodrigues, Saraiva, & Gabbard, 2005; Hirose, 2002; Stoffregen, 2000; Zwart, Ledebt, Fong, de Vries, & Savelsbergh, 2005).

BIOLOGICAL SYSTEMS THEORY

The three perspectives appropriately grouped as *developmental biodynamics* (Lockman & Thelen, 1993; Thelen, 2000), complement the developmental systems perspective by providing unique insight into the mechanisms and processes involved in the development of coordinated movement. Arguably, comprehensive understanding of the development of coordinated action requires information about the ecological surroundings.

Developmental Biodynamics

One of the most exciting and promising biological approaches to the comprehensive study of motor development emerged in the 1990s. Sparked by advances in neuroscience, biomechanics, and behavioral science, developmental biodynamics represents an interdisciplinary attempt to integrate promising theories and findings related to the behavioral study of perception and action (Bertenthal & Clifton, 1998; Lockman & Thelen, 1993; Thelen, 2000). In essence, the primary attempt is to describe and explain the intimate connection between the brain and body. This approach represents a vast improvement from the more traditional maturational approach, which described change in a descriptive series of developmental milestones. Although it is generally accepted that the control of motor behavior is under the direction of some type of generalized motor program (GMP [Schmidt, 1975; Shea & Wulf, 2005]) what the program actually controls and how control develops has been two of the most active areas of contemporary motor behavior research. This general approach is based on the hypothesis that motor coordination and control emerge from continual and intimate interactions between the nervous system and the periphery, the limbs and body segments (in essence, the brain and body). From this multifaceted approach, three theories have emerged that address the complex processes and mechanisms involved in motor development (perception to action): *coordinative structures, dynamic systems and neuronal group selection theory*. Another theory that has drawn the attention of the motor development community is *Newell's Constraints Model*, which will be considered separately.

Coordinative Structures

In past years, it was generally assumed that the individual muscles were given instructions by the commands produced in the motor program. Bernstein (1967) challenged this notion. He argued there are too many independent operations for the motor program to control them all simultaneously. In more recent years researchers have supported Bernstein's initial concern (e.g., Thelen, 2000; Turvey, 1990; Vereijken, 1991). They find it difficult to consider that the nearly 650 muscles and 100 mobile joints of the body are under the control of the central nervous system in all the possible degrees of freedom (i.e., controlled action of an independent joint movement). Bernstein suggested that motor programs control groupings of muscles instead of individual muscles. These groupings of muscles with associated joints have been termed coordinative structures, dynamic structures, and *synergies*. The commands generated by the motor program are directed toward the specific coordinative structure that is constrained to act as a single functional unit. From this general notion, a new definition of the term coordination has been proposed. It is the process by which an individual constrains, or condenses the available *degrees of freedom* into the smallest number necessary to achieve a goal (Rose & Christina, 2006). Although the actual nature of how the motor program controls movement patterns is not well understood, the existence of coordinative structures has been verified (e.g., Gentilucci, Chieffi, Scarpa, & Casetiello, 1992; Katsumata, 2007; Lee, Bhat, Scholz, & Galloway, 2008; Saling, Alberts, Stelmach, & Bloedel, 1998). The coordinative structures idea has stimulated considerable inquiry in developmental research, much of which as been associated with the next and arguably most published approach – the dynamic systems perspective.

Dynamic Systems Theory

This perspective seeks to provide an understanding of how movement and control emerge and unfold developmentally. Based on highly complex principles from theoretical physics, mathematics, and ecological psychology, this theory proposes that qualitative changes in motor behavior emerge out of the naturally developing dynamic properties of the motor system and coordinative structures (Kugler, Kelson, & Turvey, 1982). Thelen and Smith (2006) describe the following features of dynamic systems:

1. Movement appears to emerge from *self-organizing properties of* the body. Individuals are composed of several complex and cooperative systems (e.g., perceptual, postural, muscular, and skeletal), with each developing at different rates; thus the intricacy *of* coordinated movement. Even the simplest skill requires a cooperative effort, with each system providing critical input. For example, muscular strength of the legs and postural control are critical controllers for walking. Supposedly, there is a rate controller for each skill that organizes the system or systems needed to execute the task.

2. Another assumption is that movement is determined not only by muscular forces, but also by mechanical interactions (e.g., body segments and joint reaction forces). The contribution of these forces may be influenced by speed of movement, body position, length and mass of body segments, and the intentions of the movement. Research in this area seeks to examine the developmental characteristics associated with the generation and apportionment of forces and the timing-based control system.

3. With regard to the question of continuity or discontinuity, the dynamic systems perspective suggests that in the transition from old movement patterns to new ones, referred to as *a phase shift,* disruptions (discontinuities) occur in performance. The major challenge is to account for these characteristics from processes that are inherently continuous.

4. In addition to the biological contexts of dynamic systems, the nature of the environment and demands of the task influence development. Dynamic systems theory suggests that individual constraints can act as rate limiters in the development of motor skills (see discussion of constraints).

Neuronal Group Selection Theory

The dynamic systems perspective provides a glimpse into self-organizing properties of developing and mature motor systems, but it does not typically identify specific underlying neural mechanisms. The study of *neuronal group selection* (Edelman, 1992; Sporns & Edelman, 1993) focuses on how changes in brain circuitry that control synergies match o developmental changes in the musculoskeletal system. During the early stages of development, neuronal circuits are not precisely wired to execute specific skills; instead the brain contains variant circuits (structural variability) with dynamic properties. That is, those circuits selectively form *neuronal groups, which* account for the brain's organization of synergies as functional units of motor control (coordinative structures). One of its merits is that it accounts for the spontaneous adaptability of coordinative structure in response to bio-mechanical and environmental changes. Therefore, as with dynamic systems theory, neuronal group selection supports the environmental influence on motor development. Refer to Hadders-Algra (2000) and Jouen and Molina (2005) for additional information on this attractive theory.

COMBINING ENVIRONMENTAL
AND BIOLOGICAL PERSPECTIVES

Newell's (Constraints) Model

Newell's (constraints) model (Newell, 1986) offers an excellent framework for the study of lifelong motor development. It combines both the biological and ecological systems perspective. This is applied by describing the constraints to behavior in reference to the individual, the task to be performed, and the environment in which it is to be executed. In this context, the term constraint refers to factors that either facilitate or restrict development. Underscoring this view is the perspective that new motor behaviors emerge as a result of changing individual (organismic), environmental, and task constraints. In essence, this model supports the developmental systems perspective.

Individual constraints referred to originally as organismic factors, can be divided into two categories: structural and functional constraints. For example, weight, height, and reach maybe structural constraints, while speed, coordination, postural stability, and strength are considered functional factors. It is not difficult to understand that, depending on the task, we could be limited to some extent by strength, flexibility, and balance.

Environmental constraints can be related to the physical environment or sociocultural factors. This may include gravity (terrain), surface, space, temperature, and characteristics of the home. For example, the space and terrain that an infant has available to move in is a constraint on the development of locomotion.

Task constraints are broadly grouped into categories of task goal, task rules, and equipment / materials used with the task. Closely associated with the first two constraints (goal and rules) are the cognitive demands of the activity. In regard to equipment - a young child may not be successful with a normal size bat or racquet, but after modification more success or a better movement pattern may emerge. The same concept applies to the infant learning to reach and grasp, in regard to object size.

Obviously, there are more specific constraints then those mentioned. Certainly, one can think of numerous situations across all age groups. And, that is the merit of the constraints model. It can be used for evaluating performance and influence the type of instructional strategies used.

CONCLUSION

A commonality among all the approaches described is the suggestion that the brain and body are not pre-wired for skilled movements; rather, they have amazing adaptable *self-organizing properties* that adjust for biological and environmental contexts. In this dynamic process, affordance, exploration and attention to the environment are critical factors. Thus, if the student, teacher, or researcher wishes to examine motor development from a broader perspective, the *Developmental Systems* framework can be most accommodating.

REFERENCES

Adolph, K. (2008). Motor and physical development: Locomotion. *Encyclopedia of Infant and Early Childhood Development.* 359-373.

Bernstein, N. (1967). *The coordination and regulation of movements.* Peragmon Press: London.

Bertenhal, B., & Clifton, R. (1998). Perception to action, In LW. Damon (Ed.), *Handbook of child psychology: Vol 2. Cognition, perception and language.* (pp. 51-102). John Wiley & Sons: New York.

Bronfenbrenner, U. (1986). Ecology of the family as a context for human development: Research perspectives. *Developmental Psychology. 22,* 723-742.

Bronfenbrenner , U. (2000). Ecological theory. In A. Kazdin (Ed.), *Encyclopedia of psychology.* American Psychological Association and Oxford University Press: New York.

Clark, C. (1995). On becoming skillful: Patterns and constraints. *Research Quarterly for Exercise and Sport. 66,* 173-183.

Clark, C., & Uzzell, D. L. (2002). The affordances of the home, neighborhood, school and town center for adolescents. *Journal of Environmental Psychology. 22,* 95-108.

de Waal, F.B.M. (1999). The end of nature versus nurture. *Scientific American, December. 94*-99.

Edleman, G.M. (1989). *The remembered present.* Basic Book: New York.

Fischer, K., & Pare -Blagoev, J. (2000). From individual differences to dynamic pathways of Development. *Child Development, 71, 850*-853.

Gabbard, C. (2008). *Lifelong Motor Development* (5th ed.). San Francisco, CA: Benjamin Cummings.

Gentilucci, M., Chieffi, S., Scarpa, M., & Casetiello, U. (1992). Temporal coupling between transport and grasp components during prehension movements. *Behavioural Brain Research, 47,* 71-82.

Gibson, E.J. (1988). Exploratory behavior in the development of perceiving, acting, and the acquiring of knowledge. *Annual Review of Psycholog, 39,* 1-41.

Gibson, E.J. (2001). Perceiving the affordances: a portrait of two psychologists. Erlbaum: Mahwah, NJ.

Gibson, J. (1979). *An ecological approach to perception.* Houghton Mifflin: Boston.

Gottlieb, G. (2000). Nature and nurture theories. In A. Kazdin (Ed.), *Encyclopedia of Psychology.* Washington, DC, & New York: American Psychological Association and Oxford University Press.

Hadders-Algra, M. (2000). The neuronal group selection theory: An attractive framework to Explain variation in normal motor development. *Developmental Medicine & Child Neurology, 42,* 566-572.

Hirose, N. (2002). An ecological approach to embodiment and cognition. *Cognitive Systems Research, 3, 289*-300.

Johnson, J. S., Spencer, J. P., & Schöner, G. (2008). Moving to higher ground: The dynamic field theory and the dynamics of visual cognition. *New Ideas in Psychology, 26*(2), 227-251.

Jouen, F., & Molina, M. (2005). Exploration of the newborn's manual activity: A window onto early cognitive processes. *Infant Behavior and Development, 28*(3), 227-239.

Katsumata, H. (2007). A functional modulation for timing a movement: A coordinative structure in baseball hitting. *Human Movement Science, 26*(1), 27-47.

Kelso, J.A . (1995). *Dynamic patterns.* MIT Press: Cambridge, MA.

Kugler, P. N., Kelso, J., & Turvey, M. (1982). On the control and coordination of naturally developing systems. In J. A. Kelso, J. E. Clark (Eds.), *The development of movement control and coordination.* (pp. 5-78). John Wiley & Sons: New York.

Lee, H. M., Bhat, A., Scholz, J. P., & Galloway, J. C. (2008). Toy-oriented changes during early arm movements IV: Shoulder–elbow coordination. *Infant Behavior and Development, 31*(3), 447-469.

Lerner, R. (2002). *Concepts and theories of human development.* (3rd ed). Erlbaum: Mahwah, NJ.

Lewis, M. (2000). The promise of dynamic systems approaches for an integrated account of human development. *Child Development, 71,* 36-43.

Lockman, J. J., & Thelen , E. (1993). Developmental biodynamics: Brain, body behavior connections - Special feature. *Child Development, 64,* 953-1190.

Michel, G. F. (2001). The developmental-psychobiological approach to developmental neuropsychology *Developmental Neuropsychology, 19,* 11- 32.

Newell, K. M. (1986). Constraints on the development of coordination In MG Wade, HT Whiting (Eds.). *Motor development in children: Aspects of coordination and control.* (pp. 341-361). Martinus Nijhoff Publishers: Amsterdam.

Rodrigues, L. P., Saraiva, L., & Gabbard, C. (2005). Development and construct validation of an inventory for assessing the home environment for motor development. *Research Quarterly for Exercise and Sport, 76,* 140-148.

Rose, D., & Christina. R. (2006). *Multilevel approach to the study of motor control and Learning* (2nd ed.). San Francisco: Benjamin Cummings.

Saling, M., Alberts, J., Stelmach, G., & Bloedel, J. (1998). Reach-to-grasp movements during obstacle avoidance. *Experimental Brain Research, 118,* 251-258.

Salmon, J., & Timperio, A. (2007). Prevalence, trends and environmental influences on child and youth physical activity. *Medicine and Sport Sciences, 50,* 183-99.

Schmidt, R. A. (1975). A schema theory for discrete motor skill learning. *Psychological Bulletin, 82,* 225-260.

Schoner, G., & Thelen, E. (2006). Using dynamic field theory to rethink infant habituation. *Psychological Review, 113,* 273-299.

Shea, C. H., & Wulf, G. (2005). Schema theory: A critical appraisal and reevaluation. *Journal of Motor Behavior, 37* (2), 85-101.

Sporns, O., & Edleman, G. M. (1993). Solving Berstein's problem: A proposal for the development of coordinated movement by selection. *Child Development, 65,* 960-981.

Stroffregen, T. (2000). Affordances and events. *Ecological Psychology, 12,* 1-28.

Thelen, E. (1995). Motor development – A new synthesis *American Psychologist. 50,* 79-95.

Thelen, E. (2000). Motor development as foundation and future of developmental psychology. *International Journal of Behavioral Development, 24,* 385-397

Thelen, E., Schoner , G., & Scheier, C. (2001). The dynamics of embodiment: a field theory of infant perseverative reaching *Behavioral and Brain Science, 24,* 1-34.

Thelen, E., & Smith, L. B. (2006). Dynamic development of action and thought. In W. Damon & R. Lerner (Eds.), *Handbook of child psychology.* (6th ed.). New York: Wiley.

Tudge, J. R. H., Odero, D. A., Hogan, D. M., & Etz, K. E. (2003). Relations between the everyday activities of preschoolers and their teachers' perceptions of their competence in the first years of school, *Early Childhood Research Quarterly, 18 (1)*, 42-64.

Turvey, M.T. (1990). Coordination. *American Psychologist. 4*, 938-953.

Vereijken, B. (1991). *The dynamics of skill acquisition.* Unpublished dissertation, Free University, The Netherlands.

Whitacre, C., & Shea, C. (2002). The role of practice variability in retention parameter transfer and effector transfer. *Research Quarterly for Exercise and Sport, 73*, 47-57.

Woolacott, M. (1993). Age-related change in posture and movement. *The Journals of Gerontology, 48*, 56-60.

Zwart, R., Ledebt, A., Fong, F. F., de Vries, H., & Savelsbergh, G. J. P. (2005). The affordance of gap crossing in toddlers. *Infant Behavior and Development, 28*(2), 145-154.

In: Handbook of Motor Skills
Editor: Lucian T. Pelligrino

ISBN: 978-1-60741-811-5
© 2009 Nova Science Publishers, Inc.

Chapter 15

OMITTED STIMULUS REACTION TIME: A NEW TOOL FOR EXPLORING COGNITIVE AND MOTOR SKILLS

Oscar H. Hernández[*1], *Muriel Vogel-Sprott*[2] *and Victor Monteón*[1]

[1] Centro de Investigaciones en Enfermedades Tropicales,
Universidad Autónoma de Campeche, Av. Agustín Melgar s/n entre
Juan de la Barrera y calle 20, Col. Buenavista,
c.p. 24039 Campeche, Campeche, México
[2] Department of Psychology, University of Waterloo,
200 University Avenue West, Waterloo,
Ontario N2L 3G1, Canada

ABSTRACT

The time between a stimulus and a response is commonly assumed to reflect the sum of the duration of a series of mental and motor processes. The source of the timing delay related to these processes has been determined by partitioning the total reaction time (RT) into premotor RT and motor RT components. The procedure of fractionating RT to the *presentation* of a stimulus has been applied to simple and choice RT tasks. However, people also commonly make a response to the *omission* of some regular stimulus. This chapter focuses on the omitted stimulus reaction time (OSRT) task, which presents a series of sensory stimuli that require an immediate response to the omission of the train of stimuli. Unlike the reaction to the presentation of a stimulus, the reaction to an omitted stimulus is triggered by an internal process and is considered to require additional cognitive loads. Research evidence suggests that during the premotor fraction, the mental processes underlying motor skills occur. The chapter describes independent changes in the two OSRT components when several factors are manipulated (e.g., sensory modality, inter-stimulus interval or training). The relation of premotor and motor components to the brain wave, known as the omitted stimulus potential (OSP), are also examined. The

---

[*] Correspondence concerning this chapter should be sent to Oscar H. Hernández at the above address, via email at ohhernan@mail.uacam.mx; by telephone: (+1-52-981) 811-9800 x62400; or fax: (+1-52-981) 813-0176

chapter address the evidence suggesting that the impairment of motor skills by a moderate dose of alcohol might be due to impaired activity located in particular brain areas related to cognition rather than actual motor processes.

TRADITIONAL REACTION TIME TASKS

Research in motor control has clearly shown that a voluntary motor action needs to be prepared just before the initiation of the response (Keele, 1968). One important tool for understanding how such movements are prepared and what mental processes are involved has been the reaction time (RT) tasks. RT has been useful in testing drivers or operators of heavy machines in order to know how fast or slow their reactions are in an emergency. Measures of RT to sensory stimuli are widely used in neuropsychology because an RT task is commonly considered to require stimulus perception, cognitive selection of a response, and response preparation and execution (Welford, 1952). The use of an RT task apparently began with the Dutch physiologist F.C. Donders, who wanted to know in 1865 whether the time taken to perform basic mental processes could be measured. The easiest procedure is the simple RT, whereby the subject receives a sensory stimulus and provides a behavioral response, such as a button press; thus, the subject only needs to detect the stimulus and execute the motor response. It is commonly assumed that a higher load in cognitive requirements and more complicated movements require more time to choose and prepare the correct response (Ito, 1997). More complex procedures in which alternative responses are required for different characteristics of sensory stimuli are known as choice RT task. Here, the subject needs not only to detect the stimulus but also to discriminate and categorize it and, prior to executing the response, he needs to select the appropriate response.

OMITTED STIMULUS REACTION TIME

To date, most research on RT has been based on simple and choice RT tasks, where the tasks require a response to the *presentation* of a stimulus. However, under some circumstances, people also make a response to the *omission* of some regular stimulus. For example, the cessation of either a flashing stop light or the regular beep sound of a heart monitor requires an immediate behavioral response. An omitted stimulus RT (OSRT) task models this situation by presenting a series of regular stimuli and an immediate response is required to the omission of the train of stimuli. Various cognitive processes that might be associated with the OSRT have been suggested, such as stimulus detection, sensory processing, attention, expectancy, mental chronometry to determine when a stimulus is expected, making decisions and execution of a response (Hernández et al., 2005, 2006, 2007; Hernández & Vogel-Sprott, 2008, 2009a,c). All of these make the OSRT an excellent tool for exploring cognitive processes underlying motor skills.

Although measurements from the stimulus to response provide great temporal neuropsychological data, researchers have tried to obtain finer information from the RT by partitioning the total time into premotor (cognitive) and motor (movement) components (e.g., Botwinick & Thompson, 1966). The RT separation in these two components has allowed a more detailed analysis and assessment of central and peripheral factors influencing total reaction time (Ito, 1997). Premotor RT (PMRT) is the amount of time required to perceive and interpret the stimulus, to make a decision and prepare the response; and motor RT (MRT) is the elapsed time associated with the execution of the response. This procedure of fractionating RT to the presentation of a stimulus has been applied to simple and choice reaction tasks (Botwinick & Thompson, 1966; Ito, 1997; Raynor, 1998; Simmons et al., 2002). More recently, the fractionation procedure was also applied to the absence of a stimulus in the omitted stimulus task, using either behavioral or physiological methods for separate premotor and motor components. When behavioral method was used, a response key (Key 1) is depressed with the thumb of one hand until the train of stimuli ceased. At this time Key 1 is released and Key 2, placed 10 cm in front of the Key 1, is depressed. PMRT was measured by the time between the first missing stimulus and the release of Key 1. MRT was measured by the time between releasing Key 1 and pressing Key 2 (Hernández et al., 2005, 2006). In the physiological method, PMRT component was measured from the due time of the first missing stimulus until the muscle activation measured by an electromiogram (EMG) at the level of deltoid muscle, and the MRT from the EMG firing to the button-press release (Hernández et al., 2007; Hernández & Vogel-Sprott, 2008).

Hernández & Vogel-Sprott have been interested in learning about how some factors affecting the simple or choice RT are able to affect the cognitive and movement components of the omitted stimulus RT task. These authors have consistently found that PMRT component is slower than MRT and that an individual's PMRT and MRT are not correlated, which means that the two RT fractions apparently detect different processes (Hernández et al., 2005, 2006, 2007; Hernández & Vogel-Sprott, 2008). As in traditional multisensory RT tasks, the auditory stimulation produces faster OSRT responses than visual and tactile stimuli (Hernández et al., 2005; Hernández & Vogel-Sprott, 2009c). Nevertheless, although the tendency was the same for both premotor and motor components, only the effects of modality on the PMRT resulted significant. The PMRT-MRT independence has been also corroborated in the three sensory modalities (Hernández & Vogel-Sprott, 2009c).

On the other hand, the motor fraction was more sensitive than the premotor to practice effects (Hernández et al., 2005). Tests on three sensory systems (visual, auditory and tactile) were repeated three times on one day (9 a.m., 11 a.m., and 1 p.m.) and once the next day (9 a.m.). Figure 1 shows that trains of the three sensory modalities produced faster Motor responses as the tests trials were repeated. Again, the tendency for auditory to be the fastest is maintained. The results on the mean PMRT showed no differences on the first three blocks of tests administered on one day and only the fourth test 24 hours later was significantly faster than the first two tests. Comparisons of the two OSRT component measures when the frequency of stimuli in a train is high (7 Hz) or low (.5 Hz) have shown that a fast stimulus frequency produces shorter premotor RT than a slow frequency, but not differences were showed to the motor RT fraction (Hernández et al., 2007; Hernández & Vogel-Sprott, 2008). PMRT was consistently slower than MRT to each stimulus frequency and the correlations between these variables were not significant for either .5 Hz or 7 Hz. The slower premotor RT to trains of low frequency suggests that more cognitive load is necessary to perceive long inter-stimulus intervals (ISI), process the information, judge whether a stimulus is missing and decide to develop a behavioral response.

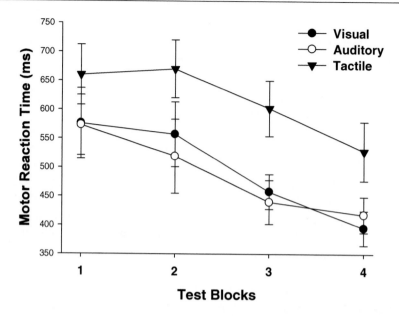

Figure 1. Motor RT to each sensory stimulus on four test blocks. Vertical bars show SEMs.

Alcohol is a good example of a centrally-acting drug that is able to impair RT to sensory stimuli. Mitchell's (1985) review of the effect of an acute dose of alcohol on simple and on choice RT observed that a low dose produce a detrimental effect on choice RT whereas simple RT is impaired at higher blood alcohol concentrations (BACs). This suggests that mental processes might be more sensitive to disruption by alcohol than are simple motor responses. Studies of the effect of alcohol on RT have primarily been based on the presentation of visual stimuli, and had not explored possible differences in the sensitivity to alcohol between fractionated measures of RT. One exception is the Liguori et al. (1999) study, where a placebo, a low (57–47 mg/100ml BACs) and a high dose (97–92 mg/100ml BACs) of alcohol were administered during declining BACS to social drinkers and tested them with visual choice RT. The total time was partitioned into "recognition" or premotor RT and motor RT. Their main findings were that the low dose had no detectable effects, but the high dose slowed the premotor RT component and did not significantly change the motor RT. In 2006 and 2007, Hernández and colleagues tested acute doses of alcohol in a within-subject design to measure premotor and motor fractions in the omitted stimulus RT task. They manipulated the stimuli applying trains of visual, auditory or tactile modalities, or fast (7 Hz) and slow (.5 Hz) frequency auditory stimuli. The results showed that comparisons of the alcohol (0.62 g/kg, or 0.8 g/kg) and placebo groups during the rising BACs slowed PMRT and had no detectable effect on MRT. More impairments occurred in visual modality than in auditory, whereas tactile was unaffected. The generality of the deleterious effects of alcohol on premotor RT was demonstrated when the inter-stimulus interval of the recurring stimuli was manipulated. These results provide valuable new information about differences in the sensitivity to alcohol to sensory modality, ISI and the cognitive and motor fractions of the OSRT. The evidence that cognitive processes are more sensitive to disruption by alcohol than are motor responses has some potentially important general safety implications. This may help to understand that a slower stop response of a person who is driving while intoxicated could be due to a slower mental processes (e.g., to make a decision to brake) whereas the time taken by the foot to release the accelerator and press the brake pedal keeps normal. In this way, social drinkers may suffer a detrimental cognitive impairment that could slow responses, even though motor functions remain unaffected.

THE OSRT IS RELATED TO OSP

The omitted stimulus paradigm is also of interest, because studies in animals and humans have shown that a special kind of event-related potential, known as omitted stimulus potential (OSP), is emitted at the end of a regular train of sensory stimuli (e.g., Bullock et al., 1994; Karamürsel and Bullock, 2000). The OSP is a slow positive wave that peaks around 500–1000 ms after the due time of the first missing stimulus and it has been considered to involve moderately high-level processing. Although the OSP and the OSRT involve cognition, no previous work relating possible associations of these measures had been examined. Just recently, studies of these two omitted-stimulus tasks have been executed manipulating the stimulus frequency (Hernández & Vogel-Sprott, 2008); the sensory modality (Hernández & Vogel-Sprott, 2009c) or applying active and passive trials (Hernández & Vogel-Sprott, 2009a). Figure 2 shows a general example of the recording method: Only the last two stimuli are shown in the horizontal axis and the first dashed line at X is the due time of the first omitted stimulus The research measured PMRT (X–Y segment) and MRT (Y–Z) of a response that released a button (Z) by lifting the arm and hand from the shoulder when the subject realizes that the train of sensory stimuli finish. Muscle activation was assessed by electromyographic signals recorded through two surface electrodes placed at deltoid muscles of the right arm (EMG). Flicking artifacts were controlled by a pair of electrodes attached to the external surface of each eye (EOG). Averaged brain recordings (EEG) were obtained until the fire of muscle action introduced artifacts in the record. Each stimulus evokes an auditory evoked potential, and the OSP onset (O) is identified by the slow positive deflection just after the due time and the OSP duration time is the segment O–Y. In both fast (7 Hz) and slow (.5 Hz) frequency of stimuli, the OSP duration time was strongly correlated with PMRT but not to MRT (Hernández & Vogel-Sprott, 2008). It also occurred for each sensory modality (auditory, visual and tactile; Hernández & Vogel-Sprott, 2009c). The slower PMRT was associated with longer OSP duration time. None of the regressions using OSP onset time were significantly related to the PMRT for each sensory modality or either frequency. Also, non-significant linear regressions were obtained of the OSP onset and the duration time on MRT for each sensory modality or stimulus frequency. Then, the correlation between PMRT and the duration time of an OSP suggested that similar cognitive processes might underlie these two measures (Hernández & Vogel-Sprott, 2008; 2009c). In order to avoid the muscle artifacts introduced by the behavioral responses, the complete waves of the OSP were recorded in passive trials (Hernández & Vogel-Sprott, 2009a . OSP parameters like onset time, rate of rise, amplitude and peak latency were obtained and tested for a possible association to PMRT and MRT. The results showed that slower premotor RT was strongly associated with a slower rate of rise in the OSP wave, but motor RT was unrelated to the OSP parameters. Because the PMRT was shown to be very sensitive to moderate doses of alcohol and this measure is closely associated with the OSP, current experiments in our lab are also showed that acute alcohol affects the PMRT and some parameters of the OSP in the same direction (Hernández & Vogel-Sprott, 2009b).

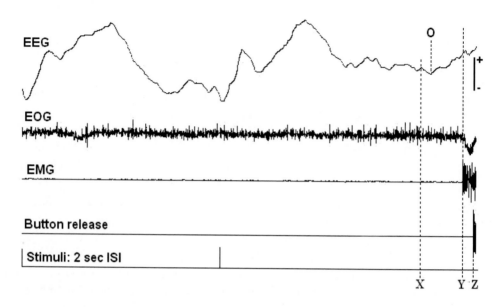

Figure 2. Illustration of a trial recording. Vertical solid line = 2.5 μV (see text for details).

One important goal in all of these studies has been to determine the main substrate (cognitive or motor) for those changes observed in traditional RT tasks due to alcohol or several manipulated factors. An increase in traditional RT is known to occur with some disturbances like neurological injuries, mental diseases or psychiatric disorders (e.g., Gauntlett-Gilbert & Brown, 1998; Leth-Steensen et al., 2000; Simmons et al., 2002; Zahn et al., 1998). However, to our knowledge, no studies have been conducted to investigate to what extent such disorders could have an impact on the premotor or motor components of the omitted stimulus task. Much more research is needed to understand which and how cognitive processes produce and modulate underlying motor skills when an expected stimulus does not come.

REFERENCES

Botwinick, J., & Thompson, L. W. (1966). Premotor and motor components of RT. *Journal of Experimental Psychology.* 71, 9-15.

Bullock, T. H., Karamürsel, S., Achimowicz, J. Z., McClune, M. C. & Başar-Eroglu, C. (1994). Dynamic properties of human visual evoked and omitted stimulus potentials. *Electroencephalography and Clinical Neurophysiology.* 91, 42-53.

Gauntlett-Gilbert, J., & Brown, V. J. (1998). Reaction time deficits and Parkinson´s disease. *Neuroscience and Biobehavioral Reviews.* 22, 865-881.

Hernández, O. H., & Vogel-Sprott, M. (2008). The Omitted Stimulus Potential is related to the cognitive component of Reaction Time. *International Journal of Neuroscience.* 118: 173-183

Hernández, O. H., & Vogel-Sprott, M. (2009a). OSP parameters and the cognitive component of reaction time to a missing stimulus: Linking brain and behavior. *Brain and Cognition*, doi: 10.1016/j.bandc.2009.04.010

Hernández, O. H., & Vogel-Sprott, M. (2009b). Alcohol slows the brain potential associated with cognitive reaction time to an omitted stimulus. *Journal of Studies on Alcohol and Drugs.* (in press)

Hernández, O. H., & Vogel-Sprott, M. (2009c). Reaction time and brain waves in omitted stimulus tasks: A multisensory study. *Journal of Psychophysiology* (in press)

Hernández, O. H., Ramón, F., & Bullock, T. H. (1999). Expectation in invertebrates: crayfish have 'omitted stimulus potentials'. *Proceedings of the Sixth Joint Symposium on Neural Computation. Vol* 9. San Diego: University of California Press. Pp 50-56.

Hernández, O. H., Huchín-Ramirez, T. C., & Vogel-Sprott, M. (2005). Behaviorally fractionated reaction time to an omitted stimulus: tests with visual, auditory and tactile stimuli. *Perceptual and Motor Skills.* 100, 1066-1080.

Hernández, O. H. , Vogel-Sprott, M., Huchín-Ramirez, T. C., & Ake-Estrada, F. R. (2006). Acute dose of alcohol affects cognitive components of reaction time to an omitted stimulus: differences among sensory systems. *Psychopharmacology.* 184: 75-81

Hernández, O. H., Vogel-Sprott, M., & Ke-Aznar, V. I. (2007). Alcohol impairs the cognitive component of reaction time to an omitted stimulus: a replication and extension. *Journal of Studies on Alcohol and Drugs.* 68: 276-281.

Ito, M. (1997). Fractionated reaction time as a function of magnitude of force in simple and choice conditions. *Perceptual and Motor Skills.* 85, 435-444.

Karamürsel, S., & Bullock, T. H. (2000). Human auditory fast and slow omitted stimulus potential and steady-state responses. *International Journal of Neuroscience.* 100, 1-20.

Keele, S. W. (1968). Movement control in skilled motor performance. *Psychological Bulletin.* 70, 387-403.

Leth-Steensen, C., Elbaz, Z. K., & Douglas, V. I. (2000). Mean response times, variability, and skew in the responding of ADHD children: a response time distributional approach. *Acta Psychologica.* 104, 167-190.

Liguori, A., D´Agostino, Jr. R. B., Dworkin, S. I., Edwards, D., & Robinson, J. H. (1999). Alcohol effects on mood, equilibrium and simulated driving. *Alcoholism: Clinical and Experimental Research.* 23: 815-821

Mitchell, M. (1985). Alcohol-induced impairment of central nervous system function: behavioral skills involved in driving. *Journal of Studies on Alcohol Supplement.* 10:109–116

Raynor, A. J. (1998). Fractionated reflex and reaction time in children with developmental coordination disorder. *Motor Control.* 2, 114-124.

Simmons, R. W., Wass,T., Thomas, J. D., & Riley, E. P. (2002). Fractionated simple and choice reaction time in children with prenatal exposure to alcohol. *Alcoholism: Clinical and Experimental Research.* 26, 1412-1419.

Welford, A.T. (1952). The "psychological refractory period" and the timing of high speed performance: A review and a theory. *British Journal of Psychology.* 43, 2-19.

Zahn, T. P., Jacobsen, L. K., Gordon, C. T., McKenna, K., Frazier, J. A., & Rapoport, J.L. (1998). Attention deficits in childhood-onset schizophrenia: Reaction time studies. *Journal of Abnormal Psychology.* 107, 97-108.

In: Handbook of Motor Skills
Editor: Lucian T. Pelligrino

ISBN: 978-1-60741-811-5
© 2009 Nova Science Publishers, Inc.

Chapter 16

MUSCLE STRENGTH TESTING IN CHILDREN: DEVELOPMENT AND EVALUATION OF A NEW MOTOR PERFORMANCE TEST

W. A. Van den Beld[*]

Human Movement Scientist and Clinical Epidemiologist;
Department of Rehabilitation Medicine (HP 898);
University Medical Centre Nijmegen St Radboud;
PO Box 9101; 6500 HB Nijmegen; The Netherlands

ABSTRACT

Most validity and reproducibility studies on instruments to test muscle strength have been done in adults. There is need for data from children, because such instruments are frequently used on children in clinical practice. Our study on the performance of muscle strength instruments in children aged 4 to 11 years showed that a new Motor Performance Test had the highest validity and highest reproducibility compared to hand-held dynamometry and the Jamar dynamometer. The child-friendly Motor Performance Test can improve the diagnostic procedure in children suspected of having myopathy and spare more children from painful muscle biopsy. Moreover, it is a suitable instrument for monitoring purposes in children.

INTRODUCTION

Many instruments have been used to test muscle strength in clinical practice. For example, hand-held dynamometry and the Jamar dynamometer are frequently used measurement instruments. However, most validity and reproducibility studies on these instruments have been done in adults, thus data from children are sparse. Too often, adult data, procedures and equipment have been used on children of various ages, with minimal

---

[*] E-mail: w.vandenbeld@reval.umcn.nl

consideration for the differences between children and adults [1]. Therefore, it is important to evaluate the performance of muscle strength instruments in children.

MOTOR PERFORMANCE TEST

We developed a new functional Motor Performance Test, because there was need for a better criterion to perform muscle biopsy in children suspected of having myopathy and to spare more of them from painful muscle biopsy [2-4]. As the indicator should discriminate between children with and without myopathy in the target population, it should aim at the general features of myopathy: loss of muscle strength and muscle endurance [5]. To encourage co-operation and motivation in children, measurement by means of a functional test would be most appropriate. Until now, no suitable functional tests have been developed for children that can measure muscle strength and muscle endurance at different muscle locations. Most of the available functional tests do not specifically measure muscle strength and muscle endurance, but other aspects, such as coordination [6]. Moreover, most tests are too difficult for the target population, for example the MOPER fitness test [7,8]. Other tests, such as Manual Muscle Strength Testing, are too insensitive or too easy for the children with suspected myopathy who are referred to a specialist centre for the first time [9-13]. If these children are tested with e.g. the functional grading system developed by Vignos et al. or the motor ability score developed by Scott et al., in all probability, they will achieve the maximum score, including the children with myopathy. Consequently, within the suspected myopathy population, the current functional tests cannot be expected to identify children with myopathy (a great many children with myopathy would have a false-negative result and the predictive value of negative results of these tests (-PV) would be too low). As far as the functional grading system is concerned, most of our patients would have achieved the maximum score due to their ability to walk and climb stairs without any assistance. The same applies to the motor ability score, i.e. most of our patients would have achieved the maximum score, because they were able to climb and descend steps correctly and they were also able to perform all the other movements [3]. Two other (non-functional) test instruments that are used to test muscle strength by many physicians and physiotherapists are the hand-held dynamometer and the Jamar dynamometer.

VALIDITY AND REPRODUCIBILITY

The performance of any test instrument depends on two important qualities: validity and reproducibility [14,15]. Validity assesses how well an instrument measures what it is intended to measure (accuracy). Reproducibility assesses the instrument's capacity to obtain the same outcome with repeated measurements (precision). The validity of the Motor Performance Test, hand-held dynamometry and the Jamar dynamometer was assessed by analysing their power to discriminate between patients with and without myopathy [3,4,16,17]. Ideally, validity should be established by comparing the measurement to a 'golden standard'. Some previous studies used technical examinations as a reference standard for the presence or absence of myopathy. Unfortunately, patients with negative (normal) results on technical examinations were considered to be myopathy-free. Evidence that this is incorrect and leads to unreliable results and conclusions was found in our prior investigation in which, despite negative results on technical examinations, 32% of the children proved to have myopathy in the muscle biopsy. Comparisons with an imperfect reference standard might also yield favourable results, although the test is not valid at all [15]. Therefore, in our studies, the result of muscle biopsy served as the golden standard for myopathy. Biopsy specimens can be analysed using the following techniques: histology, enzyme histochemistry, electron microscopy, biochemistry and when indicated, other investigations, such as molecular biology.

Evaluation of the three instruments showed that the Motor Performance Test had the highest validity and highest reproducibility. In children suspected of having myopathy, the child-friendly Motor Performance Test can improve the diagnostic procedure and spare more children from painful muscle biopsy.

MUSCLE STRENGTH TESTING

Muscle strength depends on age, gender and body size [18-20]. Therefore, the patient's muscle strength outcomes should be corrected for these variables. Hand-held dynamometry and the Jamar dynamometer reference values that account for multiple variables (multiple regression prediction equations) were only available for adults. Multiple regression prediction equations are also needed in children to correct the individual patient's muscle strength outcomes for age, gender and body size. Correction is necessary to determine the presence and extent of muscular weakness. Moreover, correction is necessary to make reliable assessments of validity and reproducibility, because otherwise e.g. misleadingly favourable reproducibility results will occur (see below). Therefore, we obtained multiple regression prediction equations from healthy primary-school children aged 4 to 11 years (provided by stepwise multiple regression analyses) [3,16,17]. In patients, performance of hand-held dynamometry showed wide variation in the 11 different muscle groups and helped to indicate which muscle groups can be tested most reliably by hand-held dynamometry in children aged 4 to 11 years [16]. The Jamar dynamometer gave a quick impression of muscle strength in children aged 4 to 11 years [17]. However, the diagnostic power of hand-held dynamometry and the Jamar dynamometer was not sufficient to serve as an indicator for muscle biopsy to spare more children from muscle biopsy. There were no cut-off points of muscle strength with high sensitivity (and high negative predictive value) as well as acceptable specificity.

CLINICAL EPIDEMIOLOGICAL AND METHODOLOGICAL CONCEPTS

Throughout all our studies, we paid very close attention to two important clinical epidemiological and methodological concepts. First, it is a principle of diagnostic research to enrol an appropriate study population. Until now, validity of instruments (e.g. hand-held dynamometry and the Jamar dynamometer) has frequently been investigated by comparing two 'extreme' groups who are easy to recruit, but highly selected, for example patients with (one type of) myopathy at a severe stage (severe loss of muscle strength) and healthy children. However, such a study population would only be suitable for initial test research and will automatically lead to artificially favourable results, because it is easy to discriminate between two extreme groups [21]. To investigate whether a diagnostic instrument is effective, the most appropriate population must be suspected of having the target disease [22,23]. Therefore, we investigated a population of patients suspected of having (different types of) myopathy, who underwent muscle biopsy. Evidence that it was the right choice to investigate the test in this population, instead of in extreme groups, was for example found in the outcomes of the item Jump [3]. The healthy primary-school children generally performed better (i.e. jumped further) than the patients suspected of having myopathy. This applied not only to the patients with myopathy, but also to those without myopathy. Thus, the enrolment of extreme groups would have led to misleadingly good validity (and reproducibility [24,25]), because of wide differences in outcome.

Second, the patients' muscle strength outcomes needed to be corrected for other characteristics, such as age, gender and body size, for the clinical interpretation of muscle strength data obtained from individual children (determination of the presence and extent of muscular weakness) and to evaluate validity and reproducibility. Therefore, we obtained external reference values (multiple regression prediction equations) from healthy primary-school children. In our evaluation of validity, corrected outcomes made it possible to compare the patients with myopathy to the patients without myopathy, although they differed, for instance, in age: a certain outcome could be good for a 4-year-old patient, but very poor for an 11-year-old patient. In our evaluation of reproducibility, corrected outcomes were used to avoid inflated results caused by other variables (age, gender, body size) that have a strong influence on test/retest and cause misleadingly high reproducibility [26]. The strong influence of these variables on reproducibility (assessed by the intraclass correlation coefficient: ICC) was confirmed in the publication on hand-held dynamometry, in which we calculated the ICCs of the non-corrected outcomes and the ICCs of the corrected outcomes [16]. For example, without correction, the ICCs of the elbow flexors (mean of two efforts) on the dominant side and nondominant side were as high as 0.94 and 0.95, instead of 0.85 and 0.90, respectively. Similarly, without correction, the ICCs of the shoulder abductors were as high as 0.94 and 0.91, whereas after correction, these values were 0.82 and 0.77, respectively. In previous studies, such influences have hardly been realized, or have not been taken into account.

MONITORING

There is also great need for an objective and non-invasive instrument to monitor the course of myopathy in children. In search of a suitable measurement instrument to monitor myopathy in children, one dilemma is that none of the existing tests form a reliable and sensitive reference standard. For example, hand-held dynamometry cannot be used as a reference standard to assess sensitivity to change (responsiveness[15]) of the Motor Performance Test. This would lead to incorrect results and conclusions, because the validity and reproducibility of hand-held dynamometry were found to have shortcomings in children. In addition, it can never be proven that the new measurement instrument is more powerful than the reference standard. Consequently, the real power of the new instrument would be underestimated by using an imperfect reference standard.

The Motor Performance Test was developed as a child-friendly functional means to measure the general features of myopathy in children with (early stage) myopathy. Our study design was not based on two extreme groups (i.e. healthy versus severe myopathy), but on a population of patients who were all suspected of having myopathy. Validity of the Motor Performance Test remained high in this population, which provides strong evidence that the test will be sufficiently sensitive to monitor changes in muscle strength and muscle endurance in children [3,4,23]. Very high reproducibility was also found, which is a necessary condition for good sensitivity to change.

When we administered the three instruments to the same population, the Motor Performance Test had the highest validity and the highest reproducibility. Up to now, hand-held dynamometry and the Jamar dynamometer have been used by many physicians and physiotherapists to monitor myopathy in clinical practice. Our results showed that the Motor Performance Test can serve as an objective and non-invasive instrument to monitor the course of myopathy in children. Thus, quantification of the patient's disease status and disease process can form a basis on which to evaluate and adjust therapeutic interventions. This information is expected to be beneficial to the clinician, the patients and their parents, e.g. for prognostic purposes. With the availability of more specific details, the 'status quo' in the patient's medical record might not prove to be the status quo at all. For research purposes, the Motor Performance Test forms a reliable and sensitive outcome measure to obtain meaningful data (e.g. in randomized clinical trials).

CO-OPERATION AND MOTIVATION

One very important aspect is that a simple game was incorporated into the straightforward functional items to achieve high levels of co-operation and motivation in the children. Co-operation and motivation are very relevant to the validity and reproducibility of instruments that measure maximum muscle strength and muscle endurance in children. Thus, the Motor Performance Test items should be administered strictly according to the standardized protocol and include simple games to motivate the children.

COST-BENEFIT CONSIDERATIONS

Motor Performance Test cost-benefit considerations were positive: the benefit was high (as mentioned above, the performance of the Motor Performance Test was high) and the cost was low. The Motor Performance Test is strikingly simple: it is inexpensive, easy to apply (e.g. by a physiotherapist), only takes a short time to administer (about 25 minutes), there is no burden on the child, it is non-invasive and very attractive to children. The standardized protocol of the Motor Performance Test has been translated into English. Currently, the Motor Performance Test is being prepared for publication and distribution.

CONCLUSION

According to our rigorous assessment, the Motor Performance Test is very powerful: it has good feasibility, high diagnostic power and high reproducibility. Five items make up the final Motor Performance Test: Stairs, Heels, Jump, Gowers and Circuit. The child-friendly Motor Performance Test can improve the diagnostic procedure in children suspected of having myopathy and is a suitable instrument for monitoring purposes in children.

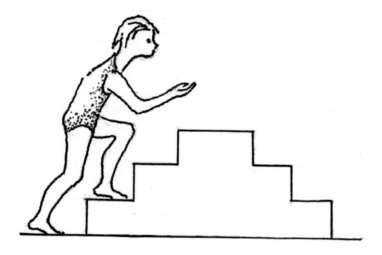

Figure 1. Stairs.

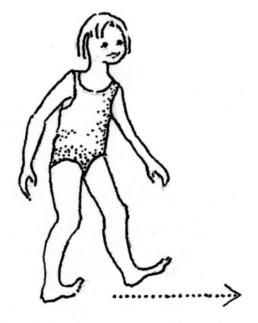

Figure 2. Heels.

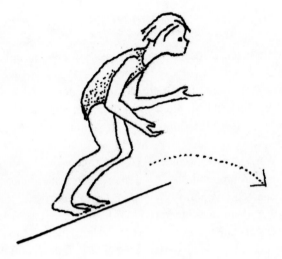

Figure 3. Jump.

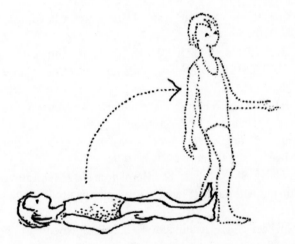

Figure 4. Gowers.

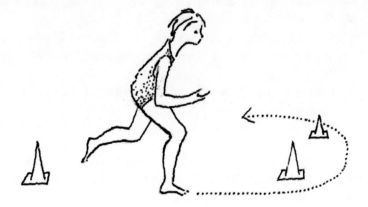

Figure 5. Circuit.

REFERENCES

[1]   Jones MA, Stratton G. Muscle function assessment in children. *Acta Paediatr.* 2000;89:753-61.

[2]   Van der Schouw YT, Van den Beld WA, Van der Sanden GAC, Binkhorst RA, Gabreëls FJM, Verbeek ALM. Item assessment in the development of a diagnostic motor performance test for myopathy in children. *Dev. Med. Child Neurol.* 1993;35:608-13.

[3]   Van den Beld WA, Van der Sanden GAC, Sengers RCA, Verbeek ALM, Gabreëls FJM. Validity and reproducibility of a new diagnostic motor performance test in children with suspected myopathy. *Dev. Med. Child Neurol.* 2006;48:20-7.

[4]   Van den Beld WA, Van der Sanden GAC, Feuth T, Janssen AJWM, Sengers RCA, Verbeek ALM, Gabreëls FJM. A new motor performance test in a prospective study on children with suspected myopathy. *Dev. Med. Child Neurol.* 2006;48:739-43.

[5]   Brooke MH. *A clinician's view of neuromuscular diseases.* Baltimore: Williams and Wilkins; 1977.

[6]   Wiart L, Darrah J. Review of four tests of gross motor development. *Dev. Med. Child Neurol.* 2001;43:279-85.

[7]   Bovend'eerdt JHF, Bernink MJE, Hijfte T van, Ritmeester JW, Kemper HCG, Verschuur R. *De MOPER fitness test: onderzoeksverslag.* Haarlem: De Vrieseborch; 1980.

[8]   Bovend'eerdt JHF, Kemper HCG, Verschuur R. *De MOPER fitness test: handleiding en prestatieschalen.* Haarlem: De Vrieseborch; 1980.

[9]   Medical Research Council. *Aids to the investigation of peripheral nerve injuries.* London: Her Majesty's Stationery Office; 1976.

[10]   Brussock CM, Haley SM, Munsat TL, Bernhardt DB. Measurement of isometric force in children with and without Duchenne's muscular dystrophy. *Phys. Ther.* 1992;72:105-14.

[11]   Vignos PJ, Spencer GE, Archibald KC. Management of progressive muscular dystrophy of childhood. *JAMA.* 1963;184:89-96.

[12]   Brooke MH, Griggs RC, Mendell JR, Fenichel GM, Shumate JB, Pellegrino RJ. Clinical trial in Duchenne dystrophy. I. The design of the protocol. *Muscle Nerve.* 1981;4:186-97.

[13]   Scott OM, Hyde SA, Goddard C, Dubowitz V. Quantitation of muscle function in children: a prospective study in Duchenne muscular dystrophy. *Muscle Nerve.* 1982;5:291-301.

[14]   Dawson B, Trapp RG. *Basic and clinical biostatistics.* 3rd ed. USA: Lange Medical Books/McGraw-Hill; 2001, p. 312-13.

[15]   Fletcher RH, Fletcher SW. *Clinical epidemiology, the essentials.* 4th ed. Lippincott Williams and Wilkins; 2005.

[16]   Van den Beld WA, Van der Sanden GAC, Sengers RCA, Verbeek ALM, Gabreëls FJM. Validity and reproducibility of hand-held dynamometry in children aged 4 to 11 years. *J. Rehabil. Med.* 2006;38:57-64.

[17] Van den Beld WA, Van der Sanden GAC, Sengers RCA, Verbeek ALM, Gabreëls FJM. Validity and reproducibility of the Jamar dynamometer in children aged 4 to 11 years. *Disabil. Rehabil.* 2006;28:1303-9.

[18] Beasley WC. Quantitative muscle testing: principles and applications to research and clinical services. *Arch. Phys. Med. Rehabil.* 1961;42:398-425.

[19] Edwards RHT, Young A, Hosking GP, Jones DA. Human skeletal muscle function: description of tests and normal values. *Clin. Sci. Molec. Med.* 1977;52:283-90.

[20] Sanjak M, Belden D, Cook T, Brooks BR. Muscle strength measurement. In: Lane RJM, editor. *Handbook of muscle disease.* New York: Marcel Dekker Inc; 1996, p. 19-34.

[21] Moons KGM, Biesheuvel CJ, Grobbee DE. Test research versus diagnostic research. *Clin. Chem.* 2004;50:473-6.

[22] Sackett DL, Rosenberg WMC, Gray JAM, Haynes RB, Richardson WS. Evidence-based medicine: what it is and what it isn't. *BMJ.* 1996;312:71-2.

[23] Van den Beld WA. Quantitative assessment of calf circumference in Duchenne muscular dystrophy patients. *Neuromuscul. Disord.* 2003;13:426-7.

[24] Altman DG. *Practical statistics for medical research.* London: Chapman and Hall; 1992.

[25] Bland JM, Altman DG. Statistics notes: Measurement error and correlation coefficients. *BMJ.* 1996;313:41-2.

[26] Colton T. *Statistics in medicine.* Boston: Little, Brown and Company; 1974, p. 214.

In: Handbook of Motor Skills
Editor: Lucian T. Pelligrino

ISBN: 978-1-60741-811-5
© 2009 Nova Science Publishers, Inc.

Chapter 17

MOTOR DEVELOPMENT IN CHILDREN WITH AUTISM SPECTRUM DISORDERS

Michelle Pope[1], Amy Lynch[2], Ting Liu[1] and Nancy Getchell[2]
[1]Texas State University-San Marcos, TX, USA
[2]University of Delaware, Newark, DE, USA

ABSTRACT

In 2007, the Centers for Disease Control and Prevention (CDC) estimated that approximately 1 in 150 children have an autism spectrum disorder (ASD) or a pervasive developmental disorder (PDD). In addition, autism ranked as the sixth most common category for children to receive services. These findings by the CDC suggest that ASD is no longer the rare condition it was once thought to be, but rather, many practitioners, both in medical and educational fields, will encounter children with suspected ASD in their practices. While the Diagnostic and Statistical Manual for Mental Disorders IV (DSM IV, American Psychiatric Association, 2000) criteria focus on the social and communication impairments of children with ASD, clinical practice and emerging literature indicate children with ASD also demonstrate a variety of motor impairments and deficits. However, a sparse number of studies have been conducted in the area of motor development and control in the past 30 years for children with ASD. The purpose of this chapter is to review literature exploring motor development and motor control abilities of people with ASD towards advancing our understanding of motor aspects in children with ASD. First, we review the existing motor related experimental and descriptive studies on motor disorder symptoms in children with ASD. Second, we will discuss both motor development and control in autism. Finally, we suggest directions for future research that integrate each of these areas. From this chapter, clinicians and researchers alike may be able to gain insights and frameworks upon which they may base clinical intervention and future research methodology.

INTRODUCTION

Within the United States and world wide, the incidence of autism is on the rise. In 2007, the Centers for Disease Control and Prevention (CDC) estimated that approximately 1 in 150 children have an autism spectrum disorder (ASD) or a pervasive developmental disorder (PDD), which was a substantially higher rate than had been previously recorded. In fact, in this same report, autism ranked as the sixth most common category for children to receive services. Historically, autism has been classified as an 'emotional disturbance' with behavioral characteristics. Autism was first identified in a case study of 11 children with autism (Kanner, 1943). In his early work, Kanner noted the emotional detachment of children from their parents and their seeming interest in being alone. In addition, Kanner noted the coldness of parents and their seeming lack of affection. More recently, autism has been defined as a neurodevelopmental disorder that appears in the International Classification of Diseases (World Health Organization - WHO, 2007) and the Diagnostic Statistics Manual of Disorders (DSM-IV, American Psychiatic Association, 2000) under the broad definition of PDD. In addition to autism, other pervasive developmental disorders include Asperger Syndrome (AS), Rett Syndrome (RS), and disintegrative disorder.

Both ICD-10 (WHO, 2007) and DSM-IV identify common characteristics of children with a PDD. These characteristics include impaired reciprocal social interactions, delayed communication skills, and the presence of stereotyped interests or behaviors. However, only the ICD-10 discusses motor characteristics of children on the autism spectrum specifically for Aspergers Syndrome:

> A disorder that differs from autism in that there is no general delay in language or cognitive development. Most individuals with autism are of normal general intelligence, but it is common for them to be markedly *clumsy*. (Italics added by authors)

The ICD-10 definition falls short of providing diagnostic criteria for clumsiness in autism. For years researchers have commented on the apparent clumsiness of children with autism (e.g., Cox, 1991; Mawson, Grounds, & Tantam, 1985; Tantam, 1988). Despite frequent claims in the literature that motor impairment is a diagnostic feature of AS, this assumption has not been assessed systematically.

Children with ASD have typically been studied in the aspects of atypical language development and social interaction. As a result, children with ASD are not diagnosed until 3 years of age or later. Research indicates, however, that early intervention in an appropriate educational setting can result in significant improvements for many young children with ASD. More importantly, movement behaviors play an important role in both the diagnosis of ASD, and the intervention. The pediatricians and health care providers informally use evidence of a delay in motor milestone attainment to screen an infant's motor development in childcare visits (e.g., Smith, 1978). Therefore, as numbers of children being diagnosed with ASD have increased drastically for the past 20 years, the authors believe that it is critical to review the literature in the motor domain. The authors believe that because ASD are considered a Pervasive Developmental Delay, it is critical that we review the literature to summarize the findings, as well as identify the inconsistencies and the gaps in the literature with respect to the motor domain. In fact, we believe that the motor domain is an overlooked and understudied area that could potentially provide insight into ASD and possibly could assist in early identification and diagnosis of autism.

The purpose of this chapter, therefore, is to review the literature with respect to the development of motor skills in children with ASD. Authors examine the early motor development in infancy, gross and fine motor skills, and gait patterns for children with autism. We believe an examination of the literature in motor domain on children with ASD is critical to advance future study in this area.

MOTOR DEVELOPMENT

Early Motor Milestones

The appearance and onset of early motor milestones and protective reflexes is often screened by physicians to determine the overall neurological development of an infant. The motor milestones often include rudimentary skills such as independent sitting, standing, rolling, and the onset of walking. The age of onset of these important indicators as well as the qualitative features of the movements need to be fully examined in children with ASD

The importance of assessing early motor development in infancy can not be underestimated in children with ASD. The appearance or atypical development motor milestones, persistence or absence of protective reflexes may be important indicators and possible red flags in the initial diagnosis and screening of children with ASD. In fact, it is possible, that the development of motor milestones may be one of the first indicators in the diagnosis of ASD appearing before delays in communication. Several studies conducted on the early motor development children are beginning to provide ample evidence to suggest that the onset of many motor milestones is delayed.

Qualitative observations of early movement patterns and reflexes during the first year of life have been studied using videotape techniques. Researchers have investigated the persistence of early protective reflexes and abnormal movement patterns. For instance, using the Eshkol-Wachman Movement Analysis System in combination with videotape analysis, Teitlebaum, Teitelbaum, Nye, Fryman, and Maurer (1998) concluded delays in the persistence of the asymmetrical tonic neck postural reflexes and rudimentary skills of lying, sitting, crawling, and walking in 17 infants with autism. Teitlebaum and associates argued that movement abnormalities in early infancy were an intrinsic part in autism, and they could be used to diagnose autism in early infancy.

Qualitative analysis of early movement patterns have also been examined during infancy using retrospective videotape analysis (Adrein et al, 1992; 1993). Baranek (1999) studied the home videos of 10 infants with ASD and 11 typically developing infants. In this study, Baranek examined the sensory motor behavior of infants 9-12 months old. It was reported that ASD infants showed salient sensory motor deficits as evidenced by poor visual orientation, excessive mouthing of objects and social touch aversions.

Another qualitative aspects of movement that is often reported in the literature to appear early in the first year of life is hypotonia or the absence of muscle tone. Early case studies in the original paper by Kanner (1943) reported:

'The average infant learns during the first few months to adjust his body to the person that holds him. Our children were not able to do so. In one instance, a mother was observed picked up her son Herbert. He remained completely passive as if he were a sack of potatoes. It was the mother who had to do all of the adjusting.'

Hypotonia has also been reported by researchers in studies investigating retrospective home videos of children during the first year of life (Adrien et. al, 1992; 1993). Researchers in the aforementioned study noted postural abnormalities and low tone in muscles in reviewing several videotapes of children.

Ozonoff et al. (2007) examined the early movement behavior of children later identified as ASD. Researchers investigated differences in the onset of motor milestones using a coded videotape technique. In this study researchers reported a delay in the onset and appearance of the rudimentary skills of walking, prone, supine, rolling, sitting, and crawling behaviors of infants with autism. Of all these skills, it should also be noted that the most significant delay in motor behavior occurred in onset walking. Ozonoff and colleagues suggested that a significant delay in the onset of walking may be one of the first signs that the motor system is delayed. Researchers in this study, however, did not note the absence of protective reflexes or abnormalities found in earlier studies.

In addition, researchers have detected qualitative differences in walking patterns of infants. Early walking pattern of autistic children demonstrated developmental abnormalities such as 'toe-walking.' The differences in the upper and lower extremities have also been documented in the early walking patterns of children with ASD. Using historical reports from clinicians and parents, Ming, Brimacombe, and Wagner (2007), determined that nearly 20% of children with ASD used this pattern. In a separate study, Esposito and Venturi (2008) have investigated early walking patten of autistic children using an observational scale and retrospective videotape analysis. In this study 42 children walking at least for 6 months were divided into three groups. The children with autism exhibited differences in upper and lower extremities as well as global differences in their early walking patterns. The greatest abnormalities reported in this study were reported in use of the arms.

Early motor milestones have been examined via self reports of parents. Mayes and Calhoun (2003) studied the onset motor milestones of children with autism during the first year of life. In a questionnaire, parents were asked to report on the appearance of milestones during the first year of their child's life. Mayes and Calhoun reported that parents did not indicate significant differences in the delay of motor milestones during the first year. These findings should be interpreted with caution as self-report data does not always provide an accurate view of development. Furthermore, self-report occurring in a retrospective fashion only captures the 'gross presentation' of the skill without reflection upon the quality in which the skill emerged or was utilized during daily activities.

Standardized testing has also been used to determine delays in motor milestones in early childhhod. Provost, Lopez, and Heimel (2007) assessed that appearance of motor development in children before the age of three. In this study, 19 children, ages 21-41 months with ASD were examined using the Bayley Scales of Infant Development II (BSID II, Bayley, 1993) and the Peabody Developmental Motor Scales-2 (PDMS-2, Folio & Fewell, 2000). In this study, 84% of the children were determined to be significantly delayed on the BSMD II and the PDMS-2.

It should be noted that the studies above have rarely captured the quality of movement as it appears in the early motor milestones. Furthermore, it is apparent that the qualitative appearance of these motor milestones may be among the first red flags to appear in the initial detection of ASD. In many cases the impairments noted are the subtle differences in quality of movement, not necessarily the actual achievement reflected on a standardized test. While there is overwhelming accumulating evidence to suggest that children with ASD may have delays in the onset of motor milestones, it is also apparent that the quality of movements merit further consideration.

Fine Motor Skills

In addition to studying emerging motor milestones in early childhood, a careful examination of motor development during early years is also necessary. Fine motor skills are important to children's development during the childhood years. Difficulties with prehension and manual dexterity can be problematic in many functional activities for children. Activities such as handwriting, buttoning, zipping clothing, or putting toys together can pose problems for children with ASD.

The reach to grasp (i.e., prehension) is a fine motor movement that has been widely studied in children (e.g., Kuhtz-Bushbeck et al., 1998; von Hofsten, 1984, 1991). Kuhtz-Bushbeck et al. (1998) studied the kinematics of the reach to grasp movement in children of six to seven years of age under several different experimental conditions. The findings indicated that grip formation is not yet mature at 6-7 years of age. Children tend to rely more on visual feedback than adults.

Mari, Castiello, Marks, Marraffa, and Prior (2003) focused on the examination of prehension movement in children with ASD. In this study, researchers determined that children with ASD showed a generalized slowness in prehension movement and planning and execution. Specifically, children with ASD demonstrated a different trajectory path with decreased efficiency, smoothness, and overall accuracy in reaching a target compared to peers. The findings supported the notion that motor impairment might be an intrinsic part of autism. Furthermore, this study also supports the idea that the quality and refinement of movements may underlie the motor impairments of children with ASD.

Children with ASD often demonstrate delays in fine motor movements necessary for performance in elementary school. Evidence of fine motor movements is identified in the poor graphomotor skills demonstrated by preschool and elementary aged children. Using the Developmental Visual-Motor Integration (VMI; Beery, 1997) to assess graphomotor skills, researchers detected significant delays in 164 autisic children ages 3-14 (Mayes & Calhoun, 2003). This finding is significant, given that graphomotor skills are a necessary component of early and later handwriting skills.

Similarly, Miyahara and colleagues identified problems in manual dexterity for children with ASD between the ages of 8-12 years old (Miyahara et al., 1997). Using the Movement Assessment Battery for Children (Movement ABC, Henderson & Sugden, 1992), researchers found a significant delay in skills involving manual dexterity of children with ASD, such as tracing, manipulation of pegs, and cutting.

Children with autism tend to have late onset of hand preference and differ qualitatively in their performance. A lack of hand dominance by age 5-7 years is associated with incoordination, visual impairments, and deficits in daily living activities (Larkin & Cermak, 2001; Sigmundson & Whiting, 2002). Early pioneers studying prehension have determined differences in dominant and non-dominant hand in children's performance (Knights & Norwood, 1979). More recently, high levels of left handedness have been reported in children with ASD (Dane & Balci, 2007; McManus, Murray, Doyle, & Baron-Cohen, 1992).

Together, these studies demonstrate mild to moderate impairments in fine motor skills among children with ASD. Most importantly, several studies demonstrated that children differ qualitatively in their performance which may not appear in a criterion referenced test that only captures the "gross presentation" of the skill. These studies suggest that further exploration of fine motor skills is warranted in the qualitative aspects of the skill.

Gross Motor Skills

The ability to move efficiently is important during childhood. The inability to move in a coordinated manner can often disadvantage children socially with peers. In addition, children who do not learn to move efficiently during childhood, abnormalities in gait, object-control skills, or locomotor skills can prevent children from participation in many important activities during the childhood.

Several researchers have demonstrated that motor impairments in gait patterns persist into childhood years. Kinematic dimensions of gait parameters have been studies in children with ASD compared to normally developing peers. Recently, Vernazza-Martin and colleagues (2005) compared various gait parameters in 15 children aged 4-6 years (9 diagnosed with ASD and 6 typically developing). Of the various gait parameters, shorter step length differed significantly between the two groups, with children with ASD demonstrating the most differences. Another finding was that children with ASD demonstrated the most irregularity in vertical translation and significant differences from the typically developing children.

Several studies have identified other qualitative gait abnormalities in children with ASD. Early researchers have demonstrated that many children with ASD demonstrate abnormal limb movements, shortened steps, and persistent toe-walking (Damasio & Mauer, 1978; Vilensky, Damasio, & Maurer, 1981). More recently, Woodward (2001) reported that children with autism between the ages of 3 and 10 years exhibited walking patterns similar to patients with Parkinson's disease. Specifically, children with autism walked more slowly and with shorter steps than children without autism.

A recent study compared children with ASD, DCD, ADHD and typically developing children on motor performance using a standardized motor skills test (Bruininks-Oeretsky Test of Motor Proficiency), as well as gestural performance using the Gestures test (examining object and non-object based gestures such as waving; Dewey, Cantell, & Crawford, 2007). The researchers examined 49 children with ASD, 38 children with DCD, 27 children with ADHD only, and 78 typically developing children. Their results indicated that, although all atypical groups displayed significant impairment on motor skills, children with ASD were significantly more impaired that their cohorts with specific motor skill deficits, and also were the only group to show impairment on gestural skills. These findings indicated that children with ASD showed a greater impairment in gestural command and imitation, which suggests that motor deficits may not lie exclusively in the realm of "motor". We explore these motor control issues in greater detail in the following section.

MOTOR CONTROL ISSUES IN CHILDREN WITH ASD

Current research suggests that in the population of children with ASD, issues of motor control accompany issues in motor development. Motor control relates to the processes involved in skilled movement, which can be neurological as well as sensory, central processing, neuromuscular, and the like. The fact that children with ASD demonstrate impaired sensory integration suggests that their ability to control movement may be affected as well. Research bears this out in two specific areas, that of anticipation deficits and motor imitation.

Anticipation Deficits

Typically developing children can successfully move in a sensory-rich environment by interpreting and attending to relevant environmental cues and then appropriately selecting the most appropriate motor response. In this fashion, anticipatory function occurs with the environmental interpretation of known cues with flexibility regardless environmental distractions or novel stimuli. However, children with autism with poor motor skills have lack of ability to attend and orient to peripheral attention cues compared to autistic children who do not have poor motor skills and with typically developing peers (Renner, Klinger, & Klinger, 2006). Because children with autism have deficits in anticipation skills, it may be possible that their decreased attention orienting and sensory processing skills negatively impact anticipatory during novel tasks or in unfamiliar environments. This reduced capacity of anticipatory guidance, in turn, may yield motor control problems.

Research suggests that, when participating in skills requiring anticipation, children with and without ASD differ in their central processing. Challenges identified include domains of auditory, visual, and proprioceptive sensory systems, all of which may impact motor control. Processing auditory stimuli appears to pose difficulties for children with ASD. For example, several studies indicated that children with ASD differed from their typically developing peers in brain activity after receiving an auditory stimulus (Gomot et al., 2006; Minshew & Williams, 2007). Further, processing unfamiliar verbal information on context is difficult for children with autism (Lopez & Leekam, 2003). Functionally, an autistic child's difficulty with motor actions upon verbal command may reflect these differences in processing auditory stimulus both with and without task specificity.

In addition to auditory processing differences, children with ASD also have difficulty processing visual stimuli. Research suggests that as the complexity of visual stumuli increases, children with ASD experience reduced integrity in both stimuli processing and motor response (Bertone, Motron, Jelenic, & Faubert, 2005). In addition, decreased visual perceptual processing may impact or be impacted by decreased integrity of a neurological observation-execution matching system (Lepage & Theoret, 2006). Detection, interpretation, and response to optical components of biological motion may also impede motor motor control in children with autism (Frietag, et al., 2008; Hubert, et al., 2007). Adolescents and young adults with ASD showed difficulty with perception and neurological response to imposed biological motion (Frietag, et al, 2008). In addition, autistic children had difficulty on impacting timing and coordination of movements in response to actual environmental motion, as well as by perceived motion with optic flow changes as the child with autism moves through the environment. Finally, research from one study suggests that children with ASD appear to have difficulty processing proprioceptive feedback as muscles contract during a bimanual lifting task (Schmitz, Martineau, Barthelemy, & Assainte, 2003). Further support for central processing difficulties contributing to motor control impairments exists in literature finding more rigid movement selection with self-generated versus advanced information movements (Glazebrook, Elliot, and Szatmari, 2008). Overall, it is possible that anticipatory deficits, influenced by central processing impairments, contribute to the establishment and integrity of gross motor plans by children on the autistic spectrum, thus lending to their presentation of motor impairments on standardized assessment tools.

Motor Imitation Issues

Another motor control area in which children with ASD show deficits is that of motor imitation. Children with ASD have deficits in motor imitation which may enable prediction of play and language deficits (Stone, Ousley, & Littleford, 1997). Children developing typically perform better when imitating motor gestures that have contextual meaning (e.g., a smile or wave) and are non-object oriented than those that have no meaning or are object oriented. Conversely, children with ASD have a more difficult time with non-object oriented imitation than they have with object oriented (Stone, et al, 1997; Vanvuchelen, Roeyers, & De Weerdt, 2007).

Children with ASD appear to be deficient in their ability to interpret contextual meaning. Deficits in action production or in action perception may explain these differences. Difficulty with body movement imitation appears early in development and extends through at least adolescents (Freitag, Kleser, & Von Gontard, 2006). Another study examining imitation skills of children with ASD who were either high or low functioning supported the notion of motor imitation issues (Vanvuchelen, et al, 2007). In this study, children with autism, regardless level of functioning, eventually achieved some resemblance of imitation. However, both groups of children required more effort in trial number to attempt to imitate 24 gestures and demonstrated errors in targeting and position accuracy in final imitation stance compared to typically developing children and those with learning disabilities. Such findings suggest challenges in action production may underlie motor impairments (Bernabei, et al, 2003; Dewey, et al, 2007). Furthermore, these findings suggest that practice, feedback and feedforward systems may need more attention. Not all research shows that children with ASD perform better in object oriented than non-object oriented imitation. Mostofsky et al. (2006) examined 8 – 12 year old children with ASD on a variety of imitation tasks, found that children were less successful with object oriented imitation than body movement orientation. They suggested that these deficits may represent a deviance in developmental pattern of motor imitation.

The differences in motor imitation in children with ASD have two possible explanations. One explanation is that there exists a developmental transition in motor imitation impairments. In this scenario, younger children with ASD have problems with non-object oriented (i.e., body movement) imitation. As they age, they transit to have more difficulty with object using perception of object imitation. In other words, initial motor imitation issues are related to action production, and across development to become more related to perception action deficits. An alternative explanation suggests that these differing findings may reflect the wide range of phenotypes of children on the spectrum of autism. Some children may display delayed development of action production systems (i.e., body imitation is harder than object imitation) while other children may have a different pathology contributing to an actual difference in action perception systems (i.e., when object imitation is harder than body imitation). In other words, it may be possible that some children have action production as a primary impairment such as poor body awareness affecting imitation of body movements. Primary impairments in internal and environmental feedback systems during motor action may influence this group. Meanwhile, other clusters of children have action perception (i.e., object oriented) related impairments, with deficits in feed forward systems influencing motor action. Longitudinal studies following children from late infancy through adolescence may help advance explanation of motor imitation deficits in autism.

CONCLUSIONS AND FUTURE DIRECTIONS

As the number of children with ASD continues to rise, more research needs to be performed to understand the complex nature of the disorder. We have focused on an area that has received limited empirical and clinical attention, that of motor skill impairment. It is clear based on the extant literature that, although not explicitly included in the diagnosis of ASD, impairments exist across a range of developing motor skills. Differences in motor development and control appear as early as infancy, with infants ultimately diagnosed with ASD displaying such differences as hypotonia and abnormal reflexes. As children with ASD approach school age, they may demonstrate poor prehension and graphomotor skills, which translate into difficulty drawing and writing. Children with ASD may also demonstrate difficulty with gross motor skills such as gait, bilateral coordination, and visuomotor control. Motor control issues include problems with motor imitation as well as anticipation deficits.

The difficulty in motor skills research with children with ASD is multidimensional. Standard research designs tend to be ineffective, owing to individual differences among children with ASD. Even children labeled as "high functioning" may differ a great deal from each other in terms of their reactions to testing situations, responses to researchers, and ability to comprehend and/or perform motor tasks. A researcher attempting to provide a uniform procedure for all participants will no doubt encounter many problems, all of which will negatively impact both internal and external validity of the results. Therefore, researchers must approach the study of motor skills in children with asd with both caution and an open mind. For example, one can not assume that a child with ASD who has difficulty performing a gross motor task has motor coordination issues; that child may perform the exact same task in an environment that has reduced sensory stimuli in several modalities. One should not be discouraged by the range of individual differences in ASD. In fact, research in the future should include creating a database related to motor proficiency on a variety of motor skills tests, such as the Movement Assessment Battery for Children (Henderson & Sudgen, 1992) and Test of Gross Motor Development II (Ulrich, 2000). Research should consider similarities and differences in performance within a variety of contexts, such as home, school, community centers, and research laboratory. The manner in which the tests are administered should be critically examined, to avoid the spurious conclusions on motor skill impairment that are actually related to inability to understand or imitate the task. Finally, researchers should attempt to create a unique developmental trajectory for motor development for the population of children with asd, which may some day be used to help identify the presence of this condition at a younger age than currently now possible.

REFERENCES

Adrien, J. L. Lenoir, P., Martineau, J., Perrot., A., Hameury, L., Larmande, C., & Sauvage, D. (1993). Blind ratings of early symptoms of autism based upon family home movies. *Journal of the American Academy of Child and Adolescent Psychiatry*, 32, 617-626.

Adrien, J. L., Perot, A., Sauvage, D., Ledder, El., Larmande, C.,Hammeury, L., & Berthelemy, C., (1992). Early symptoms in autism from family home movies: evaluation and comparison between first and second year of life using I.B.S.E. scale. *Acta Paedopsychiatrica*, 55(2), 71-75.

American Psychiatic Association. (2000). *Diagnostic and Statistical Manual of Mental Disorders*. (5th. ed.) Washington, DC: American Psychiatric Association.

Baranek, G.T. (1999) Autism during infancy: a retrospective video analysis of sensory motor and social behaviors at 9-12 months of age. *Journal of Autism and Developmental Disorders*, 29, 213-224.

Bayley, N. (1993). *Bayley Scales of Infant Development* (2nd ed.). San Antonio, TX: The Psychological Corporation.

Beery, K. (1997). *The Beery-Buktenica developmental test of visual-motor integration* (4th ed.), Parsippany, NJ: Modern Curriculum Press.

Bernabei, P., Fenton, G., Fabrizi, A., Camaioni, L., & Perucchini, P. (2003) Profiles of sensorimotor development in children with autism and with developmental delay. *Perceptual Motor Skills*, 96, 1107-1116.

Bertone, A., Motron, L., Jelenic, P. & Faubert, J. (2005). Enhanced and diminished visual spatial information processing in autism depends on stimulus complexity. *Brain*, 128, 2430-2441.

Centers for Disease Control and Prevention (2007). Retrieved October 12, 2008, from *http://www.cdc.gov/ncbddd/autism/asd_common.htm*

Cox, A.D. (1991). Is Asperger's syndrome a useful diagnosis? *Archives of Disease in Childhood*, 66, 259-262.

Damasio, A. R., & Maurer, R. G. (1978). A neurological model for childhood autism. *Archives of Neurology*, 35, 777-786.

Dane, S. & Balci N. (2007), Handedness, eyedness and nasal cycle in children with autism. *International Journal of Developmental Neuroscience*, 25(4), 223–226.

Dewey, D., Cantell, M., & Crawford, S.G. (2007) Motor and gestural performance in children with autism spectrum disorders, developmental coordination disorder, and/or attention deficit hyperactivity disorder. *Journal of International Neuropsychology*, 13(2), 246-256.

Esposito, G. & Venturi, P. (2008). Analysis of toddlers'gait after six months of independent walking to identify autism: A preliminary study. *Perceptual and motor skills*, 106, 259 – 269.

Folio, M. K, & Fewell, R. (2000). *Peabody Developmental Motor Scales: Examininer's Manual*. 2nd ed. Austin, Tex: PRO-ED, Inc.

Freitag, C. M., Kleser, C. & Von Gontard, A. (2006). Imitation and language abilities in adolescents with autism spectrum disorder without language delay, *European Child and Adolescent Psychiatry*, 15, 282–291

Frietag, C.M., Konrad, C., Haberlen, M., Kleser,C., von Gontard, A., Reith, W., Troje, N.F., & Krick, C. (2008) Perception of biological motion in autism spectrum disorders. Neuropsychologia. 2008 Apr;46(5):1480-1494.

Glazebrook, C.M., Elliot, D., and Szatmari, P. (2008) How do individuals with autism plan their movements? Journal of Autism and Developmental Disorders, 38(1): 114 – 126.

Gomot, M., Bernard, F., Davis, M., Belmonte, M., Ashwin, C., Bullmore, E., & Baron-Cohen S. (2006). Change detection in children with autism: an auditory event related fMRI study. *NeuroImage*. 29:475-484.

Henderson , S. E., & Sugden, D. A. (1992) *Movement Assessment Battery for Children* (Movement ABC). London: The Psychological Corporation.

Hubert, B., Wicker, B.,Moore, D.G., Monfardini, E., Duverrger, H., Da Fonseca, D., and Deruelle, C., (2007). Brief report: recognition of emotional and non-emotional biological motion in individuals with autistic spectrum disorders. Journal of Autism and Developmental Disorders, 37(7):1386 – 1392.

Kanner, L. (1943). Autistic disturbances of affective contact. *Nervous Child, 2*, 217- 250.

Knights, R. M. & Norwood, J. A. (1979). Revised smoothed normative data on the neuropsychological test battery for children. Ottawa, Ontario, Canada: Dept. of Psychology, Carleton University.

Kuhtz-Bushbeck, J. P., Stolze, H., Boczek-Funcke, A., Johnk, K., Heinrichs, H., & Ilert, M. (1998). Kinematic analysis of prehension movements in children. *Behavioural Brain Research*, 93, 131-141.

Larkin, D. & Cermak, S. (2001). Issues in identification and assessment of Developmental Coordination Disorder. In: S. Cermak and D. Larkin, Editors, *Developmental Coordination Disorder* (pp. 86–102). Albany, NY: Delmar,

Lepage, J. F. & Theoret, H. (2006). EEG evidence for the presence of an action observation-execution matching system in children. *The European Journal of Neuroscience*, 23(9), 2505-2510.

Lopez, B., & Leekam, S. (2003). Do children with autism fail to process information in context? *Journal of Child Psychology and Psychiatry*, 44(2), 285-300.

Mari, M., Castiello, U., Marks, D., Marraffa, C., & Prior, M. (2003). The reach-to-grasp movement in children with autism spectrum disorder. *Philosophical Transactions of the Royal Society of London, Series B, Biological Sciences*, 358, 393–403.

Mawson, D., Grounds, A., & Tantam, D. (1985). Violence and Asperger's syndrome: A case study. *British Journal of Psychiatry*, 147, 566-569.

Mayes, S. D., & Calhoun, S. L. (2003). Ability profiles in children with autism: influence of age and IQ. *Autism, 7*, 65–80.

McManus, I. C., Murray, B., Doyle, K., & Baron-Cohen, S. (1992). Handedness in childhood autism shows a dissociation of skill and preference. *Cortex*, 28, 373-381.

Miyahara, M., Tsujii, M., Hori, M., Nakanishi, K., Kageyama, H., & Sugiyama, T. (1997). Brief report: Motor incoordination in children with Asperger's syndrome and learning disabilities. *Journal of Autism and Developmental Disorders*, 27, 597-603.

Minshew, N. J. & Williams, D. L. (2007). The new neurobiology of autism: Cortex, connectivity, and neuronal Organization. *Archives of Neurology*, 64, 945 - 950.

Ming, X., Brimacombe, M., & Wagner, G. C. (2007). Prevalence of motor impairment is autism spectrum disorders. *Brain & Development, 29,* 565-570.

Mostofsky, S. H., Dubey, P., Jerath, V. K., Jansiewicz, E. M., Goldberg, M. C., & Denckla, M. B. (2006). Developmental dyspraxia is not limited to imitation in children with autism spectrum disorders. *Journal of International Neuropsychology Society*, 12(3), 314-326.

Ozonoff, S., Young, G., Goldring, S., Greiss-Hess, L., Herrera, A. M., Steele, J., Macari, S., Hepburn, S., & Rogers, S. (2007). Gross motor development, movement abnormalities, and early identification of autism. *Journal of Autism and Developmental Disorders*, 38, 644-656.

Provost, B., Lopez, & Heimel, S. (2007). A comparison of motor delays in young children: Autism Spectrum Disorder, Developmental Delay, and Developmental concerns. *Journal of Autism and Developmental Disorders,* 37, 321-328.

Renner, P., Klinger, G. L., & Klinger, M. R. (2006). Exogenous and endogenous attention orienting in autism spectrum disorders. *Child Neuropsychology,* 12, 361-382.

Schmitz, C., Martineau, J., Barthelemy, C., & Assainte, C. (2003). Motor control and children with autism: deficit in anticipatory function? *Neuroscience Letters,* 348, 17-20.

Sigmundson H, & Whiting, HTA. (2002). Hand preference in children with developmental co-ordination disorders: cause and effect? *Brain and Cognition,* 49, 45-53.

Smith, R. D. (1978). The use of developmental screening tests by primary care pediatricians. *Journal of Pediatrics*, 93, 524-527.

Stone, W. L., Ousley, O. Y., & Littleford, C. D. (1997). Motor imitation in young children with autism: What's the object? *Journal of Abnormal Child Psychology*, 25(6), 475-485.

Tantam, D. (1988). Annotation: Asperger's syndrome. *Journal of Psychology and Psychiatry*, 29, 245-255.

Teitelbaum, P., Teitelbaum, O., Nye, J., Fryman, J., & Maurer, R. G. (1998). Movement analysis in infancy may be useful for early diagnosis of autism. *Proceedings of the National Academy of Sciences of the United States of America*, 95, 13982–13987.

Ulrich, D.A. (2000). *Test of Gross Motor Development–2*. Austin, TX: Pro–Ed.

Vanvuchelen, M., Roeyers, H., & De Weerdt, W. (2007). Nature of motor imitation problems in school-aged males with autism: how congruent are the error types? *Developmental Medicine Child Neurology*, 49(1), 6-12.

Vernazza-Martin, S., Martin, N., Vernazza, A., Lepellec-Muller, A., Rufo, M., Massion, J., & Assaiante, C. (2005). Goal directed locomotion and balance control in autistic children. *Journal of Autism and Developmental Disorders*, 35(1), 91-102.

Vilensky, J. A., Damasio, A. R., & Maurer, R. G. (1981). Gait disturbances in patients with autistic behavior: a preliminary study. *Archives of Neurology*, 38(10), 646–649.

von Hofsten, C. (1984). Developmental changes in the organization of prereaching movements. *Developmental Psychology*, 20, 378-388.

von Hofsten, C. (1991). Structuring of early reaching movements: a longitudinal study. *Journal of Motor Behavior*, 23, 280-292.

Woodward, G. (2001). Autism and Parkinson's disease. *Medical Hypotheses,* 56, 246-249.

World Health Organization. (2007). International classifications of diseases (ICD-10). Chapter 5: Disorders of psychological development (F80-F89). Retrieved on-line (October 15, 2008). *www.who.int/classifications/apps/icd/icd10online/*

In: Handbook of Motor Skills
Editor: Lucian T. Pelligrino

ISBN: 978-1-60741-811-5
© 2009 Nova Science Publishers, Inc.

Chapter 18

LANGUAGE-BASED LEARNING DISABILITIES AND MOTOR COORDINATION: ASSOCIATIONS AND APPLICATIONS

Nancy Getchell[1], Samuel W. Logan[2]
and Kevin Neeld[1,2]

[1] University of Delaware, Newark, DE, USA
[2] University of Massachusetts – Amherst, MA, USA

ABSTRACT

In this paper, we review research that examines associations between language-based learning disabilities (LD) and motor coordination. Driving this review is our belief that the theoretical concept of embodied cognition (Chiel & Beer, 1997; Thelen, 2000), which suggests a dynamic interdependence of perceptual, cognitive, and motor processes, may hold promise in providing both questions and solutions for those interested in understanding learning disabilities. Based on the literature, relationships appear to exist between language and motor development in children at risk for language-based learning disabilities, which are suggestive of motor skill acquisition delays and differences in fine and gross motor coordination. The relationship between learning disabilities and movement disorder suggest that decrements in motor coordination may indicate a child may be at risk for LD; potentially, standardized motor tests may be used as part of a battery of tests to identify young children at risk for language-based learning disabilities . We believe this line of inquiry holds promise, and calls for more empirical research into the quantitative nature of the learning disabilities-motor coordination association, and for more theoretical consideration into the heuristic value of embodied cognition as applied to language-based learning disabilities.

INTRODUCTION

Within the United States, the number of children living with learning disabilities (LD) has grown over the past 20 years; currently, about 2.9 million school aged children (which represents about 5% of the population of children in public schools) have been diagnosed with a learning disability (Learning Disabilities Association of America, 2006). The most prevalent types of learning disabilities are language-based, which consist of issues with accurate and/or fluent word recognition and with poor spelling and decoding abilities (President's Commission on Excellence in Special Education, 2002; US Department of Education, 2002). Clearly, it is preferable to identify children at risk for LD as early as possible so that intervention and remediation can begin before a gap exists between a child's intellectual potential and their academic achievement in reading, writing, and/or spelling (Fawcett, 2002). Of course, this becomes difficult considering that this discrepancy between ability and achievement has been a primary criterion for identifying learning disabilities in children. In other words, children must fail in language-based skills before they can be helped. Any efforts in early identification indicating that a child is at risk, therefore, should be explored.

To this end, we believe that an investigation into the co-existence of language-based learning disabilities and motor coordination problems may suggest an additional avenue for helping to determine if a child is at risk for a language-based LD. In this paper, we review research associating language and motor development, and language-based learning disabilities with motor coordination issues. This association becomes important to consider because motor coordination can be validly and reliably measured in children as young as three or four years old using standardized tests such as the Test of Gross Motor Development II (Ulrich, 2000) and the Movement Assessment Battery for Children - 2 (Henderson, Sugden, & Barnett, 2007). This offers the potential that specific motor coordination deficits, along with other indicators, may help identify children at risk at a younger age.

Establishing an association between cognitive and motor domains would serve an additional function in that it may offer new theoretical and empirical directions in understanding learning disabilities: It may provide support, at least on a descriptive level, for the theoretical notion of *embodied cognition* (Chiel & Beer, 1997; Thelen, 2000). Theoretically, embodied cognition suggests that a dynamic relationship exists among perception, cognition, and action systems. As Thelen (2000) suggested, "cognition depends on the kinds of experience that come from having a body with particular perceptual and motor capabilities that are inseparably linked and that together form the matrix within which reasoning, memory, emotion, language, and all other aspects of mental life are embedded" (pp. 5). According to such a theory, it would be highly likely that any issues a child had in learning would be manifested across perceptual and motor domains as well. Empirically, this notion offers novel research questions and paradigms, and may provide an alternative direction in the learning disabilities research.

ISSUES IN IDENTIFYING LANGUAGE-BASED LEARNING DISABILITIES

To date, no one knows exactly what causes or constitutes a learning disability. Although there appear to be neurobehavioral etiologies, there is no clear consensus as to what these might be. For example, several researchers have hypothesized abnormalities in cerebellar activation in the dyslexic population (Nicolson, Fawcett, & Dean, 1995; Nicolson, Fawcett, Berry, Jenkins, Dean, & Brooks, 1999).

At the same time, others do not support the idea of cerebellar dysfunction as the cause of phonological and reading impairment, which are considered to be the primary deficits in dyslexic population (Ramus, Pidgeon & Frith, 2003). Still other researchers have suggested deficits in interhemispheric integration (Moore, Brown, Markee, Theberge, & Zvi, 1995). Because no one has agreed on specific causes of LD, its definition relies heavily on a description of behavioral manifestations, such as difficulties in the acquisition of reading, spelling, and writing skills. Difficulties and/or deficits in these language skills, rather than specific neurological processes, remain the clinical focus of both assessment and treatment of language-based learning disabilities, demonstrated as a discrepancy between students' ability for learning and their low level of achievement (Everatt, McNamara, Groeger, & Bradshaw, 1999).

The ability-achievement discrepancy criterion in language skills for LD identification remains problematic. McLeskey and Waldron (1991) found that, of the 790 students identified as LD based on the eligibility criterion outlined in the Indiana's statewide guidelines, one-third of students failed to meet the ability-achievement discrepancy criterion. These researchers acknowledged that teachers may label these students as LD because children needing additional attention could only attain it through being labeled as LD or because a child exhibits a behavioral problem resulting in increased energy expenditure on the part of the teacher. In 1999-2000, 2.8 million or 6% of public school students obtained some form of special education for their learning disabilities (U.S. Department of Education, 2002). However, according to the President's Commission on Excellence in Special Education (2002), up to 40% of the children receiving special education do so because of literacy issues and not learning disabilities. These findings suggest that the discrepancy criterion is not sufficient for the identification of LD. The commission also expressed concern in the fact that specific learning disabilities are not identified on the basis of physical or neurological findings, but rather by psychometric (IQ) tests. They criticized current identification practices as "an antiquated model that waits for a child to fail" (Commission, p.7). In essence, children must be school aged or older and failing to perform academically before their learning disabilities can be identified and appropriate intervention procedures can be taken.

If, at this point, we enter the notion of embodied cognition, the identification issues can be examined in a different way. In order to get to the point at which academic deficiency is recognized and measured, children proceed through the continuous, dynamic development of multiple, interdependent systems. Two points become important: First, although language-based deficiencies may be the most important result or symptom of the learning disability, they may likely be accompanied by other differences across domains. Second, differences develop over time through the interaction of cognitive, perceptual, and motor processes, and therefore should exist in some form prior to the recognition of academic problems.

By recognizing that the cause or causes of language-based learning disabilities exist prior to the initiation of formal education, practitioners may be well served in determining earlier diagnostic criteria. Using measures of academic discrepancy are problematic in early childhood. Lowenthal (1998) argued that preschool aged children have not been exposed to the formal schools settings, so it is not appropriate to conceptualize the presence/absence of a LD on academic performance. To add to the question of using the discrepancy model, questions exist about the validity and reliability of measuring intellectual potential in early childhood. Cognitive development occurs discontinuously during the preschool years (2 to 6 years), marked by frequent, rapid spurts; because changes occur frequently, measures tend to not be reliable (Smith, 1994). This suggests looking in other domains for differences. Deficiencies in academic performance come as a result of some underlying difficulty that the individual has with processing information; whatever the nature of the difficulty, it is likely that it existed well before academic training began and in motor or perceptual domains as well. As Nicolson and Fawcett (1990) argued, reading—in which one may not identify problems until a child is older than 6 years--is not an intrinsic capability, but represents an acquired cognitive skill; that is, dyslexic children have general problems in learning/skill acquisition. If these children have general problems in learning, then they would show problems in a wide range of skills, cognitive as well as motor (Nicolson & Fawcett, 1994). Hence, the best way to identify LD in early childhood may be evaluation of specific delays/deviances in the developmental domains: socio-emotional, adaptive, motor, communication and cognitive.

Of these, the motor domain offers promise as a means by which to identify individuals at risk for language-based learning disabilities at younger ages. Unlike the other domains, children obtain functional motor skills at a relatively young age. For example, research suggests that toddlers walk with adult-like spatial and temporal relationships (Bril & Breniér, 1992) and with adult-like consistency after only 3 months after the onset of walking (Clark & Phillips, 1993; Clark, Whitall, & Phillips, 1988). Another example is that of clapping, where infants generally begin clapping by or before the onset of walking and go through predictable changes in certain coordination measures as a function of development (Fitzpatrick, Schmidt, & Lockman, 1996). These motor skills exist at a point in early childhood which is well before the ability to measure academic potential or achievement.

Key to the argument of using motor coordination as an early identifier for children at risk for language-based learning disabilities is establishing that the developmental processes of language and motor domains co-vary in children at risk for learning disabilities. Although few researchers have examined these associations, several longitudinal research studies do suggest such developmental trajectories exist.

PREDICTIVE ASSOCIATIONS BETWEEN LANGUAGE AND MOTOR DEVELOPMENT

Several researchers have examined the relationship between language and motor development of children at-risk for language impairments. In 2001, Lyytinen and associates conducted a longitudinal study of children from birth to five years old. They compared children with (n=107) and without (n=93) familial risk for dyslexia on various developmental features related to language and motor domains. The researchers attempted to identify potential predictor variables for early identification of at-risk children by looking for associations within the first 2.5 years, and found early vocalization and early motor development to have predictive associations with later language development. Further, early gross motor development showed higher correlation to later language skills among the at-risk group rather than the control children. Also, fine motor skills were found to have no correlation with later language skills for children at risk of dyslexia.

Results of this study seem to suggest that gross motor performance may be important in the early screening process of motor skills as a predictor of the development of language skills. The performance of gross motor skills requires the use of the whole body and this appears to be more difficult, even in earlier childhood, for children who are at risk to eventually develop difficulties in language skills. These results fit within the embodied cognition concept because the use of the whole body in the environment requires greater integration of perceptual, cognitive, and motor processes. Implications for practice include focusing on tasks which assess gross motor skills in the early screening process to identify children who may be at risk to develop difficulties in language skills.

Following the study by Lyytinen et al. (2001), Viholainen, Ahonen, Cantell, Lyytinen, & Lyytinen (2002) conducted another longitudinal study from birth through 2 years old to look for a relationship between language and motor development in 176 children, 88 with and 88 without familial risk of dyslexia. In this study, expressive language was assessed using the Reynell Developmental Language Scales at 18 months and with the MacArthur Communicative Development Inventories at 18 and 24 months. Motor development was assessed using a structured parental questionnaire. Almost 38% of the children within the at-risk group showed delays in both fine and gross motor development. In addition, children at risk for dyslexia and with delayed motor development had a smaller vocabulary and produced shorter sentences than the controls and at-risk children without delayed motor development.

Although relatively little research has examined the association between language and motor development, the existing research is suggestive of relationships between the two. This lends some support to the notion that developmental processes may exist across domains rather than exclusively within the realm of one domain or another. Following this line of reasoning, we would predict that children who have been diagnosed with language-based learning disabilities would show some motor coordination differences from their typically developing counterparts. A further prediction would be that children with motor coordination difficulties such as Developmental Coordination Disorder (DCD) would show language-based learning difficulties. The following sections provide a review of research to see if these predictions hold up.

FINE MOTOR AND BIMANUAL COORDINATION AND LEARNING DISABILITIES

Because hand writing has been associated with academic performance, it is perhaps not surprising that researchers have investigated differences in coordination involving the hands (fine motor and bimanual skills). Several researchers have examined the relationship between fine motor functioning and cognitive learning disabilities. Lazarus (1994) looked at the existence of associated movements, or motor "overflow" in the non-active hand when 53 (37 with LD) children between the ages of 7 – 14 years were asked to produce a specific amount of force in the opposite limb by pinching an apparatus with their fingertips. The results indicated that the children with cognitive learning disabilities demonstrated greater associated movements or motor "overflow" in their non-active limb than their age-matched, typically developing peers. Lazarus (1994) determined that motor overflow occurs in young children as a normal developmental phenomenon that decreases with age both in intensity and frequency. On the other hand, LD children lacked "inhibitory control" over this motor overflow as compared to the age-matched controls. In another study looking at general cognitive learning disabilities, Woodard and Surburg (1999) found that children with cognitive learning disabilities demonstrated slower choice reaction times both in the upper and lower extremities, particularly when producing movements with the upper body that crossed the body's midline, than children without learning disabilities.

Other investigators have examined fine motor performance of children with specific language-based LD. Fawcett and Nicolson (1995) compared 3 groups of children (mean ages 8, 13, and 17 years) with dyslexia and 3 groups of controls matched for age and IQ, on different measures of motor skill. Their results revealed that children with dyslexia were significantly slower than their chronological age controls on tasks of peg moving and bead-threading. On the basis of their results, these researchers suggested that dyslexic children have severe problems in fine motor skills in even the simplest tasks, and that these deficits persist into adolescence.. In addition, researchers have found deficits in bimanual coordination in individuals with dyslexia. Moore et al (1995) found deficits in the accuracy of tactile motor coordination in dyslexic adults in a bimanual task. Another study indicated that individuals with dyslexia are more variable than controls and have particular difficulties in asynchronous, asymmetrical tapping tasks (Wolff, Michel, & Drake, 1990). Waber et al. (2000) determined similar results in children referred for learning impairment in a paced finger-tapping task (bimanual coordination) as compared to the non-learning impaired group in their study. In all, these studies point not only to the existence of deficits in fine motor coordination, but also to the heterogeneity of these deficits in the LD population. The evidence of fine motor coordination deficits leads to the next line of inquiry: Do children with learning disabilities exhibit gross motor coordination deficits?

GROSS MOTOR COORDINATION AND LEARNING DISABILITIES

One of the early studies that suggested a link between gross motor difficulties and dyslexia was by Haslum (1989), who examined data collected as a part of the British Births Cohort study in which 17,000 children were surveyed on issues of health at birth, and at 5 and 10 years. One of the purposes of the study was to identify predictors of dyslexia using these data, in children who were diagnosed with dyslexia on the basis of their scores on the Bangor Dyslexic Test and the British Span Test from the British Ability Scales. Two gross motor skills, namely, catch a ball (throw ball up-clap-catch) and walking backwards in a straight line for 6 steps were the first two among the 6 variables that could significantly distinguish between dyslexic and the normally achieving children at 10 years old.

Some other investigators have also reported deficits in balance and upper limb coordination in this population. Powell and Bishop (1992) designed a study to investigate the nature of motor difficulties of 17 specific language impaired (SLI) children (mean age: 9.3 years) and compared their motor skills to those of 17 age-matched controls. Out of the 11 variables introduced in the discriminant analysis, balance on the preferred leg, peg moving, ball-rolling with foot, clap-and-catch score, and balance on non-preferred foot were 5 of the 7 variables, in order of importance that most successfully discriminated between the language-impaired and normal children. In another study, Fawcett and Nicolson (1992) have reported problems in 'automaticity' of balance in dyslexic children. In this experiment, children with dyslexia made more balance errors in a dual task condition (balancing and a selective choice reaction time) than did typically developing age-matched children. Yap and van der Leij (1994) conducted a similar study, examining 14 children with dyslexia and comparing them to age-matched controls in a dual task paradigm (primary task: balance; secondary task: auditory choice reaction time). They found that the secondary task caused more interference in the children with dyslexia.

The results of these three studies seem to support the notion that children with dyslexia may have an automatization deficit. In other words, they may experience interference from the secondary task, which in turn inhibits the automatic production of the primary, motor task, providing evidence that these processes may not be truly automatized at all. Savage (2004) suggests that such deficits are not noticed when only the primary task is performed due to conscious compensation. In other words, children with a learning disability are able to allot additional focus on performing the tasks, allowing them to perform at levels similar to controls. The addition of the secondary task interferes with this supplementary attention and the performance on the primary task suffers. Additionally, in his review of the automaticity literature, Savage (2004) suggested that improved experimental design (e.g. using longitudinal rather than cross sectional studies) and better criteria for participant inclusion (e.g. participant screening for co-existing developmental difficulties) should allow future research to clarify the relationship between dyslexia and automaticity.

Because gross motor development is a major component of preschool programs in special education (Esterly & Griffith, 1987), some researchers have attempted to investigate gross motor problems in preschool children with LD. Merriman, Barnett, and Kofka (1993) designed a study to investigate the standing long jump performances of 30 preschool children, 3-5 years of age, with and without speech impairments on both qualitative and quantitative aspects of the skill. The developmental sequence of the standing long jump was used to evaluate the qualitative component, and the quantitative component was measured as the distance jumped. While the quantitative component revealed no differences between the groups, significant differences were found in the qualitative scores of the two groups. On the basis of their findings, these researchers supported the importance of analyzing both qualitative and quantitative aspects of a skill to evaluate the nature of the control processes involved in the production of movement in children with speech impairment.

As a sequel to the Merriman et al (1993) study, Merriman and Barnett (1995) investigated the relationship between language and gross motor skills of 28 preschool children (mean age: 4.2 years) diagnosed as speech/language impaired. Children were tested on the revised Preschool Language Scale and the Test of Gross Motor Development (TGMD). Locomotor skills were found to significantly correlate to both auditory comprehension(r=.47) and verbal ability(r=.41). These results suggested at least a moderate relationship between language and gross motor skills. One limitation to this study was that the authors reported screening for other disabilities, but did not relay how or for what disabilities they screened.

Do the characteristics of gross motor functioning differ among LD children? Miyahara (1994) designed a study to identify homogenous subtypes of students with LD based upon gross motor functions, and cluster analysis techniques. Fifty-five LD students (mean age: 11.5 years) were tested on the items from Bruininks-Oseretsky Test of Motor Proficiency. Four possible subtypes were identified: Free from motor problems, poorly coordinated, good balance, and poor balance. The poorly coordinated subtype constituted 25.5% of the LD sample and exhibited consistently poor performance in all the gross motor subtests. The poor balance group comprised 7.3% of the LD sample and demonstrated extreme deficits in balance. Thus, studies on gross motor skills in the LD population reveal the existence of these deficits early in the developmental sequence in this population, beginning at the preschool level. Also, deficits are seen in different measures of gross motor function.

LANGUAGE-BASED LEARNING DIFFICULTIES IN CHILDREN WITH MOVEMENT COORDINATION DISORDERS

Within the realm of learning disabilities, one type of learning disability relates specifically to motor coordination deficits: Developmental Coordination Disorder (DCD). If a close association exists between cognitive and motor domains, one would expect deficits in language-based processes to co-exist in children with DCD. Several researchers have discussed this association. Kaplan, Wilson, Dewey and Crawford (1998) investigated the issue of overlap between the three developmental disorders: reading disability (RD), attention deficit hyperactivity disorder (ADHD), and DCD. These researchers argued that it is more common to find children with a combination of these difficulties to a greater/lesser extent, than to find one of these as an entirely isolated problem. They describe co-morbidity in childhood disorders as a 'rule', rather than an 'exception'. To address this issue of co-morbidity, a sample of 162 children (8-18 years of age) were tested for the three disorders. A three-way classification was employed to categorize these children, and out of the 71 children identified as RD, 81 as DCD, and 81 as ADHD, 23 were found to have deficits in all three measures, 22 with a co-existing deficit in RD and DCD, 10 in ADHD and DCD, and 7 in RD and ADHD. In another study, Dewey, Kaplan, Crawford, and Wilson (2002) found problems in learning (reading, writing, and spelling) in children with DCD and children suspect for DCD.

It appears then, that children with language-based learning disabilities may show concomitant decrements in motor coordination. Further, children with DCD may show concomitant decrements in language-based performance. Although the nature of this relationship is not absolute, nor is it understood, the fact that these deficiencies do co-exist suggest that both functional and theoretical applications may exist, and are worthy of further study.

THE ROLE OF THE CEREBELLUM IN LANGUAGE IMPAIRMENTS AND MOTOR SKILLS

Abnormalities in the cerebellum have been associated with language impairments, specifically dyslexia, as well as a decreased performance in balancing (Stoodley et al, 2005). As suggested earlier, several researchers have hypothesized abnormalities in cerebellar activation in the dyslexic population (Nicolson, Fawcett, & Dean, 1995; Nicolson, Fawcett, Berry, Jenkins, Dean, & Brooks, 1999). Eckert et al studied this hypothesis at the neuroanatomical level by using MRI scans (Eckert et al, 2003). Eighteen children with dyslexia and thirty-two control children in grades 4-6 participated in the study. Researchers found that children with dyslexia exhibited "significantly smaller right anterior lobes of the cerebellum" (Eckert et al, 2003). Based on their results, the researchers concluded that in imaging studies, "the cerebellum is one of the most consistent locations for structural differences between dyslexic and control participants" (Eckert et al, 2003).

As discussed earlier, balance difficulties have been observed in the population with dyslexia suggesting that the atypical development of the cerebellum is at least partly responsible for the difficulties to perform balancing tasks (Stoodley et al, 2005). It has been suggested that an atypical cerebellum is not the cause of dyslexia but it is part of an overall group of brain abnormalities which contributes to difficulties in information processing which results in the expression of behavioral symptoms including balance and language impairments (Stoodley et al, 2005). The concept of Atypical Brain Development (ABD) has been described to account for the various underlying deficits observed in populations with various language and movement disabilities.

ATYPICAL BRAIN DEVELOPMENT: A HYPOTHESIS TO EXPLAIN LANGUAGE AND MOTOR IMPAIRMENTS

It is likely an underlying mechanism has not been proposed to explain a connection between language impairments and motor impairments because such a specific mechanism does not exist. It has been established that the comorbidity between developmental disorders is significant (Kaplan et al, 1998). A practical theory towards explaining the overlapping presentation of symptoms includes the concept known as Atypical Brain Development (ABD).

This term does not embody a set group of symptoms in an individual but may include one or several impairments in the following areas: "language, spelling or writing, motor skills, and coordination, and attention or activity" (Gilger & Kaplan, 2001). Evidence for the necessity of such a concept exists in studies which show high comorbidity between disabilities such as reading disabilities, ADHD, and DCD (Gilger & Kaplan, 2001). Research has not shown a one to one relationship between brain abnormalities and developmental learning disabilities (Gilger & Kaplan, 2001). It is suggested the interaction between genetics and the environment leads to the development of various disabilities (Gilger & Kaplan, 2001). The ABD concept attempts to account for the various underlying mechanisms which are associated with the common symptoms presented in some learning and motor disabilities.

For the purposes of research, it is suggested that specific brain abnormalities in developmental learning disabilities should still be investigated, but in exploring these relationships it is important to understand there may be various underlying mechanisms responsible for the different symptoms (Gilger & Kaplan, 2001). In addition, it may be important to shift research efforts to study symptoms rather than clinically defined syndromes (Gilger & Kaplan, 2001). If individual symptoms can be understood more completely at the brain level, then a collection of underlying mechanisms for each learning disability could be established. Based on the ABD framework, in practice it is suggested to focus on the individual differences in the presentation of symptoms.

MOTOR COORDINATION AND LANGUAGE-BASED LEARNING DISABILITIES: IMPLICATIONS FOR PRACTICE

Based on previous research examining motor coordination in children with language-based learning disabilities, it appears as though there may be some co-existence of conditions. That is, children with language-based learning disabilities may also have problems with one or several aspects of motor coordination. The conclusions of the research suggest that, just as children with learning disabilities show a decrement in academic performance, they often exhibit concomitant motor coordination decrements. That is, children who show language deficits also show coordination deficits, which appear to persist throughout adolescence and beyond. One clearly defined type of motor deficit did not emerge, however. Coordination issues ranged from motor planning to movement execution and production. In addition, different domains (e.g. fine motor, gross motor, balance, movement speed and accuracy) as well as different measures of movement (e.g. qualitative and quantitative) were affected.

We believe, based on the research reviewed, that whatever neurobehavioral issues that lead to learning difficulties in children may also be responsible for these movement deficits. This provides a unique window into early identification of children at risk for learning disabilities. This suggests that tests of motor coordination that have been validated for younger age groups may provide another tool for the early identification of children at risk for learning disabilities. There are many validated tests, such as the Test of Gross Motor Development (TGMD II; Ulrich, 2000) which is validated for children 3 – 11 years old, the Movement Assessment Battery for Children - 2 (MABC - 2; Henderson, Sugden, & Barnett, 2007), which has validated sub-tests within age bands 4 – 11 years old, or the Peabody Developmental Motor Scales, validated from 0 – 7 years old (PDMS-2; Folio & Fewell, 2000). The specific motor tasks assessed in these tests include various measures of balance, ball skills, locomotor skills (ability to run, walk, gallop, etc), and object skills (the ability to strike, underhand roll, throw, and kick a ball). Since each test only requires approximately thirty minutes for a child to complete, it is a practical way to gain information about each individual child. For example, since balance difficulties are known to exist in some children with dyslexia, poor balance performance on standardized tests would indicate further investigation into the potential development of dyslexia. Also, if a large data base of information was established for children of varying ages, after a few years of data collection, it may be more clear which motor skill deficits are associated with the development of language-based learning disabilities.

These or other validated tests could be used to assess motor coordination both within the population of children who have language based LD (in order to get a better idea of specific deficits and norms for this group), followed by testing children determined to be at risk for LD, to see if they display these deficits. ,If this strategy indicates that predictable deficits exist, the tests can then be used as part of an assessment battery for children to determine if they are at risk for LD. Perhaps a better strategy would be to test all preschoolers on motor proficiency using standardized tests and to track their progress over time (and in conjunction with scores on other, more specific tests that assess at-risk status). Of course, this would require a trained professional to administer the motor proficiency test, which would most likely occur within a structured physical activity setting. Unfortunately, physical activity for preschoolers is not mandated on the federal level and many preschools do not provided structured physical activity for their students, nor motor development or physical education training for their staff. Thus, implementing such motor proficiency testing within preschools would require a large shift in policy at all levels (school, state, federal).

MOTOR COORDINATION AND LANGUAGE-BASED LEARNING DISABILITIES: THEORETICAL IMPLICATIONS

We also wished to examine previous and current research to see if the theoretical notion of embodied cognition is supported by empirical findings in the field of language-based learning disabilities and motor coordination. Emerging from contemporary developmental psychological thought within the ecological perspective, embodied cognition suggests the dynamic interdependency of perceptual, cognitive, and motor systems within the human body (Thelen, 2000). There is an interdependence of the three systems; complete understanding of cognition relies on acknowledging the reciprocal and evolving effects towards and from perception-action systems. Following the logic of embodied cognition, any deficits we see in academic performance (cognition, per se) will be accompanied by differences in movement abilities among other domains. Further, this concept promotes the notion that change in one system may result in a qualitatively new way of functioning within and among body systems. The support of this concept would lead to an alternative way not only to think about learning disabilities, but also potentially identify and remediate them as well. By identifying a link between motor and cognitive domains within existing research, we would like to suggest that it may be fruitful to use this theory as a guide for empirical questions and predictions. There are further implications of the association between learning disabilities and gross motor coordination. Bushnell and Boudreau (1993) have emphasized the role that motor development plays in determining developmental sequences in other domains. Could remediation within the motor domain somehow assist in the overall improvement in learning ability? The idea is tempting, and theoretically supported in the concept of embodied cognition.

CONCLUSIONS

Grosshans & Kiger (2004) have suggested that the Physical Education setting is ideal for identifying children who may have certain types of language-based learning disabilities (among others) in school aged children. As Movement specialists who work at a school for children with learning disabilities, they discuss how, within physical education class, school aged children with learning disabilities may move differently than typically developing children, and that these differences may be interpreted as clues to their learning disabilities. We wish to make a similar argument here and suggest that issues with motor coordination may offer early clues regarding the potential for learning disabilities to emerge later in childhood. We see this argument as offering two distinct benefits to the study of language based LD.

First, the theoretical benefit of the association between language-based LD and motor coordination is that new questions can be asked and predictions can be made based on embodied cognition. This will offer new ways to conceptualize LD, and further, initiate innovative empirical investigations. There is a need for additional research within such a framework to examine the viability of embodied cognition as a good model with which to study language- based learning disabilities.

A clear, functional benefit of this association would be the establishment of specific motor criteria that serve as early indicators for those at risk for such learning disabilities. In order to do this, the nature of motor coordination deficits must be quantified, and performance norms for children with learning disabilities must be established on standardized motor tests. The return on this venture has great promise, though. If consistent motor coordination deficits can be identified in populations with a learning disability, then standardized motor tests can be used as part of a diagnostic strategy aimed at helping children with learning disabilities before they fail academically.

ACKNOWLEDGEMENTS

We would like to acknowledge the contributions of Priya Pabreja to earlier versions of this chapter. In addition, we would like to thank Linda Gagen, Ph.D. for taking the time to review this work.

REFERENCES

Bril, B. & Breniér, Y. (1992). Postural requirements and progression velocity in young walkers. *Journal of Motor Behavior. 24,* 105-116.

Bushnell, E. W. & Boudreau, J. P. (1993). Motor development and the mind: the potential role of motor abilities as a determinant of aspects of perceptual development. *Child Development. 64,* 1005-21.

Chiel, H.J., & Beer, R.D. (1997). The brain has a body: Adaptive behavior emerges from interactions of nervous sytems, body and environment. *Trends in Neuroscience. 20,* 553 – 557.

Clark, J.E. & Phillips, S. (1993). A longitudinal study of intralimb coordination in the first year of walking: A dynamical systems analysis. *Child Development. 64,* 1143-1157.

Clark, J.E., Whitall, J. & Phillips, S. (1988). Human interlimb coordination: The first 6 months of independent walking. *Developmental Psychobiology. 12,* 445-456.

Dewey, D., Kaplan, B. J., Crawford, S. G., & Wilson, B. N. (2002). Developmental coordination disorder: associated problems in attention, learning, and psychosocial adjustment. *Human Movement Science. 21,* 905-918.

Eckert, M.A., Leonard, C.M., Richards, T.L., Aylward, E.H., Thomson, J., & Berninger, V.W. (2003). Anatomical correlates of dyslexia: frontal and cerebellar findings. *Brain. 126,* 482-494.

Esterly, D. L. & Griffith, H. C. (1987). Preschool programs for children with learning disabilities. *Journal of Learning Disabilities. 20,* 571-573.

Everatt J., McNamara, S., Groeger, J. A., & Bradshaw M. F. (1999). Motor aspects of dyslexia. In J. Everatt (Ed.), *Reading and dyslexia: visual and attentional processes.* (pp. 122-136). New York: Routledge.

Fawcett, A.J. (2002). Evaluating therapies excluding traditional reading and phonological based therapies. London: DfES SEN Publications. Available at http://www.dfes.gov.uk/sen

Fawcett, A. J. & Nicolson, R. I. (1992). Automatisation deficits in balance for dyslexic children. *Perceptual and Motor Skills. 75,* 507-529.

Fawcett, A. J. & Nicolson, R. I. (1995). Persistent deficits in motor skill of children with dyslexia. *Journal of Motor Behavior. 27,* 235-240.

Fitzpatrick, P., Schmidt, R.C. & Lockman, J.J. (1996). Dynamical patterns in the development of clapping. *Child Development. 67,* 2691-2708.

Folio, M. R & Fewell, R. R. (2000).*Peabody Developmental Motor Scales, Second Edition.* Austin, TX: Pro-Ed.

Gilger, J.W., & Kaplan, B.J. (2001). Atypical brain development: A conceptual framework for understanding developmental learning disabilities . *Developmental Neuropsychology. 20,* 465-481.

Grosshans, J. & Kiger, M. (2004). Identifying and teaching children with learning disabilities in general physical education. *Journal of Physical Education, Recreation, and Dance. 75,* 6, 18 – 21, 58.

Haslum, M. N. (1989). Predictors of dyslexia? *The Irish Journal of Psychology, 10,* 622- 630.

Henderson, S.E., Sugden, D.A., & Barnett, A.L. (2007). *Movement Assessment Battery for Children –2.* London: Harcourt Assessment.

.Kaplan, B. J., Wilson, B. N., Dewey, D., & Crawford, S. G. (1998). DCD may not be a discrete disorder. *Human Movement Science. 17,* 471-490.

Lazarus, J. C. (1994). Evidence of disinhibition in learning disabilities: The associated movement phenomenon. *Adapted Physical Activity Quarterly. 11,* 57-70.

Learning Disabilities Association of America (2006). LD at a glance. http://www.ldaamerica.org

Lowenthal, B. (1998). Precursors of learning disabilities in the inclusive preschool. *Learning disabilities: A Multidisciplinary Journal. 9,* 25-31.

Lyytinen, H., Ahonen, T., Eklund, K., Guttorm, T. K., Laakso, M. L., Leinonen, S., et.al. (2001). Developmental pathways of children with and without familial risk for dyslexia during the first years of life. *Developmental Neuropsychology. 20,* 535-54.

McLeskey, J. & Waldron, N. L. (1991). Identifying students with learning disabilities: the effect of implementing statewide guidelines. *Journal of Learning Disabilities. 24,* 501-506.

Merriman, W. J., Barnett, B. E., & Kofka, J. B. (1993). The standing long jump performances of preschool children with speech impairments and children with normal speech. *Adapted Physical Activity Quarterly. 10,* 157-163.

Merriman, W. J. & Barnett, B. E. (1995). A preliminary investigation of the relationship between language and gross motor skills in preschool children. *Perceptual and Motor Skills. 81,* 1211-1216.

Miyahara, M. (1994). Subtypes of students with learning disabilities based upon gross motor functions. *Adapted physical Activity Quarterly. 11,* 368-382.

Moore, L. H., Brown, W. S., Markee, T. E., Theberge, D. C., & Zvi, J.C. (1995). Bimanual coordination in dyslexic adults. *Neuropsychologia.* 33, 781–793.

Nicolson, R. I. & Fawcett, A. J. (1990). Automaticity: A new framework for dyslexia research? *Cognition. 35,* 159-182.

Nicolson, R. I. & Fawcett, A. J. (1994). Comparison of deficits in cognitive and motor skills among children with dyslexia. *Annals of Dyslexia. 44,* 147-164.

Nicolson, R. I., Fawcett, A. J., Berry, E. L., Jenkins, H., Dean, P., & Brooks, D. J. (1999). Association of abnormal cerebellar activation with motor learning difficulties in dyslexic adults. *The Lancet. 353,* 1622-1667.

Nicolson, R. I., Fawcett, A. J., & Dean, P. (1995).Time estimation deficits in developmental dyslexia: Evidence of cerebellar involvement. *Proceedings: Biological Sciences. 259,* 43-47.

Powell, R. P. & Bishop, D. V. M. (1992). Clumsiness and perceptual problems in children with specific language impairment. *Developmental Medicine and Child Neurology. 34,* 755-765.

President's commission on excellence in Special education. (2002). *A new era: Revitalizing special education for children and their families.* Washington, D.C.: US Department of Education Office of Special Education and Rehabilitative Services. Available online at: http://www.ed.gov/inits/commissionsboards/whspecialeducation/reports/index.html

Ramus, F., Pidgeon, E., & Frith, U. (2003). The relationship between motor control and phonology in dyslexic children. *Journal of Child Psychology and Psychiatry. 44,* 712-722.

Savage, R. (2004). Motor skills, automaticity and developmental dyslexia: A review of research literature. *Reading and Writing: An Interdisciplinary Journal. 17,* 301-324.

Stoodley, C.J., Fawcett, A.J., Nicolson, R.I., & Stein, J.F. (2005). Impaired balancing ability in dyslexic children. *Experimental Brain Research. 167,* 370-380.

Thelen, E. (2000). Grounded in the world: Developmental origins of the embodied mind. *Infancy. 1,* 3-28.

Ulrich, D. A. (2000). *Test of Gross Motor Development-Second Edition, Examiner's Manual.* Austin, Texas: Pro-ed.

United States Department of Education, National Center for Education Statistics, *Digest of Education Statistics.* 2002, Table 52.

Viholainen, H., Ahonen, T., Cantell, M., Lyytinen, P., & Lyytinen, H. (2002). Development of early motor skills and language in children at risk for familial dyslexia. *Developmental Medicine and Child Neurology. 44,* 761-9.

Waber, D. P., Weiler, M. D., Bellinger, D. C., Marcus, D. J., Forbes, P. W., Wypij, D., & Wolff, P.H. (2000). Diminished motor timing control in children referred for diagnosis of learning problems. *Developmental Neuropsychology. 17,* 181-97.

Wolff, P. H., Michel, G. F., & Drake, C. (1990). Rate and timing precision of motor coordination in developmental dyslexia. *Developmental Psychology. 26,* 349–359.

Woodard, R. J. & Surburg, P. R. (1999). Midline crossing behavior in children with learning disabilities. *Adapted Physical Activity Quarterly. 16,* 155–166.

Yap, R. & van der Leij, A. (1994). Testing the automatization deficit hypothesis of dyslexia via a dual-task paradigm. *Journal of Learning Disabilities. 27,* 660–665.

In: Handbook of Motor Skills
Editor: Lucian T. Pelligrino

ISBN: 978-1-60741-811-5
© 2009 Nova Science Publishers, Inc.

Chapter 19

THE DEVELOPMENT OF THE ADULT-LIKE STRATEGY FOR REACHING MOVEMENTS IN CHILDHOOD

Marco Favilla[*]

Dipartimento di Scienze biomediche e terapie avanzate,
Sezione di Fisiologia umana, Università di Ferrara, Ferrara, Italy

ABSTRACT

The present study was undertaken to follow the development of the capability to produce fast and precise movements reaching to visual targets, during childhood. One child (male) was tested repeatedly since age 6, until age 9. Accuracy increased progressively, while reaction and movemet times decreased, eventually approaching those typical of the adult. The most prominent finding is that our subject changed the strategy adopted for reaching to targets at different distances, from "width control" to "height control": when youngest, he scaled movement times of trajectories mainly (width control); when older, he scaled peak velocity of a stereotyped bell-shaped trajectory (height control), thus adopting a fully adult-like strategy. The results were confirmed in two groups of 5 children each, aged 6 and 9 respectively. It is concluded that, between age 6 and 9, children become capable of producing both quick and accurate trajectories to target, by implementing the optimized "height control" strategy typical of adults.

Keywords: Motor control, Reaching, Development, Childhood.

INTRODUCTION

The development of reaching has been well studied in children of different ages: for example hand trajectories become smoother and less variable with age and interjoint coordination becomes more consistent [10]; the ability to rely on visual feedback information

---

[*] e-mail: marco.favilla@unife.it; Fax n° +39-0532-291242

evolves with age too, as well as precision and rapidity of response [5], many of such changes taking place around age 7. However, the development of the strategy adopted to scale reaching trajectories to targets has not been studied. Adult normal human subjects reach visual targets at different distances, quickly and accurately, by using a simplified strategy. Mainly, they scale peak velocity and acceleration of a stereotyped bell-shaped trajectory (height control strategy), while scaling movement time (width control strategy) to a lesser extent [7,9]. The present study was undertaken to follow such development in time. In this study, one child has been tested repeatedly. Recordings began at age 6 and have been followed up to age 9. Two groups of 5 children each, aged 6 and 9 respectively, have also been tested to verify and extend the findings obtained in the one longitudinal follow-up study, to a larger population. A control group of normal adult subjects has been tested too. Subjects were typically required to reach for visual targets at different distances in one of two directions, producing simple, quick, uncorrected movements.

MATERIALS AND METHODS

One child (S1), male, was tested starting at the age of 6 till to the age of 9. Control subjects were 5 (3 males and 2 females) adults (age: 20-40 years). Two groups of 5 children each, aged 6 and 9 respectively were also tested. The study was approved by the ethics committee. All subjects and/or their parents signed an informed consent form prior to their inclusion in the study. The apparatus is described in detail elsewhere [1,2,3,4]. Very briefly, subjects sat viewing the screen of a computer and moved a hand-held cursor on a digitizing tablet (size 42 cm X 30 cm, resolution 0.0025 cm, Numonics model 2200), positioned at waist level. The position of the hand-held cursor on the tablet (x and y coordinates) was sampled by the computer at 200 Hz and displayed on the computer monitor with a reduced gain (2.4=1). Subjects were requested to slide the cursor on the tablet to reach a visual target. At the start of a trial, the position of the cursor on the tablet was displayed on the computer monitor together with a circle representing the starting location. After subjects had positioned the cursor inside the start circle and maintained it there for two seconds, the visual target appeared. Subjects were then to make an "accurate, single, quick, uncorrected movement" to the target, as soon as possible. Knowledge of result was provided by displaying the movement path on the screen after the end of the movement. Targets were presented in different locations on the screen and required movements of the hand on the tablet in different directions. Directions are described with reference to the starting position, 0° being the horizontal direction to right (3 o'clock) and angles progressively increasing in a counter-clockwise direction. Two directions were used: 45° and 135°. The number of the possible targets was always four, two for each direction, at distances of 3.2, 9.6 cm from the start point. Targets were round and their diameter increased as target distance increased. In previous experiments we found that, with equal target diameters, target requiring a larger movement extent were too difficult to hit consistently. An empirical formula was developed to approximately equalize the number of target hits (target radius = 0.64 cm + target distance/15) [8]. When trajectories ended inside the target circle, the response was considered as a successful hit. In each experiment 128 trials were run, 64 in each direction. Targets were presented 32 times each, in a pseudo-random sequence. Due to the inertial anysothropy of the arm [8], in this paper we will focus on the responses produced in one only of the two directions: 135°. Automatic computer programs marked movement onset, peak velocity and movement end point of each trial. These critical Movement extent was computed as the length of a straight line from the starting point to the end point of the movement. Trials with responses showing more than one peak in the velocity profile or those with evident changes in direction were assumed to show voluntary corrections and were rejected (total of rejected trials < 5%). The arrays of trajectory variables were then subjected to statistical analyses including mean, standard deviations and correlations between trajectory and target values. The regression coefficients (r) and their squares (r2) between the extents of the responses and movement times or peak velocities were calculated. We used the percentage of variance (r2 x100) as the measure of the strategy adopted, mainly width control for higher correlations with movement time, mainly height control for higher correlations with peak velocities.

RESULTS

Our main subject, S1, was tested once a year, at the age of 6, 7, 8, 9. Average reaction time decreased, while accuracy, as measured by the percentage of succesful hits, increased. As it can be seen in table 1, these changes were progressive. Around the age of 7, there was an impressive shortening of reaction time. Afterwards, at the age of 8, accuracy increased noticeably and, like reaction time, it attained values comprised within those of controls.

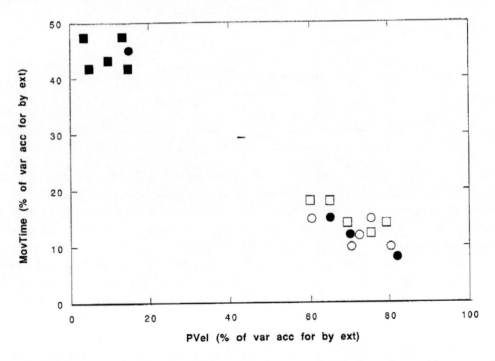

Figure 1. Correlations of movement duration on the y axis and peak velocity on the x, with movement extent, for S1, the adult control group and the two groups of children tested. The filled circles show the correlations obtained for S1, from left to right, at the age of 6, 7, 8, 9. Empty circles, control group. Filled squares, 6 years old children. Empty squares, 9 years old children.

Table 1. Percentages of hits and reaction times (means and standard deviations), from top to bottom, for S1 at the tested ages, for the two tested groups of 5 children (6 and 9 years old respectively) and for the 5 adults (A1-A5)

Age(years)	% of hits	RT +SD (ms)
6	25	585+55
7	20	390+35
8	44	372+20
9	45	335+19

Age(years)	% of hits	RT +SD (ms)
6	27	590+57
6	20	565+53
6	18	637+62
6	22	583+60
6	24	570+51

Age(years)	% of hits	RT +SD (ms)
9	40	340+27
9	42	355+22
9	44	328+19
9	48	375+30
9	37	387+22

Adults	% of hits	RT +SD (ms)
A1	50	380+28
A2	45	327+20
A3	44	338+22
A4	34	324+18
A5	39	367+26

This capability was confirmed when S1 was 9 years old. From 6 to 9 years movement time decreased too, while peak velocity increased. These two parameters reached adult-like level at the age of 7 and they maintained it when S1 was 8 and 9 years old. To assess and quantify the strategy mainly adopted, width or height control, we correlated these two parameters, movement time and peak velocity, with extent. The percentage of variance accounted for by extent obtained are plotted in figure 1, on the y axis for movement time, on the x axis for peak velocity. As it can be seen, control subjects (empty circles) used a predominantly height-control strategy by mainly scaling trajectory's velocity to the targets and only minimally modulating movement time. S1 modulated more movement time and less peak velocity, using a mainly width-control strategy, when he was 6. Then, with age, mode of controlling movement reached the adult standard. Such a strategy (mainly height control) is represented by a percentage of variance accounted for by extent > 60% for peak velocity (p < 0,0001) and < 20% for movement time. Thus, height control strategy appears very well established in S1, especially at the age of 9, when he uses it even more than adult controls. As it can be seen in table 1 and in figure 1, all the main results obtained from S1 are confirmed by the two groups of children tested, aged 6 and 9 respectively.

CONCLUSION

In the present study, to follow the development of motor capabilities, we recorded arm motor trajectories aimed at visual targets, as they were produced by a child (S1), at different ages (6 to 9). Normal young adults were taken as controls. Two groups of children aged 6 and 9 respectively were also tested.

In this study, subjects were requested to aim at visually presented targets, starting to move as soon as possible, with a single, quick, uncorrected trajectory. We focussed on reaction time, accuracy and strategy adopted to scale the trajectories up to different distances. S1 showed a progressively decreasing mean reaction time, while his precision increased, over the years. By the age of 8-9, in this task, S1's reaction time and accuracy had become undistinguishable from those typical of adults. The two groups of 5 children each tested showed similar changes. These findings are consistent with previous reports on motor development in children [see introduction and 5 for a review].

The major new finding of this work concerns the development of the adult-like strategy for producing reaching trajectories. Adult normal human subjects reach visual targets at different distances mainly by scaling peak velocity of a stereotyped bell-shaped trajectory (height control strategy), while scaling movement time (width control strategy) to a lesser extent [7, 9]. This height control policy allows responses of different amplitudes to be produced by proportional scaling of a stereotyped waveform, whose time to peak is regulated. Such a strategy simplifies accurate control of responses amplitude by reducing the number of variables that must be controlled. This is in accord with the need for the nervous system to simplify the control of the many degrees of freedom in the motor system. Our results show that 6 years old children adopt a width control policy. This strategy allows the same advantage as the height control as far as having to control one parameter only out of two (peak velocity and movement duration). At the same time width control permits more correction during execution, even though at the expense of speed. Such strategy could be advantageous during development, when the nervous system has to learn to organise the coordinated control of a great number of degrees of freedom. The acquisition of new skills is driven both by the development of the nervous system in itself and its interaction with the perception of the environment (dynamic system approach, see 6). Once developing subjects have learned to deal with variability of environment as well as the many variables of their own musculoskeletal apparatus, after age 7, they learn to rely on feedforward or internal feedback mechanisms progressively better and shift to height control, which gives the great ecological advantage of speed.

ACKNOWLEDGEMENTS

This research was supported by a Grant from the Italian MIUR.

REFERENCES

[1]   Favilla, M. & De Cecco, E. Parallel direction and extent specification of planar reaching arm movements in humans. *Neuropsychologia.* 34, 609-613, 1996.

[2]   Favilla, M. Reaching movements: programming time course is independent of choice number. *Neuro. Rep.* 7, 2629-2634, 1996.

[3]   Favilla, M. Reaching movements: concurrency of continuous and discrete programming. *Neuro. Rep.* 8, 3973-3977, 1997.

[4]   Favilla, M. Reaching movements: mode of motor programming influences programming time by itself. *Exp. Brain Res.*, 144, 414-418, 2002.

[5]   Ferrel-Chapus, C; Hay, L; Olivier, I; Bard, C; Fleury, M. Visuomanual coordination in childhood: adaptation to visual distortion. *Exp. Brain Res.* 144, 506-517, 2002.

[6]   Gibson, JJ. The ecological approach to visual perception. Houghton-Mifflin, Boston, 1979.

[7]   Gordon, J & Ghez, C. Trajectory control in targeted force impulses. II. Pulse height control. *Exp. Brain Res.* 67, 241-252, 1987

[8]   Gordon, J; Ghilardi, MF; Ghez, C. Accuracy of planar reaching movements: I. Independence of direction and extent variability. *Exp. Brain Res.* 99, 97-111, 1994a.

[9]   Gordon, J; Ghilardi, MF; Cooper, SE; Ghez, C. Accuracy of planar reaching movements: II. Systematic extent errors resulting from inertial anisotropy. *Exp. Brain Res.* 99, 112-130, 1994b.

[10] Schneiberg, S; Sveistrup, H; Mc Fadyen, B; McKinley, P; Levin, MF. The development of coordination for reach-to-grasp movements in children. *Exp. Brain Res.* 146, 142-154, 2002.

In: Handbook of Motor Skills
Editor: Lucian T. Pelligrino

ISBN: 978-1-60741-811-5
© 2009 Nova Science Publishers, Inc.

Chapter 20

MOTOR SKILLS:
DEVELOPMENT, IMPAIRMENT, AND THERAPY

A. M. Keane[*]

Psychology, University of Bolton, England

ABSTRACT

The often held view that motor control occurs largely as the final stage of cognitive processing is something that still needs to be dispelled. Granted that while there is a final level of motor control, all-be-it a lower level of motor control, this is only one level in the motor control hierarchy. Some inroads have been made in clarifying the different stages of motor control and its lateralization, however there is still a way to go with regards to delineating the various levels of motor control from the very highest or early inception/goal level to the final level of movement execution, as well as how each of these levels contributes to bimanual control, hand preference, hand proficiency and overall motor skill. Also, how exactly posture figures within the motor control hierarchy and its influence on final motor skill needs to be taken into account. Motor control is not separate from cognitive functioning, the two are intimately linked, and so the challenge within this area and one of the main directions for future research is the need to find the cognitive and language functioning associated with each respective level of motor control, thus clarifying the cognitive – motor skills link.

COMMENTARY

There is often a general-held view that we do all our thinking – and then we move, leading to movement being perceived as an "add on" to cognitive processing. While there is this final, thought to be contralaterally controlled (Lawrence & Kuypers, 1968a, 1968b) movement execution level, there are also several other levels of motor control prior to this final level, that appear to be hierarchically organized and also differ in the way in which they

---

[*] Mailing address for all correspondence: Dr Anne Maria Keane; Psychology; University of Bolton; Deane Road; Bolton BL3 5AB; ENGLAND; Telephone No.: +44 (0) 1204 – 903677; E-mail: A.Keane@bolton.ac.uk

are lateralized within the brain. For example, my own research (Keane, 1999) has shown that lateralization of one of the highest levels of motor control, namely general motor programming, varies according to a person's degree of hand preference irrespective of direction, in that those who consistently have a preference for one hand over the other have the general motor programmer lateralized in the left hemisphere, while those who have a strong hand preference but less consistently favour one hand seem to have a general motor programming capacity in both hemispheres. The general motor programming level precedes the whole concept of a right and left hand, as the general programmer is not specific to the programming of just hand movements in that this mechanism also appears to be required for some aspect of verbal processing as well. The concept of right and left does not seem to arise until a more intermediate level of motor control, which is more specific to programming movements of the hands. The movement execution level, the part often equated with movement is then just the final stage of movement, the point where the movement is actually carried out, and is the lowest level in the motor control hierarchy.

It is thought that the earlier general motor programming level, which is probably involved in determining the goal of the movement, feeds into subsequent more specific levels of motor control for not just the hands, but for all movement, including for example the specific motor control of speech (Kimura, 1982). So it is at this intermediate level of motor control, that is, below general motor programming and above final motor execution that there is the more specific motor control of the hands, each hand right and left, and it is likely that hand preference is also associated with this level of motor control, but how exactly is not yet known. It could be that that the specific control of each hand determines the proficiency of each hand which in turn culminates in a person's final hand preference. Or it could be that proficiency is the end product of hand preference and the specific programming of the hands. This is the whole, as yet unresolved area, of whether it is proficiency that determines hand preference or whether instead it is hand preference that determines proficiency. Alternatively, it could be that hand preference is a separate dimension altogether and is more associated with some aspect of language processing. It is also important to distinguish between direction and degree of hand preference as the motor control hierarchy may be contributing differently to these two dimensions. Therefore, there is still a way to go in deciphering how each level of motor control contributes to the direction and degree of handedness and also how hand preference, hand proficiency and overall motor skill are associated.

An interesting development in the handedness literature, with studies on nonhuman primates leading the way, are the findings with regards to posture where differential use of the hands for reaching for food has been found to be dependent on postural stance. For example, in chimpanzees and orangutans (Hopkins, 1993) a right hand preference in reaching for food from an upright posture has been found, whereas there is an absence of this right hand preference for reaching from a quadrapedal posture. Westergaard et al. (1998) also report an increase in right hand responding associated with an increase in postural demands, although this was not equally so for all primates. Geschwind (1985), too, was aware of the importance of posture on hand usage in humans when he remarked on seven individuals who wrote on paper with their left hand but used their right hand to write at the blackboard. Therefore, postural control must also be accommodated within the motor control hierarchy, with the extent to which it influences hand skill and hand preference requiring further future exploration, especially in humans.

That the general motor programming mechanism, a structure involved in bimanual control (Keane, 2008), is the same mechanism used to perceive certain aspects of speech (Keane, 1999), shows how intimately linked cognitive functioning and motor control actually are with each other. Other levels of motor control also appear to share neural mechanisms with cognitive functioning. For example Keane (2002) found an association between the hand preference level and an aspect of speech processing (i.e., perception of consonant vowels when they were the same). The more specific motor control of each hand in each of the hemispheres was found to be associated with an aspect of tonal processing (Keane, 2001). In this same vein, Bryden et al. (1994), from correlations between hand preference/skill and language lateralization, found that the largest correlations were not with the expected writing hand but with such activities as striking a match, holding a needle and cutting bread. This suggests that only certain aspects of hand preference are related to certain aspects of language lateralization. Exactly what these aspects of hand control that are related to language processing are, needs to be teased out. Ultimately, of course, if we can find how each level of motor control is related to cognitive processing then this should also lead to greater clarity as to what exactly each level of motor control contributes to an individual's overall handedness. A move away from the consideration of skilled action in isolation from cognitive processing towards a greater emphasis on trying to determine what specific aspects are shared by both will likely find that perception and production share the same or similar neural substrate (MacKay, 1987). It will probably turn out to be the case that at certain levels within the motor control hierarchy, not only do action and language share the same or similar neural components, but that common components underlie perception and production for all cognitive functioning.

In summary then, apart from final execution of movement, the mechanisms and structures of the brain involved in the planning and programming of movement also seem to be the very same structures involved in language and probably many other cognitive tasks as well. The planning and programming of movement is hierarchically organized, with the different levels of motor control related to different aspects of cognitive processing. The challenge now, and one of the main directions for future research, is to try to ascertain how each specific level of motor control is related to each specific aspect of cognitive processing and how in turn each of these levels determine degree and direction of hand preference, and overall motor skill.

REFERENCES

Bryden, M.P., Singh, M., Steenhuis, R.E., & Clarkson, K.L. (1994). A behavioral measure of hand preference as opposed to hand skill. *Neuropsychologia. 32*, 991 – 999.

Geschwind, N. (1985). Implications for evolution, genetics, and clinical syndromes. In S. D. Glick (Ed.), *Cerebral lateralization in nonhuman species*. New York: Academic Press.

Hopkins, W. D. (1993). Posture and reaching in chimpanzees (Pan troglodytes) and orangutans (Pongo pygmaeus). *Journal of Comparative Psychology. 107*, 162 – 168.

Keane, A.M. (1999). Cerebral organization of motor programming and verbal processing as a function of degree of hand preference and familial sinistrality. *Brain and Cognition. 40*, 500 – 515.

Keane, A.M. (2001). Motor control of the hands: The effect of familial sinistrality. *International Journal of Neuroscience. 110*, 25 – 41.

Keane, A.M. (2002). Direction of hand preference: The connection with speech and the influence of familial handedness. *International Journal of Neuroscience. 112*, 1287 – 1303.

Keane, A.M. (2008). What aspect of handedness is general motor programming related to? *International Journal of Neuroscience. 118*, 519 – 530.

Kimura, D. (1982). Left-hemisphere control of oral and brachial movements and their relation to communication. *Philosophical Transactions of the Royal Society of London: B: Biological Sciences. 298*, 135 - 149.

Lawrence, D.G., & Kuypers, H.G. (1968a). The functional organization of the motor system in the monkey. I. The effects of bilateral pyramidal lesions. *Brain. 91*, 1-14.

Lawrence, D.G., & Kuypers, H.G. (1968b). The functional organization of the motor system in the monkey. II. The effects of lesions of the descending brain-stem pathways. *Brain. 91*, 15-36.

MacKay, D. G. (1987). *The organization of perception and action: A theory for language and other cognitive skills.* New York: Springer-Verlag.

Westergaard, G.C., Kuhn, H.E., & Suomi, S.J. (1998). Bipedal posture and hand preference in humans and other primates. *Journal of Comparative Psychology. 112*, 55 – 64.

INDEX

B

E

H

I

J

Japan, 42, 93, 223, 224, 234
Japanese, 234
jobs, 103
joints, xi, 12, 129, 211, 212, 215, 263
joystick, 143, 149
judge, 271
judgment, 97
jumping, 7, 9, 10, 17, 24, 95, 97, 98, 104, 226
Jun, 58

K

kappa, 49
kindergarten children, 108
kinematics, 66, 93, 291
kinesthesis, 34
kinesthetic, 108, 250
kinetic energy, 82, 134
kinetics, 34, 66
King, 89
knee, 6, 8, 120, 121, 122, 126, 127, 129, 130, 134, 201, 202, 206, 239, 247
knees, xi, 7, 211, 212, 214, 242
Kolmogorov, 77, 91

L

laboratory studies, 163
lack of confidence, 13
lactation, 46
language, xiv, 15, 17, 19, 26, 45, 46, 105, 108, 114, 118, 130, 141, 145, 229, 239, 253, 266, 288, 294, 297, 299, 300, 301, 302, 303, 304, 305, 306, 307, 308, 309, 311, 312, 319, 320, 321, 322
language acquisition, 229
language delay, 297
language development, 288, 302
language impairment, 118, 302, 306, 307, 312
language lateralization, 321
language processing, 145, 320, 321
language skills, 301, 302, 303
laparoscopic, 114
latency, x, 172, 177, 179, 181, 182, 183, 184, 273
later life, 7
lateral epicondylitis, 114
laterality, 235
law, 220
laws, 66, 174
LD score, 15
learners, 16
learning difficulties, 38, 44, 303, 308, 312
learning disabilities, xiv, 14, 15, 16, 17, 32, 33, 34, 35, 43, 48, 59, 182, 183, 294, 297, 299, 300, 301, 302, 303, 304, 306, 307, 308, 309, 310, 311, 312

learning outcomes, 2
learning process, 142
learning skills, 102
learning styles, 103
learning task, 145, 151, 153
left hemisphere, 46, 320
left-handed, 45, 46
leg, 6, 7, 8, 15, 76, 84, 87, 91, 104, 125, 127, 128, 132, 304
lending, 294
lesions, 45, 46, 199, 322
lesson plan, 2
life experiences, 9
life span, 36
lifespan, vii, 2, 31, 34, 35
lifestyle, 215
lift, 196, 213, 214
Likert scale, 189, 252
limitation, 12, 124, 125, 165, 212, 217, 219, 253, 254, 305
limitations, xi, 3, 12, 49, 115, 118, 126, 134, 135, 187, 188, 211, 213, 246, 254
Lincoln, 96, 104, 114
linear, 78, 142, 273
linear regression, 78, 273
linguistic, 230
links, xiii, 123, 125, 131, 143, 164, 218, 219, 257, 259
literacy, 301
loading, 48, 91
local anesthesia, 206
localization, 152
location, 88, 118, 143, 145, 147, 148, 217, 225, 230, 314
locomotion, 6, 7, 24, 66, 68, 83, 90, 92, 106, 265, 298
locus, 151
London, 54, 55, 56, 58, 89, 91, 94, 111, 134, 154, 169, 184, 266, 284, 285, 297, 311, 322
long distance, 85, 86, 91
long period, 18, 206
longitudinal studies, 38, 126
longitudinal study, 60, 129, 153, 169, 209, 298, 302, 303, 310
long-term retention, 16
Los Angeles, 58
losses, 27, 159
low birthweight, 48, 60
lying, 1, 26, 95, 97, 289

M

M1, 149
machines, 270

N

right hemisphere, 45, 46

rigidity, 41

risk, vii, xi, xiv, 37, 38, 39, 43, 46, 49, 51, 53, 54, 55, 59, 60, 62, 105, 118, 124, 188, 206, 207, 213, 216, 221, 251, 299, 300, 302, 303, 308, 310, 311, 312

risk factors, 43, 46, 54, 55, 58, 59, 124

robustness, 144, 146

rolling, vii, 6, 26, 95, 97, 289, 290, 304

rotator cuff, 213

routines, 24, 26, 42

Royal Society, 297, 322

S

saccadic eye movement, 151

SAD, 139

safety, 31, 99, 261, 272

saliva, 207, 208

sample, 24, 49, 50, 88, 108, 120, 129, 160, 162, 165, 204, 206, 242, 252, 254, 260, 306

sampling, 176, 242

satisfaction, 40

scaling, 314, 316, 317

scalp, 176, 184

scalp topography, 184

scarcity, viii, 37

schema, 267

schizophrenia, 41, 46, 275

school, vii, xi, 2, 14, 17, 31, 37, 38, 39, 41, 42, 43, 47, 49, 51, 53, 55, 58, 60, 62, 63, 64, 100, 102, 103, 110, 113, 206, 211, 214, 260, 261, 266, 268, 279, 280, 291, 295, 298, 299, 301, 309

school adjustment, 43

school failure, 38

school performance, 100

school work, 214

schooling, 47

scientific method, 50

sclerosis, 102

scoliosis, 206

scores, x, 47, 48, 51, 62, 63, 64, 98, 114, 123, 157, 158, 160, 161, 162, 164, 165, 166, 167, 168, 169, 195, 204, 205, 240, 252, 253, 254, 304, 305, 308

screening programs, 58

SDT, 103

search, 5, 57, 213, 215, 219, 249, 261, 280

searching, 215, 219

sedentary, 124

sedentary lifestyle, 124

seed, 221

segmentation, 154

seizure, xi, 187

selecting, 102, 123, 293

self, viii, 37, 39, 49, 53, 64, 168, 169, 251, 254, 256

self-concept, 16

self-confidence, xii, 43, 249, 250, 251, 252, 253, 254, 255, 256

self-efficacy, 55, 250, 256

self-esteem, 14, 17, 38, 42, 48, 60, 245

self-organization, 91

self-organizing, 260, 264, 265

self-perceptions, 61

self-regulation, 153

self-report data, 290

sensation, xi, 105, 127, 128, 129, 184, 187, 237, 244

sensitivity, 24, 49, 52, 59, 64, 111, 112, 114, 272, 279, 280, 281

sensory modalities, 44, 271

sensory modality, xiii, 269, 272, 273

sensory systems, 240, 271, 275, 293

sentences, 107, 303

separation, 270

sequencing, 105

sequential behavior, 145

series, vii, xiii, 10, 11, 144, 161, 163, 173, 174, 176, 220, 262, 269, 270

serotonin, 46

services, xiii, 14, 40, 209, 285, 287, 288

severe intellectual disabilities, 12

severity, 19, 27, 118, 131, 136, 188, 206, 207, 208

sex, 48, 92, 124, 177

sex differences, 48

shape, 76, 175, 176, 227, 228

sharing, 23, 243

short period, 39, 183

shortage, 243

short-term, 105, 114

short-term memory, 105

shoulder, xi, 75, 104, 106, 189, 211, 213, 215, 241, 273, 280

shoulders, xi, 8, 211, 212, 214, 215, 216

sibling, 23

sign, 19, 43, 166, 226

signal transduction, 183

signaling, 56

signals, xi, 46, 211, 217, 273

significance level, 202, 253

signs, 17, 26, 43, 99, 290

similarity, xii, 70, 223, 229

simulation, 218, 257

sine, 143

Singapore, 42, 55, 57

sites, 176, 218

skeletal muscle, 133, 285

skill acquisition, xiv, 3, 140, 149, 221, 238, 240, 268, 299, 302